GLOBAL HEALTH POLICY, LOCAL REALITIES

Directions in Applied Anthropology: Adaptations and Innovations

Timothy J. Finan, Series Editor
BUREAU OF APPLIED RESEARCH IN ANTHROPOLOGY,
UNIVERSITY OF ARIZONA, TUCSON

Editorial Board

Beverly Hackenberg
UNIVERSITY OF COLORADO, BOULDER

Robert Hackenberg
BUREAU OF APPLIED RESEARCH IN ANTHROPOLOGY,
UNIVERSITY OF ARIZONA, TUCSON

Evelyn Jacob
GEORGE MASON UNIVERSITY

Peter Van Arsdale
COLORADO MENTAL HEALTH INSTITUTE
FT. LOGAN, DENVER

Linda M. Whiteford
UNIVERSITY OF SOUTH FLORIDA, TAMPA

GLOBAL HEALTH POLICY, LOCAL REALITIES

The Fallacy of the Level Playing Field

EDITED BY
Linda M. Whiteford
Lenore Manderson

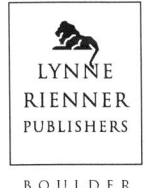

LYNNE
RIENNER
PUBLISHERS

BOULDER
LONDON

Published in the United States of America in 2000 by
Lynne Rienner Publishers, Inc.
1800 30th Street, Boulder, Colorado 80301

and in the United Kingdom by
Lynne Rienner Publishers, Inc.
3 Henrietta Street, Covent Garden, London WC2E 8LU

© 2000 by Lynne Rienner Publishers, Inc. All rights reserved

Library of Congress Cataloging-in-Publication Data
Global health policy, local realities : the fallacy of the level playing field /
  edited by Linda M. Whiteford and Lenore Manderson.
    p. cm. — (Directions in applied anthropology)
  Includes bibliographical references and index.
  ISBN 978-1-55587-874-0 (alk. paper)
    1. World health—Social aspects—Case studies. 2. Medical policy—
Social aspects—Case studies. I. Whiteford, Linda M. II. Manderson,
Lenore. III. Series.
RA441.G57 2000
362.1—dc21   99-056616

British Cataloguing in Publication Data
A Cataloguing in Publication record for this book
is available from the British Library.

Printed and bound in the United States of America

 The paper used in this publication meets the requirements
of the American National Standard for Permanence of
Paper for Printed Library Materials Z39.48-1992.

Contents

Introduction: Health, Globalization, and the Fallacy
of the Level Playing Field   1
   Lenore Manderson and Linda M. Whiteford

Part 1   International Health Policy and Issues of Localization

1. The Politics of Child Survival   23
   Judith Justice

2. Administering the Epidemic: HIV/AIDS Policy,
Models of Development, and International Health   39
   Richard Parker

3. Local Identity, Globalization, and Health in Cuba
and the Dominican Republic   57
   Linda M. Whiteford

4. Health Care from the Perspectives of Minahasa Villagers,
Indonesia   79
   Peter van Eeuwijk

Part 2   The Global Pharmacy

5. The King's Law Stops at the Village Gate:
Local and Global Pharmacy Regulation in Vietnam   105
   David Craig

6 The Business of Medicines and the Politics of Knowledge
   in Uganda   127
   Susan Reynolds Whyte and Harriet Birungi

Part 3 Relocating Bodies and Body Parts

7 Bodies Transported: Health and Identity Among
   Involuntary Immigrant Women   151
   Lenore Manderson, Milica Markovic, and Margaret Kelaher

8 Poverty, Pity, and the Erasure of Power:
   Somali Refugee Dependency   177
   Christina Zarowsky

9 Ethical Issues in Human Organ Replacement:
   A Case Study from India   205
   Patricia A. Marshall and Abdallah Daar

Part 4 Globalizing Mothering

10 Does Authoritative Knowledge in Infant Nutrition
   Lead to Successful Breast-Feeding? A Critical Perspective   233
   Arachu Castro and Lauré Marchand-Lucas

11 Reforming Routines: A Baby-Friendly Hospital in
   Urban China   265
   Suzanne Zhang Gottschang

Part 5 Conclusion

12 International Health Research: The Rules of the Game   291
   James Trostle

Selected Bibliography   315
The Contributors   319
Index   325
About the Book   333

Introduction: Health, Globalization, and the Fallacy of the Level Playing Field

Lenore Manderson and Linda M. Whiteford

This book is born of our common and contradictory experiences. Our work as anthropologists and our personal histories cause us to cross continents on numerous occasions and, in so doing, to reflect on who we are, what we do, and where we are going. We meet primarily in two ways. Most expensively, reflecting the privilege of most of us, we attend professional meetings around the globe, where the Hilton hotel in which we stay might be a Hilton anywhere else. The point of globalization, in one respect, is precisely this—the "local" is the color that adds a slight frisson to travel, a variation on the menu or an item in the gift shop. Otherwise, but for the plane trip, we are always at home, wherever we are. More often, we meet via the information technology we increasingly take for granted. It is through this media too that we maintain contact with our research sites, our colleagues in other countries and communities, our students, and our friends. We participate in international health debates and programs, attend workshops, and discuss how health policies might be implemented in different places. We help to develop the tools to ensure that this occurs, we undertake field visits to explore local conditions, we advise bilateral and international agencies, and we work with colleagues to translate the ideas developed (centrally) for their local delivery.

Globalization captures the transcendence of geopolitical boundaries. The term is used widely to refer to the political, economic, and demographic processes that occur within and between nations. Health experience, status, policies, and programs also transcend national boundaries and are carried out in the nexus between global forces and socially constructed local identities. Too often, international health planners design programs based on the assumption that "all else is equal" and that each recipient

1

nation shares the same "level playing field." The assumption of uniformity of context may be necessary to the process of planning global health programs but also may create needless barriers to their effective execution. This book addresses the intersections and tensions between global processes and local identities as they affect health.

Intergovernmental agencies, nongovernmental organizations, and individual countries filter and mediate between local realities and global categorizations of health, illness, and risk. This volume uses as its focus an analysis of how socially constructed local identities understood in the context of the globalization of health render the playing field uneven. The authors of the chapters in this book challenge the assumption of the "level playing field" by analyzing the consequences of the globalization of humanitarian and health-related projects that fail to recognize local ethnic and national identities. An "economy of knowledge" perspective explores the process by which various types of knowledge and ideology are transformed into cultural capital and examines the dynamic tensions between international health agencies' mandates and guidelines and powerful centralized governmental agendas, supports, and sanctions. We look at the way in which ideologies of best practice—such as advocating bottom-up programs and community-based interventions—are often introduced where the basic social preconditions for success are lacking, or where community structures and resources are inadequate to respond to such program goals. We discuss how the HIV/AIDS epidemic and other international health crises, such as those related to child survival, force us to reexamine the construction of dominant discourses, power, and authority.

As anthropologists, we are also well aware of the discordance between center and periphery, global ideal and local reality. The anthropological creed of "culture" insists on the importance of context. Particular economic, political, and social systems that evolve in one place and time do not "naturally" transfer to a different setting. Hence the democratic ideals of government of Western Europe are not easily or happily translated into, for instance, a Southeast Asian setting; the values of capitalism transmogrify in the villages of China; notions of freedom have very different meanings in France, Nigeria, or El Salvador. Yet many of us involved in international health have worked toward goals for human well-being—"health for all" optimistically by the year 2000 as though the transfer were complete—yet the economic inequalities of nations mean that poorer countries lack resources and are strained even to meet the most basic health needs. Social, economic, and political circumstances result in different priorities for health and welfare, diverse national and local objectives, time lines, goals and targets, and very different structures and institutions. While we have worked with both international agencies and local communities toward public health and the public good, we have been aware—or have gained awareness—of the importance of the local setting and the constraints and difficulties in the local translation of knowledge.

Global forces are not acultural or supracultural. They are, rather, historical artifacts that derive from Western domination; they reflect Western values of rationality, competition, and progress, in which context there is an implicit assumption that with modernization, local "traditional" institutions and structures will be replaced by Western systems and patterns. As B. Geddes notes (1997a:2), globalization is neither the result of industrialization nor market dominance alone, although our evidence of globalization tends to have an economic take: consider the introduction of multi-country currency such as the euro (without apparent irony in the choice of name of the currency), or continuous mergers of national and multinational companies across continents as well as more proximate borders. The structural, fiscal, and strategic links between industrial centers and peripheries highlight how economic globalization—the production and distribution of goods—is tied to issues of world governance. But this is accompanied with a cultural dominance, best illustrated, perhaps, by the resistances that occur in contradiction to these apparent homogenizing trends: the development of local identities, the reemerging importance of ethnicity, the demands for autonomy, self-government, and independence, or the civil wars in Asia, Africa, and Europe, for example.

At the same time, it behooves us to remember that globalization is merely an old book in a new cover: imperialism and colonialism had the same purposes and encouraged the same eclecticism and synchrony. Not surprisingly, the issues that we explore in this volume have a historic resonance. International health policies, for example, date not from the most recent priorities of the World Bank, but from the efforts of nineteenth-century colonial powers to control the spread of disease that would threaten their economic well-being. The use of wireless systems nearly a century ago for epidemiological surveillance differs from optic fiber and internet communications today by virtue of technical difference but not by virtue of intent (Manderson 1995).

Globalization ignores national boundaries. Its superficial face, tied to the flow of commodities, is one of taste and market manipulation—the pervasiveness of Coca-Cola and Hershey's chocolate in Manila as well as in New York. But this is not a one-way traffic of cultural products: San Miguel Beer and Durian are available in New York as well as in Manila. In this context, globalization conceptually accommodates both postmodern notions of syncretism and the underlying principles of the political economy of late monopoly capitalism. In this context, it is worth highlighting the way in which the global economy both engineers and ignores political groupings. As we wrote this introduction, the war in Kosovo continued. Hundreds of thousands of people were homeless; NATO continued to drop bombs in an attempt to force a change in Serbian policy against people then categorized as "ethnic Albanians" (as opposed, for instance, to "displaced Kosovars"). The international aid machinery worked overtime to provide the most rudimentary food and medical supplies to people in camps. Televisions carry news of the war as it happens; and we are now old hands as real-time witnesses of the dropping of bombs and the discovery of corpses, and updates of events of the "theater of war" are precisely that—"theater" (see Kleinman and Kleinman 1997). Families keep each other informed—and keep hope alive—between nations, via the Internet. And McDonald's has reopened three fast-food outlets in Belgrade War notwithstanding, globalization respects no boundaries.

Hence globalization is not only about commerce or the construction of taste. It is also about local politics, international government, strategic alliances, power and force, and communication systems. In the case of the wars of the former Yugoslavia, it provides the rhetorical and moral basis for intervention from other, outside forces. In more benign contexts, globalization is a process that blurs or renders irrelevant national identity, while forging transnational and transcultural identities (Altman 1994). The dramatic changes in international communication systems and the constant movement of people as tourists and workers facilitate this process, or the creation of what in the 1940s to 1950s was called "the third culture"—an international culture (Nancy O. Lurie, personal communication).

The discourse on globalization's impact on cultural form and practice in international health is still limited. In this book, we want to inject the insights of globalization theory into international public health practices. Common agendas and definitions of health and well-being, operationalized in specific policies and programs, are set nationally or at a state level. But even these are very much influenced and increasingly shaped by wider governmental purposes. The eradication of smallpox is the best historical example; the worldwide adoption of the Expanded Programme on Immunization, global efforts to eradicate polio by the year 2000, to control malaria within and between countries, and so on, are all contemporary examples. Indeed, even practices that are supposed to counter the homogenizing effects of globalization are advocated and implemented through global governance: WHO (World Health Organization) programs, for instance, promote community participation and bottom-up approaches to agendas that have, after all, been predetermined and prioritized at the center (Fisher 1997).

Within countries, there is ongoing tension between local cultural demands and national goals and targets. Policies of multiculturalism designed to accommodate difference respond to this tension, superficially privileging the cultural over the epidemiological. To some degree, too, under a cloak of pragmatism, even international government acknowledges that real differences need to be addressed and valued. Hence the efforts of WHO programs to develop instruments, protocols, and procedures that acknowledge and work with, not against, local practice. The World Health Organization's (1978) advocacy of the use of traditional practitioners and therapies in primary health care is an early instance. So too are more recent developments of focused ethnographic instruments to identify local lexicon for the incorporation into health education material to prevent life-threatening illness (e.g., Gove and Pelto 1994).

A similar example was the work conducted following the change of international organizational leadership in HIV/AIDS, from the Global Programme on AIDS (GPA) to the combined program of the WHO, United Nations Development Programme (UNDP), and World Bank known as United Nations AIDS (UNAIDS). UNAIDS was distinguished from GPA as having an "expanded response" to HIV/AIDS, and in this context took steps to tailor national AIDS programs to local circumstances (see Chapter 2). Yet, exactly how this was to occur in the context of a vast and centralized network of experts, committees, and funding agencies was left undetermined. The resulting approach was to support strengthening institutional capacity in policy and planning, and to enhance the administrative processes and structures required to translate policy into programs. This has led, inter alia, to advocating a policy of contextual assessment and program review as components of the national strategy. This enlightened policy encouraged countries to assess the suitability of the national programs in light of national social, economic, and political changes, and in light of epidemiological changes relating to HIV/AIDS. In sum, local factors deemed relevant to understanding and responding to the transmission of infection included population issues (migration, fertility, and mortality rates), social structure, political and economic systems, education and communication, the institutional environment, and human rights issues (Aboagye-Kwarteng, Manderson, and Msiska 1997). However, the mechanisms by which to transform the enlightened policy into actions were not provided, and failing that, the policy was rendered void of effect.

Even the most well intentioned of these approaches assumes at some point a level playing field—or, at least, it is not explicit how policies might be both locally and internationally comparable. For over twenty years now the WHO has advocated primary health care as a means of improving the access of the poor to basic medical care and treatment, and there is a substantial literature on the introduction of primary health care and on translating disease control programs locally. But the descriptions of these processes largely gloss over the tensions in the implementation of centrally generated, vertical programs (which remain the primary means by which countries attempt to reduce infectious disease) and adaptations to distinctive, localized realities (critical to program sustainability).

Accordingly, much of the policy work in the area of primary health care and community participation is idealistic. The enthusiastic literature advocating a strong role of people in conceiving, contributing to, and sustaining quality health services often overlooks that fact that the pilot projects along these lines have been highly resource intensive and, in the long term, nonsustainable. In particular, arguments for community participation have often overlooked the impediments to partnerships between central government authorities and local bodies, and have ignored the resource, structural, institutional, and personal preconditions for improved health. Most elusive and ephemeral, and therefore easiest to overlook, are the local histories and local identities that allow community participation programs to become actualized within their institutional and political contexts. The complex and problematic reality of contextualizing policy in the arena of international health programs is the focus of Part 1.

The chapters in Part 1 focus on the localization of international health policy. In Chapter 1, Judith Justice reviews the development and history of child survival programs and compares their efficaciousness across countries. She notes that child survival strategies had enormous political appeal through the 1980s and 1990s and, in consequence, were able to attract substantial resources and sustained input from both the WHO and UNICEF. The interventions were simple: full immunization and oral rehydration therapy for diarrhea disease, with other adjunct programs such as monitoring child growth and breastfeeding. Immunization had an immediate appeal, promising to drive down infant and child mortality in poor countries. Other interventions were attractive because of their simplicity and cost-effectiveness. As Justice illustrates, however, this approach was selective and by-passed major problems in the delivery of primary health care. In addition, the approach proceeded without community participation to establish local health priorities and implement programs, despite the WHO's commitment to this model. The themes in this chapter anticipate those of succeeding contributions: tensions between donors and recipients, providers and clients, and the global and the local.

Chapter 2 addresses the globalization of HIV/AIDS policies and programs as international agencies themselves have queried how to translate worldwide policies of prevention, control, and care to local circumstances. Richard Parker sets forth a series of paradoxes derived from his analysis of the processes of globalization, capitalist development, and international health. According to Parker, the spread of HIV infection has been along fault lines created by the structures of oppression, social cleavage, and inequality. The paradoxes Parker identifies embeds his analysis in the world arena of international lending practices, development agendas, and the dynamics of power. Parker elegantly articulates the concern with a policy process dominated by the most powerful of the players—international banking and its connected institutions—and the inability of such a process to alleviate human suffering rather than to administer it.

Parker's paradoxes are based on international HIV/AIDS policies and highlight the contradictions and dilemmas between priorities of prevention or administration, legitimizing local or international concepts, and standardized or individualized programs within the political economy of international health. The continued colonization of health is manifested in Parker's analysis of the structure of oppression crystallized in the HIV/AIDS epidemic.

Chapter 3, by Linda M. Whiteford, examines how the political and economic histories of nations shape local identities, which in turn influence the effectiveness of disease prevention and control activities. Citizen responses to dengue fever control programs in Cuba and the Dominican Republic demonstrate how local identities shape community members' willingness to participate in government-initiated health programs, and to see the utility of such initiatives in the longer term. Her chapter on local identities, globalization, and the commodification of health takes as its starting point Michael Kearney's definition of globalization, which refers to "social, economic, cultural and demographic processes that take place within nations but also transcend them, and which places local processes, identities, and units of analysis in a global context" (Kearney 1995:548). Whiteford notes, however, that the focus on global processes may blind health planners to local differences and circumstances with self-defeating consequences. Whiteford's attention to local identities and their idioms of hope and despair illuminates the leitmotif running throughout the book: the ways in which global economic, political, and communications systems vibrate with and against local circumstances, contingencies, and contexts. In health, the local circumstances are environmental, ecological, and epidemiological as well as political, social, and ideological, and for this reason single solutions are rarely appropriate. Vector habitat and behavior are critical in malaria control, for example, and the practice of indoor house spraying by malaria control programs in many countries makes no sense when the primary vector is exophilic and exophagic and disease transmission is in the forest, not the village. And as Whiteford illustrates with respect to dengue fever, public health planners continually struggle with the intersection of global agendas and local settings, and communities struggle to understand the kinds of programs that they are being offered and in which they are expected to participate.

In Chapter 4, Peter van Eeuwijk explores issues of state and local discourse further in his discussion of globalization and its meanings to villagers in Minahasa, Indonesia. Here, issues of development, the incursion of the cash economy, the role of multinational organizations, and the relationship of the nation-state to local communities are all corralled as evidence of *globalisasi*. He makes an important point about these processes. Even in relatively isolated areas of Indonesia, the term *globalization* has been incorporated into everyday parlance, but there is a local nuance to understandings of the relationships of international economic, political, and cultural relations to local circumstance.

The economic transitions that have occurred in north Sulawesi—and in other settings described in this volume such as Uganda and Vietnam—highlight the nature of the deregulated market with globalization. Countries, communities, and individuals participate as producers and consumers in an increasingly interdependent, internationalized economy that takes little responsibility for their welfare, and nation-states have little leverage in minimizing the exploitations that occur via this process. Further, as Geddes (1997b) argues, the weaker the bargaining power of the country, the greater its vulnerability to transnational business and multinational forces either with respect to access to resources or production (e.g., conditions of employees in off-shore industries) or with respect to trade. As Unwin and colleagues argue (1998), while tobacco companies are being prosecuted in the United States and Australia, they continue to expand their markets in low-income countries (many of which are also tobacco-producing countries that are reluctant, therefore, to follow developed nations' leads to inhibit tobacco use). The examples of the marketing of drugs and infant formula in this volume provide further evidence of the contradictions that exist in promoting "free trade" that enhances the profits flowing to the largest, most powerful and richest multinational corporations. Poor countries and communities service an internationalized economy without the political leverage of economic power to protect their citizens.

Minahasan villagers' readiness to use *globalisasi* as a catch-all explanation of the twists and turns of economics and politics locally and nationally is enhanced by their access to global communication (notwithstanding that television sets sit unused, in the absence of electricity). But there are, as many of the authors in this volume illustrate, strong trends also to (re)assert cultural difference, to establish the autonomy and integrity of cultural communities, and to reject the homogenizing demands of "global culture," although, paradoxically, often via the media of global communication.

In Part 2, "The Global Pharmacy," David Craig for Vietnam and Susan R. Whyte and Harriet Birungi for Uganda describe how multinational corporations impact people's daily health practices. In most poor countries worldwide, drugs prescribed by local professionals are available over-the-counter or on the street. These drugs—designed to deal with unpleasant symptoms of illness, to control pain, to prevent the development of certain conditions and ailments, or to control underlying causes of discomfort—are produced, distributed, and marketed primarily by multinational drug companies. This governs the choice, cost, and availability of various drugs, influences prescription patterns, and encourages self-medication and overuse of drugs. Often the consequences are serious for both public and personal health, including the development of iatrogenic ailments and drug resistance of pathogens and the use of unnecessary and dangerous substances (see, for example, Silverman 1976; Van der Geest and Whyte 1988; Kanji et al. 1992; Rozemberg and Manderson 1998).

The response by the World Health Organization (1987) was to regulate marketing by drug companies, to insist upon standard labels and pricing, and to improve the control of distribution, registration, and manufacturing. This resulted in identifying "essential drugs," deemed basic or vital to primary health care, and in developing policies to control the availability of other pharmaceuticals. In addition, policies were developed to control the use of drugs through polypharmacy (e.g., the prescription of two, three, or four drugs, often similar in clinical effect) and prescribing drugs for symptomatic relief only (e.g., as is the case with cough medicines). As Whyte and Birungi and Craig suggest, these codes and national generic drug laws have had limited impact on people's use of pharmaceuticals, and multinational companies continue to market their products in ways that affect prescribing practices, pharmacy provision of drugs, and consumer expectations and behavior.

In Chapter 5, "The King's Law Stops at the Village Gate: Local and Global Pharmacy Regulation in Vietnam," David Craig explores the workings of multinational drug companies, and how the marketing and availability of pharmaceuticals fit with local ideas of the management of illness in Vietnam. In Part 1, current neoliberal economic policies are manifest through decentralization and deregulation; Part 2 provides case studies from Vietnam and Uganda that revisit the consequences of decentralization in the global marketplace. Craig provides powerful examples from the highly contested arena of globalization of pharmaceutical regulation, and its equally complex local-level application. As Craig points out, modes of regulation promoted globally are at considerable odds with national and local political and regulatory forms and where the local modes of regulation are too often overlooked. Yet these local regulatory modes can be seen as local development and a sign of active participation, itself a reflection of a move away from governmental responsibility and a shift toward greater individual and community responsibility. Effective decisionmaking, however, is dependent upon the provision of sufficient and appropriate data, often provided by extralocal authorities. As the Vietnam case demonstrates, data come in many forms, not the least of which is practice knowledge derived from personal experience, and if local and global understandings of drug use are to be symbiotic, they will, as Craig writes, have to be reconciled primarily at the household level.

In each country setting, the nature of pharmaceutical business and its impact on people's health take on rather different turns. In Chapter 6, "The Business of Medicines and the Politics of Knowledge in Uganda," Susan Reynolds Whyte and Harriet Birungi write about their involvement in a project on international drug policy and the local context of action. They situate their analysis in the global discourse on rational use of drugs and the tension between the arguments for standardization of drug policies—as promoted by the WHO under the rubric of the Drug Action Programme and competing forces that propose that local use is always right. Whyte and Birungi write that they hope to offer a more differentiated and pragmatic approach to anthropological assessments of the commodification of health. This chapter moves forward, with their careful and thought-provoking analysis, the discussion of applied medical anthropology, globalization, and international health policies.

Part 3, "Relocating Bodies and Body Parts," is concerned with the movement and location of people as permanent settlers and as refugees, and—through a quirk in our own imaginations—the immigration of technological know-how to enable the transplantation of body organs. Chapters 7 and 8 focus on the global displacement of people, their dislocation/resettlement, and the public health issues that are implicit in this process. Migration has become an increasingly important phenomenon in recent years, and its ease is indeed an example of globalization. Affluent nations increasingly find their borders difficult to police, as recognized de facto in Europe via changes in citizenship and "community membership." Everywhere illegal immigration is an increasingly common problem; people slip across national boundaries and/or overstay tourist or student visas. Other people move around to meet the labor force needs of different sites, working often for poor pay and in substandard conditions to earn hard currency that is then remitted to support families in their homelands. The personal health costs of this movement of bodies—a modern take on an old form of slavery—has yet to be calculated. However, in most places, whether employed legally or illegally, in the formal or informal sector (e.g., as construction laborers, domestic servants, soldiers, or sex workers), migrants are highly vulnerable, lack civil rights protection, and are subject to racism and other structural discriminations. Further, as Bruenjes suggests (1997:134), the official ideologies of temporary migration, including those that provide the policy context for the care of refugees, create an expectation of return that may be unrealistic for refugees. They also provide a rationale for host countries to ignore human rights and public health obligations.

At the same time, ethnic and religious tensions, and environmental disasters, displace millions of people on a daily basis. Geddes (1997a:5) suggests that population movement is without regard for "lines drawn on maps" where poverty is endemic, and where "displaced people, often despairing and hopeless, search for somewhere less threatening and less devastated than their home environments" to reorder their existence. People move now not because of the "bright lights" that characterized such movement in the 1960s and 1970s, but because the social, political, economic, and environmental conditions in their home communities often make flight the surer option (Bruenjes 1997).

In Chapter 7, Lenore Manderson, Milica Markovic, and Margaret Kelaher demonstrate the fallacy of the level playing field when refugee women are treated as though they were all the same, ignoring ethnic identities among immigrant women from Bosnia and Herzegovina. The authors focus on women who have moved on a permanent basis to a different country because of the politics "at home"—local politics very much under an international microscope and subject to global political forces.

Late-twentieth-century war has been highly localized. The responses to it have been global, however, mediated by intergovernmental agencies, nongovernment organizations, and individual countries that negotiate the borders of war and the politics of identity to provide relief to those requesting and demonstrating the need for rescue. In this context, notions of risk have been developed and incorporated in United Nations and country guidelines on gender, and adapted to facilitate the targeted emigration of women from difficult circumstances, particularly war and/or flight. In Australia, Women at Risk and other special visa categories are used to facilitate the immigration of single women and women with children whose partners have been killed or are missing. The political circumstances precipitating immigration are often present also in the country of receipt, however, and this has implications for the provision and delivery of support services and for the physical and mental-health status of the immigrants. Drawing on data from women who have migrated to Australia from the former Yugoslav republics from 1991 to 1996, this chapter raises questions about the globalization of humanitarian projects, the lack of attention in such projects to ethnic and national identities, the ways in which these impinge on migration experience, and the implications for women's health.

In Chapter 8, Christina Zarowsky furthers our insight into the personal costs of migration and flight through her examination of the way in which the provision of temporary care to refugees creates relations of dependence. Zarowsky argues that increasing global mobility, ranging from voluntary repatriation, to settlement in the host country, to third country resettlement, is based on models developed in the West. These are embedded in a long tradition that emerges from a European discourse of charity and are challenged in their non-Western applications. The Office of the United Nations High Commissioner for Refugees (UNHCR) maintains that there are more people today forcibly living outside their home countries than at any time in the past. Zarowsky's chapter is based on her sixteen months of research among various groups of Somali refugees and returnees, during which she paid particular attention to the rhetoric of refugee dependency, suffering, and mental health. She situates her discussion of Somali discourse in an analysis of the historical antecedents of both the Somali idioms and the practices of modern humanitarian aid. Her intention, Zarowsky writes, is to facilitate practitioners and scholars of the Western tradition to revisit some of the assumptions at play in the global discourses of refugees and of refugee suffering and mental health.

By placing the refugee discourses within the institutional idioms of "empowerment" and centering them both in the historical context of aid, charity, and pity, Zarowsky provides a powerful and disturbing example of how humanitarian aid is used to hide the political and economic agendas of refugee relief.

Chapter 9, by Patricia Marshall and Abdallah Daar, shows how globalization operates on multiple levels: goods, policies, experts, and organizations, but also on bodies and technologies of the body. Marshall and Daar explore the way in which access to resources and technological capacity are imported without account of local context, and how materials—including parts of the human body—are traded to enhance the well-being of those wealthy enough to take advantage of such global knowledge. The harvesting of bodies for an international market is perhaps the most vulgar and extreme example, when organs are taken from dead bodies in poor countries and exported to high-technology tertiary hospitals in rich settings to extend others' lives. Alternative patterns are the movement of people between countries to buy technological capacity not locally available: Japanese patients who travel to Australia and the United States for transplants are an example in this case. One might reflect, too, on the "export" of babies for adoption between poor and rich nations. Bodies and body parts are market commodities.

Even in poor countries, technical capacity and demand have outpaced supply, and there is a shortage of cadaver organs and public money to pay for organ transplants. In highly industrialized as much as in poor countries, as Fox and Swazey (1992:75) suggest, access to transplantation is not equal: poor people, women, and minority group members are all less likely to receive organ donations and are less likely than middle-class men to afford transplants or other, similar high-technology medical care. In this context, again, the very poor are victims of globalization. Marshall and Daar examine this as the demand for organ transplants grows in India. Marshall and Daar compellingly situate the international practice of organ transplantation in the constitutive elements of personal beliefs about human identity and moral agency, conventional forms of healing, and technological resources. They suggest that these elements, along with the production of biomedical knowledge regarding organ replacement therapies, shape the lived experience of social suffering and the embodiment of pain. This chapter raises disturbing and provocative questions about the process of decisionmaking and the moral dilemmas surrounding the allocation of scarce human and nonhuman resources, and the power differential between countries. In addition, Marshall and Daar explore the following three factors and how they affect the distribution of organ and tissue replacement: resources and technology available for organ transplantation; cultural construction of beliefs about the body and personhood; and the articulation of biomedical authority and the negotiation of power relationships in the particular social and political contexts.

Globalization enables knowledge and authority to be exported in ways that extend a process established under colonial rule, where local behaviors, belief systems, values, and practices were subject to colonial rule and scrutiny, and deemed inferior. A hierarchy of knowledge is implicit in the representation of biomedical advances, the organization and delivery of medical care, and the production and dissemination of and rewards for knowledge (see also Chapter 12).

Maternal and child health policies and programs provide a superb example of this. Social welfare and public health programs serve as cultural agents or forces, agents of Western expansion in colonial settings. Middle-class and imperial values predominate, and state authorities through the activities of home nurses, inspectors, police, and welfare workers transport these values to poor workers in colonies and imperial centers (Manderson 1996). The rules and regulations that are introduced, from those that govern access to medical care and provide "poor relief" and "single mothers' benefits," to divorce laws, adoption, baby welfare, schooling, "deserted mothers' benefits," maternity leave, and so on, in the past were all—and still are—ideological weapons. Categories of people based on characteristics such as age, sex, ethnicity, and socioeconomic status were once identified as an extension of state intervention under colonialism and required acquiescence to a particular knowledge base, values, behavior, and institutions. Those at a distance from European settlement, whose illnesses were least likely to affect colonial economic life or the health of others, had little access to medical and hospital services, and the geographic and cultural distance between the hospitals and populations in need was sometimes significant. In the center, such factors operated on a socioeconomic class basis—as they still do.

The establishment of public health and social welfare programs occurred through the state, inserting itself into private lives. Whereas some behaviors and practices were defined as "natural," sanitary officers, home visitors, and hospital attendants sought to introduce change and replace "cultural" (reflecting ideas of the nondominant group) practices with "proper" (as defined by the dominant group and thought to be culturally neutral) practices. Public health was concerned with domestic, personal, and women's domains of the household: food, sex, and their by-products. As the Cuban dengue fever example demonstrates, it was women and their commitment to making changes in the domestic environment that led to the success of the control project. The need to intervene in personal matters took the state literally into the home. As part of this move, women everywhere were subject to contemporary European views of "proper" mothering, and to extraordinary levels of monitoring, surveillance, and education in order to change their practices to align with the practices of the colonial elite.

Bottle feeding of infants is a case in point. This practice was introduced in various colonial as well as industrialized settings from the late nineteenth century and was followed quickly by maternal and child health programs, home visiting, and "mothercraft" nursing aimed at educating women in the science of infant care and the medicalization of feeding (Manderson 1982; Robinson 1986; Ram and Jolly 1997; and see Chapter 10). For much of the twentieth century, milk companies played a major role in eroding breast-feeding rates worldwide. Ironically, international nongovernmental organizations such as the La Leche League and multilateral agencies such as the UN Children's Fund (UNICEF) now positively encourage (and teach) women to breast-feed through policy, programs, and individual counseling. What came naturally once is now a learned behavior, resulting in the development of a professional expertise (lactation consultants, for example) and in a range of internationally endorsed policies that challenge multinational hegemony over the diets of infants.

In Chapter 10, "Does Authoritative Knowledge in Infant Nutrition Lead to Successful Breast-Feeding? A Critical Perspective," Arachu Castro and Lauré Marchand-Lucas examine how the underlying discourse, legislation, and practices effectively curtail breast-feeding in France. They compare their data on cultural ethnic groups living in France (French, North African, and Southeast Asian women) with the results of a qualitative survey of French general practitioners, and contextualize these results with an analysis of discourse style and content found in French publications aimed at physicians and parents. Their analysis is organized around the factors that undermine breast-feeding promotion such as the medicalization of infant feeding. Because France has one of the lowest rates of breast-feeding at birth in the world, simultaneously with enlightened social policies to encourage reproduction and provision of family support, the Castro and Marchand-Lucas findings take on a poignancy and power, as well as practical and applied consequences.

In Chapter 11, "Reforming Routines: A Baby-Friendly Hospital in Urban China," Suzanne Zhang Gottschang pursues this ironic twist further when she examines how Chinese mothers in a "baby-friendly" hospital, so-called via a UNICEF initiative, struggle to decide "what's best for baby." Conflict arises between the attraction to globally constructed emphasis on breast-feeding, and the local realities for women whose lives have changed economically in ways that make prolonged breast-feeding extremely difficult.

The direction of our arguments in this introduction, and in the various contributory chapters of this book, is to caution against global realities and to bring to others' attention the ways in which global trends—economic, political, and intellectual—take advantage of powerlessness and poverty. Current debate at the center of public health discourse suggests that this is only one possible perspective, and we want to explore the alternative reading, offered by C. P. Howson and colleagues as we move toward a conclusion. The overarching lesson of the chapters in this volume is that globalization brings mixed blessings and hidden costs. In contrast, in a recent issue of the *Lancet*, Howson et al. (1998) begin with the premise that globalization everywhere brings benefits, that economic development and industrialization lead to an improvement in all people's health and well-being, and that it is in the interests of industrialized countries to invest in global health—this is an argument entirely in sympathy with the World Bank Report of 1993, *Investing in Health*. It is consistent with the more recent pronouncement of the Board of International Health of the Institute of Medicine of the National Academy of Science of the United States, that investing in global health would allow the United States to protect its own people, improve its economy, and advance its international interests. Without apparent irony, Howson et al. extend this argument to maintain that all developed countries will gain in the same way:

> International trade and labour markets, deepening poverty, political instability, and environmental degradation have increased the movement of people across national borders to 1 million per day. Consequently, the industrialised countries face new threats, including emerging infectious diseases, reflecting, in part, the increasing prevalence of drug-resistant pathogens; exposure to dangerous substances, such as contaminated foodstuffs; and violence, including chemical and bioterrorist attack. (Howson et al. 1998:586)

These problems, the authors argue, are neither caused nor can be dealt with nationally. The incidence of infectious diseases has increased because of increased mobility, worldwide, and the growing movement of goods and services—no site is too remote, no person too removed, and no organism too isolated to guarantee safety from infection. Second, they point to the inappropriate and indiscriminate use of antimicrobials in both developed and less developed countries, leading to drug resistance. Third, they point to rapid urbanization, as a result of population displacement due to war and civil disorder and increasing economic needs that people perceive might be resolved in cities. The costs to human health in these patterns in poor countries have repercussions in the industrialized world also: "The health of cities in the developed world depends in some measure on developing nations' efforts to control new diseases and drug-resistant strains of old ones incubating in their slums" and, accordingly, the developed world "ignores at its peril the problems of Third World cities." But, Howson et al.

argue, the logic of investing in poor countries is not only defensive, for "healthier populations in the developing world also provide more vibrant markets for the goods and services of industrialised countries. Investment in health, such as education, can help break cycles of poverty and political instability worldwide, and thus contribute to national economic development and the growth of such markets." Further, they argue, the global market has untapped potential for vaccines, drugs, and medical devices (Howson et al. 1998:587).

Although this approach might seem like a cynical argument against changes in the structural, economic, and political relations of North and South, the authors also argue against the governmental role of investment and institutional strengthening. Governments, they argue, "are no longer the sole agents in the global-health arena." Instead, they argue for a multisectoral approach that would include the private or commercial sector (including multinational corporations); the independent sector of nongovernmental organizations, universities, and private foundations; the multilateral sector, including the WHO and other United Nations agencies; the World Bank, regional development banks, and other Bretton Woods institutions such as the International Monetary Fund and the World Trade Organization; and the bilateral sector (aid agencies). Gill Walt suggests that, in this company of investors in global health, international health organizations have lost moral ground, and that among those who remain committed, in whatever ways, to global cooperation, there is a need to avoid being dominated by a "handful of countries, or by being blinded by conventional wisdom" (Walt 1998:437). This "conventional wisdom" might include, we suggest, a disregard for context and local circumstance, an assumption that the social and personal costs of ill health are everywhere the same (as implied, for example, by the use of DALYs (Disability Adjusted Life Years; see Kleinman and Kleinman 1997:12–15), and a further assumption that the solutions to health problems could be the same. The homogenization of human experience, and of problem solving, continues despite the gestures to heterogeneity that are captured in the discourses of the global. In addition, the economic commodification and capitalization of health results in the moral scarcity of health as measured by quality of life and well-being (Whiteford 1997, 1998).

The *Lancet* incorporates issues at the heart of both the production of knowledge and the political economy of global inequality. "Scientific and economic capabilities," they maintain, "provide a practical basis for coordinated improvement of the health of all people," global surveillance and communication networks (including epidemiological surveillance) help to confine disease, and health services are improved by sharing data—such as, they suggest, comparative studies of health financing, and the acquisition of knowledge from collaboration in international research programs (such as clinical trials) (Howson et al. 1998:588; also Walt 1998). Scientists in developed countries, they continue, should study health issues in poor countries, with the investment of this amply returned as untapped markets of people needing drugs are uncovered.

> If people in developing countries are to have a greater access to essential drugs, vaccines, and medical devices, and if industrialised countries are to take advantage of the expanding markets in these nations, national governments and international agencies must undertake certain measures in response. Mechanisms to increase incentives for industries to invest in research and development on products that would primarily benefit poor populations are needed most. Incentives could include reduced regulatory barriers to product development. (Howson et al. 1998:589)

Industrialized countries have the scientific and technological capability to reduce disease and social and economic inequities, but, the authors argue, increased investment in biomedical research is needed on major global health problems; incentives need to be created for medical advances in poor countries; governments and other international donors need to share the costs of this work; and there needs to be greater investment in the education and training of physicians, researchers, and health care workers. Collaboration is essential between the WHO, the World Bank, and regional development banks to support industry to develop drugs and vaccines for poor countries (Howson et al. 1998:589–590), and by investing in global health, developed nations will be able to improve the health of their own populations, advance their respective economies, and promote humane values and moral leadership in a world of opportunities and profound health needs.

This is not an unreasonable argument. As Walt (1998) also points out, there are now many players in global health, including multinational corporations and other private sector investors, yet still, everywhere, most money spent on health is generated nationally and the "investment in health" is concordant with other national economic investments in social welfare programs (e.g., education) and the general healthiness of the state treasury.

In Chapter 12, James Trostle casts his eye on intellectual imperialism, the paradigms of science, and the issues involved in institutional strengthening and developing research capability in poor countries. In his chapter, "International Health Research: The Rules of the Game," Trostle uncovers "hidden" rules that are too often either not explored or not clarified, leaving the unenlightened reader to assume that the playing field for publishing international health research is level and therefore the same for everyone. Trostle explores the local systems of professional prestige and ranking that help to define who has expertise, what types of questions are seen as appropriate for research and publication, who is an appropriate audience, and what kinds of scientific writing and analysis are valued. As he points out, understanding these views may force readers to evaluate the rationales for supporting researching differently: because it is valued, and because it is labeled high quality.

The chapters in this volume represent diverse sociocultural, political, and economic experiences in our attempt to provide a scholarly investigation of how global processes and local identities commodify health. The book draws on examples related to the appropriate use of drugs and the political economy of pharmaceuticals; on reproductive, child survival, and HIV/AIDS prevention policies and programs; on population movement and the health crises of refugees within and between nations; on breast-feeding and the conflicts of global marketing, global health policies, advocacy, and modernity; on the ethics and distribution of body parts; on local ideological frameworks that interpret health policies and outcomes; and on the politics of knowledge and notions of universal science. In so doing, the authors challenge conventional assumptions often used in international health planning about the means by which health standards might be improved, mortality rates reduced, and well-being enhanced. There are, the authors argue, no easy solutions, no global answers to bring about changes in health behavior, to address structural inequalities that strip people's access to health and medical services, or to overcome the trade imbalances that result in the term *investing in health* having very different meanings according to whether the view is from New York or Tokyo, Yaoundé or Yangon.

References

Aboagye-Kwarteng, T., L. Manderson, and R. Msiska. 1997. "Reviews and Strategic Planning for HIV/AIDS Prevention and Care: Anthropology and the Expanded Response to AIDS," *AIDS and Anthropology Bulletin* 9(2): 1, 8–10.

Altman, D. 1994. *Power and Community: Organizational and Cultural Responses to AIDS.* London: Taylor and Francis.

Bruenjes, A. 1997. "Patterns of Migration." In *Global Forces, Local Realities, Anthropological Perspectives on Change in the Third World,* B. Geddes and M. Crick, eds. Geelong, Australia: Deakin University Press.

Fisher, J. 1997. "Doing Good? The Politics and Antipolitics of NGO Practices," *Annual Reviews in Anthropology* 26: 439–486.

Fox, R. C., and J. P. Swazey. 1992. *Spare Parts: Organ Replacement in American Society.* New York and Oxford: Oxford University Press.

Geddes, B. 1997a. "Introduction." In *Global Forces, Local Realities, Anthropological Perspectives on Change in the Third World,* B. Geddes and M. Crick, eds. Geelong, Australia: Deakin University Press.

———. 1997b. "Third World Nations: Global Demands, Local Political Realities." In *Global Forces, Local Realities, Anthropological Perspectives on Change in the Third World,* B. Geddes and M. Crick, eds. Geelong, Australia: Deakin University Press.

Gove, S., and G. H. Pelto. 1994. "Focused Ethnographic Studies in the WHO Programme for the Control of Acute Respiratory Infections," *Medical Anthropology* 15(4): 409–424.

Howson, C. P., H. V. Fineberg, and B. R. Bloom. 1998. "The Pursuit of Global Health: The Relevance of Engagement for Developed Countries," *Lancet* 351: 586–590.

Kanji, N., A. Hardon, J. W. Harnmeijer, M. Mamdani, and G. Walt, eds. 1992. *Drugs Policy in Developing Countries.* London and New Jersey: Zed Books.

Kearney, Michael. 1995. "The Local and the Global: The Anthropology of Globalization and Transnationalism," *Annual Reviews in Anthropology* 24: 547–565.

Kleinman, A., and J. Kleinman. 1997. "The Appeal of Experience, the Dismay of Images: Cultural Appropriations of Suffering in Our Times." In *Social Suffering*, A. Kleinman, V. Das, and M. Lock, eds. Berkeley and Los Angeles: University of California Press.

Manderson, L. 1982. "Bottle Feeding and Ideology in Colonial Malaya: The Production of Change," *International Journal of Health Services* 12(4): 597–616.

———. 1995. "Wireless Wars in the Eastern Arena: Epidemiological Surveillance, Disease Prevention and the Work of Eastern Bureau of the League of Nations Health Organisation, 1925–1942," In *International Health Organisations and Movements, 1918–1939,* P. Weindling, ed. Cambridge, England: Cambridge University Press.

———. 1996. *Sickness and the State: Health and Illness in Colonial Malaya.* Cambridge, England, and Melbourne: Cambridge University Press.

Ram, K., and M. Jolly, eds. 1997. *Maternities and Modernities: Colonial and Post-Colonial Experiences in Asia and the Pacific.* Cambridge, England: Cambridge University Press.

Robinson, K. 1986. "Australia's Got the Milk, We've Got the Problems." In *Shared Wealth and Symbol: Food, Culture and Society in Oceania and Southeast Asia,* L. Manderson, ed. New York: Cambridge University Press.

Rozemberg, B., and L. Manderson. 1998. "'Nerves' and Tranquilizer Use in Rural Brazil," *International Journal of Health Services* 28(1): 165–181.

Silverman, M. 1976. *The Drugging of the Americas.* Berkeley: University of California Press.

Unwin, N., G. Alberti, T. Aspray, R. Edwards, J. C. Mbanya, E. Sobngwi, F. Mugasi, S. Rashid, P. Setel, and D. Whiting. 1998. "Economic Globalisation and Its Effect on Health," *British Medical Journal* 316: 1401–1402.

Van der Geest, S., and S. R. Whyte, eds. 1988. *The Context of Medicines in Developing Countries: Studies in Pharmaceutical Anthropology.* Dordrecht: Kluwer Academic Publishers.

Walt, G. 1998. "Globalisation of International Health," *Lancet* 351: 434–437.

Whiteford, Linda M. 1997. "Children's Health as Accumulated Capital: Structural Adjustment in the Dominican Republic and Cuba." In *Small Wars: The Cultural Politics of Childhood,* Nancy Scheper-Hughes and Carolyn Sargent, eds. Berkeley and Los Angeles: University of California Press.

———. 1998. "Sembrando el Futuro: Globalization and the Commodification of Health." In *Crossing Currents: Continuity and Change in Latin America,* Michael B. Whiteford and Scott Whiteford, eds. Englewood Cliffs, NJ: Prentice Hall.

WHO (World Health Organization). 1978. *Alma Ata Statement.* Geneva: World Health Organization.

———. 1987. *The Rational Use of Drugs.* Geneva: World Health Organization.

PART 1

International Health Policy and Issues of Localization

1

The Politics of Child Survival

Judith Justice

In the 1980s and 1990s the political appeal of international initiatives dealing with child survival were unprecedented in development assistance, garnering broad-based bipartisan support among governments, international agencies, and nongovernmental organizations (NGOs), and resulted in successful mobilization of funds and resources for child health. These initiatives were designed to reduce mortality rates among infants and children under the age of five, principally by providing oral rehydration therapy to combat dehydration from diarrhea, and immunization to protect against early childhood diseases. This international success at mobilization raises the question: How did the political appeal of the focus on child survival at the global level fit with national policies and local priorities in developing countries?

This chapter draws upon multicountry collaborative research in Egypt, India, Indonesia, and Uganda to examine the full spectrum of the international health policy process from the initiation of health priorities by donor countries, to the level of international organizations, to recipient governments, and ultimately to implementation and the impact upon beneficiaries at the local level.

By studying the international child survival initiatives within a broader political and cultural context, including bureaucratic politics and organizational factors in foreign aid policy, together with the influence of domestic politics and the underlying cultural values of donor countries, it is possible to investigate powerful but often unrecognized effects of the formulation of international health policy and its appropriateness for recipient countries. The current trends and priorities of international health, starting with the exceptional support for the child survival initiatives, cannot be understood without taking such factors into account. Among the many lessons learned is that despite the impressive gains, particularly in reducing infant mortality, such global policies often create problems and confusion at the national and local levels.

International Initiatives for Child Survival

The child survival initiatives are unique among international development programs for the exceptional mobilization of global support for child health. In fact, these initiatives were so successful that they progressed from initiatives to a global Child Health Revolution. This revolution provides an excellent opportunity to examine the relationship between global forces and local identities.

By the late 1970s, children's health was given increasing attention by the international health community. At that time, the focus was on factors contributing to infant mortality rates and the high number of deaths from diarrheal-related diseases. The result was the infant diarrheal-disease control program, which utilized a simple technology for rehydration called oral rehydration solution (ORS) (Phillips et al. 1987; Coreil and Mull 1990). ORS is a solution of salt, sugar, and water, to be mixed at home or available in factory-made packets, and distributed at low cost through local health services and marketplaces. Although ORS quickly became an international priority, it was developed in a local context in Bangladesh at the International Cholera Research Centre.[1]

Many international organizations supported programs promoting ORS. For example, the U.S. Agency for International Development (USAID) provided large-scale, long-term support to establish the wide use of ORS in Egypt—and quickly learned that what in Bangladesh had appeared to be adoption of a simple technology nevertheless initially encountered many problems among Egyptian health professionals and in local communities (Langsten and Hill 1995; Miller and Hirschhorn 1995). Yet despite unanticipated problems when global child health programs met local realities, children continued to be the focus of international health. By the early 1980s, infant survival began receiving priority attention at international conferences and in the development literature (Arora 1980; Gwatkins 1980; Mosley and Chen 1984).

UNICEF Steps In: The Child Survival Revolution

In 1982 the United Nations Children's Fund (UNICEF) launched the global international Child Health Revolution (UNICEF 1985; Goodfield

1991; Black 1996). By the mid-1980s, the international health community had mobilized resources in the developed and developing world to address the health needs of children worldwide. The objective of the Child Survival Revolution was to reduce mortality rates among infants and children under the age of five. This goal was to be accomplished by providing life-saving treatment using two principal methods: oral rehydration therapy (defined previously) to combat dehydration from diarrhea, and immunization in early childhood against such major infectious diseases as tuberculosis, diphtheria, pertussis, tetanus, measles, and poliomyelitis. In promoting and implementing Child Survival initiatives, international development agencies varied the definition of this term to suit their individual viewpoints, but the two technological interventions—oral rehydration and immunization— emerged as the twin-engine approach to child health and reducing infant mortality. The logic underlying these two selected interventions was that they attacked the primary causes contributing to infant death: dehydration from diarrheal diseases and infectious diseases of early childhood.

Although the Child Survival Revolution as initially promoted by UNICEF advocated the adoption of a number of cheap, accessible, and simple technologies including growth monitoring, oral rehydration therapy, breast-feeding, and immunization (which were referred to as GOBI), the 1984 Bellagio Conference, "Protecting the World's Children," shifted attention to mortality from childhood diseases that could be prevented through immunization (Rockefeller Foundation 1984). The result was a program called Universal Childhood Immunization (UCI), which became the core of the Child Survival Revolution. A goal was set to immunize 80 percent of the world's children by 1990. However unrealistic this target seemed at the time, it has reportedly been met in some countries. Even in countries where it was not possible to meet the global target, the immunization coverage rates improved dramatically (UNICEF 1990; World Health Organization 1991a).

Debate, Competition, and Collaboration

With the Child Survival Revolution, UNICEF became a major player in the health field, a position seen by some as challenging the World Health Organization's role of formulating international health policy. Because of UNICEF's high visibility from its aggressive media campaign to promote universal childhood immunization, it was falsely credited with creating the child immunization initiative (LaFond 1994). In fact, in 1974 the World Health Organization initiated the Expanded Program on Immunization (EPI) to prevent the six major childhood diseases by immunization (Jamison and Saxenian 1994). This was in the wake of the success of the smallpox eradication program. Because smallpox eradication was such a demonstrable success, a fact widely cited as one of the great health achievements of the twentieth century, the founders of the Expanded Program on Immunization were determined that the lessons learned from the smallpox experience should benefit a broader program of disease control through vaccination (Henderson 1994).

Although the media and literature reflected the public debate between the executive directors of the WHO (Halfdan Mahler) and UNICEF (James Grant) over the WHO's more horizontal approach of EPI within Primary Health Care and UNICEF's vertical approach through its UCI program, it was quickly recognized that the collaboration of the global health community was necessary to garner the necessary technical, financial, and political support needed to achieve international and national immunization goals. The broad range of partners included international organizations such as the WHO and UNICEF, bilateral development agencies, and nongovernmental organizations such as the Rockefeller Foundation and Rotary International (Henderson 1994). Rotary International's role in providing financial support for polio and the active involvement of local Rotary members in the promotion of national immunization campaigns have established a model of collaboration for other NGOs and service organizations such as the Lions Clubs (Foreman 1991; Skolnick 1993).

Together with individuals well known in the international community such as Ken Warren with the Rockefeller Foundation, Jonas Salk, and Robert McNamara (former president of the World Bank who viewed child survival as a key to population control), the international organizations were instrumental in forming the prestigious Task Force for Child Survival to spearhead the immunization effort, coordinate support, and develop country programs and research aspects of accelerated immunization activities. This task force, officially established in 1984, was located in Atlanta, Georgia, and directed by William Foege, one of the architects and leaders of the smallpox eradication campaign. The original members of the Task Force were UNICEF, the WHO, the Rockefeller Foundation, the United Nations Development Programme, and the World Bank (Guerrero 1995; Bowles 1998). Task force members and their representatives were among the inner circle of people (with almost no women) who had met in public and private meetings over the years to formulate the child survival strategy.

The Child Survival Revolution culminated in the 1990 World Summit for Children, which brought together an unprecedented number of heads of state. The summit, organized by UNICEF and held in New York, gave the highest-level recognition to the tremendous accomplishments of the child immunization campaign (UNICEF 1990). The impressive list of participants at the Children's Summit confirmed the claim of UNICEF's executive director, James Grant, that through the promotion of child immunization, every president, prime minister, and other head of state knew about the needs of children in their countries (personal communications, 1988–1990). Many of these national leaders had been personally involved in media campaigns in their countries, appearing on TV and radio, attending immunization sessions, and being photographed for posters showing the president or first lady immunizing children. Thus, child immunization was politically attractive at the national level, as well as internationally.

Following the Children's Summit and the much publicized reported achievement in reaching the targeted 80 percent immunization goal, the Task Force on Child Survival changed its name to the Task Force on Child Survival and Development to reflect its expanded mandate, to add other immunizations such as hepatitis B, to extend the target to include eradication of diseases such as polio, and to begin to looking at the health needs of children beyond immunization. The task force was also active in developing the Children's Vaccine Initiative (CVI), established in 1990 by many of the task force's original member organizations. The ultimate objective of CVI was the development of a single vaccine that could protect against all infectious diseases with a single oral dose administered any time after birth (Mitchell et al. 1993; Muraskin 1998). As the CVI developed, an even greater concern about the need to build a truly global system of high-quality vaccine supply was added (Henderson 1994).

Criticism and Concerns

Despite the universally recognized achievements of the child immunization campaign and other child survival interventions, the approach is not without its critics (Banerji 1988, 1990). Many of these concerns relate to the ongoing debate between comprehensive and selective primary health care (Rifkin and Walt 1986; Unger and Killingsworth 1986; Newell 1988; Wiener 1988). The earlier international approach to improving health, primary health care, was characterized as concerned with a developmental process by which people improve both their lives and their lifestyles. Good health was seen as a key factor to this process. Child immunization and diarrheal disease control programs were categorized as selective primary health care and described as being concerned with medical and/or technological interventions aimed at improving the health status of the most individuals at the lowest cost (Walsh and Warren 1979). From this perspective, child immunization programs are regarded as technical interventions, similar to the earlier vertical health programs, and therefore "selective" rather than "comprehensive" health care. An Indian critic (Banerji 1988,

1990) of the global focus on child immunization summarized the following from a country perspective: The Universal Child Immunization Program

1. Negated the concept of community participation with programs planned from the "bottom up."
2. Gave allocations only to people with priority diseases, leaving the rest to suffer.
3. Reinforced authoritarian attitudes.
4. Had a fragile scientific basis.
5. Had a questionable moral and ethical value in which foreign and elite interests overruled those of the majority of the people.

Others compared primary health care and child immunization:

> PHC was crystallized as an approach at a time when there was wide agreement that the causes of poverty were non-natural and that social justice was a requisite for health. UNICEF locates health action wholly outside the realm of socioeconomic rights and responsibilities. Appropriate technologies have become a substitute for social transformation. The Children's Revolution is a minimal package in the face of the failure of parents to achieve a revolution in the power relations determining health. (Wiener 1988:965)

Even major donors to the child immunization initiative voiced concerns about the narrow focus to child immunization. Although the Scandinavian countries were among the largest donors to UNICEF, they registered complaints at UNICEF's board meetings about the need to support more comprehensive approaches to maternal and child health (personal communications 1989, 1990). Bilateral donor organizations such as USAID and U.S.-based NGOs quickly realized the political appeal of child survival to obtain funds from the U.S. Congress, but then used the funds to support a broader range of interventions, including ORS, vitamin A, and birth spacing programs.

UNICEF was widely criticized by many in the international community as being irresponsible because of its careful crafting of the Universal Childhood Immunization Initiative, avoiding any reference to the negative impact of large family size on children's health or the need for family planning, in order to obtain support of the Catholic Church and leaders in Catholic countries (personal communications 1988–1990; Basch 1990). At the country level, some governments questioned whether child immunization addressed their priority health needs (Banerji 1988, 1990). Many expressed concern about the need to shift financial and human resources from other health programs to meet the expectations of the latest international health priority—child immunization.

Questions of Long-Term Sustainability: The Research

Along with such criticisms, a number of people involved at the international, national, and local levels have recognized that there are problems relating to the long-term sustainability of child survival programs. Such issues take us back to the relationship between the global, national, and local and the level playing field.

What is the sustainability and long-term effectiveness of such global programs, even one as successful as universal childhood immunization, that are conceived and implemented from the top down with very little local input from the bottom up? For example, how can child immunization move from a high-profile campaign approach, promoted through aggressive social moblization, to the institutionalization of immunization as part of routine health services (Dietz and Cutts 1997)?

How Were Child Survival Initiatives Promoted at the Global Level?

Research carried out from 1985 to 1998 on child survival[2] addressed these and other issues, building upon the growing interest of anthropologists and other social scientists in studying the impact of globalization in a cultural context (Nader 1974; Kleinman 1995; Gupta and Ferguson 1997). The research studied the history of child survival initiatives from the initial formulation of this policy to the implementation of programs in recipient countries. The first phase of this research investigated how the initiatives were promoted, what factors made child survival politically attractive, how it reflected domestic politics and values, and its significance for the international health policy making process. The study found that the child survival initiatives were vigorously advocated in the United States by a strong grassroots mobilization of constituent pressure and lobbying from special interest groups and nongovernmental organizations such as Bread for the World and Results (Quinley and Baker 1986). The grassroots promotion of specialized foreign aid issues suggests a new politics of international health in which domestic politics and values have a greater impact on foreign aid. Although child survival initiatives were international from the start, the early strategy for promotion of the child survival concept was developed to fit the U.S. policy context in order to acquire congressional support and funding. Gaining active support from U.S. constituents is one way in which child survival was unique, as foreign aid is rarely a priority issue with members of Congress or their constituents. Yet nongovernmental organizations mobilized Americans to use traditional lobbying techniques in convincing their representatives to support child survival (Quinley and Baker 1986). In fact, one of the ironies of the Child Survival

Revolution is the willingness of U.S. citizens to advocate support for children's health in other countries while neglecting the health of children in the United States.

The grassroots support in the United States for Child Survival resulted in congressional funds being allocated for programs through USAID and United States–based nongovernmental organizations, and also for increased funding for UNICEF and other international organizations promoting childhood immunization (Nowels 1991). Thus, child survival initiatives quickly became the international priority. But what was happening at the same time at the national and local level in countries targeted for child immunization campaigns? What was the impact of increased funding from international organizations and an influx of intense manpower support in many cases?

How Were Child Survival Initiatives Promoted at the National Level?

The second phase of this research studied the relationship between the international Child Survival Revolution, the role of donors and nongovernmental organizations, and the recipient country's health priorities. A series of country case studies was developed to examine recipient country responses to Child Survival. The countries, including Egypt, India, Indonesia, and Uganda, were selected to provide a comparison of national responses to child survival initiatives.[3] By examining national approaches to child health prior to and during the 1980s and early 1990s, the case studies have documented how the child survival policies and funding have affected the way governmental, international, nongovernmental, and recipient-level health organizations function and deliver child health services. Each study was designed to assess child survival policies and programs within the national context, and this information was related back to the broader policy issues.[4]

The case studies were also designed to document the child survival/child health priorities as defined by each participating country. The research focused on the cultural appropriateness of services that have resulted from the international child survival policy. In order to study the impact of this policy on local health services, including reproductive health, the research looked at how international and national agencies have translated the child survival policy and resources into programs and services. How was child survival packaged in the bureaucratic context of the health agencies? How were child survival policies translated from the international to the national level? In recipient countries, were international child survival priorities incorporated into national child health policies? What impact have child survival initiatives had upon ongoing health services?

How do these services fit with local cultures, priorities, needs, and resources? Was there any consideration of the appropriateness of child survival programs to local conditions? How did local communities perceive the initiative, and were they involved in the planning of programs? How were child survival programs implemented and evaluated at the country level? A particular focus of the country studies was also on the sustainability of child survival and child immunization programs in view of reduced support from international organizations in the 1990s, as the international health community has already moved on to other priorities (Pan American Health Organization 1995; UNICEF 1996; Werner and Sanders 1997).

Realities at National and Local Levels

In spite of the tremendous achievements improving immunization rates, many of the gains were receding in the 1990s as national and local governments struggled to continue earlier programs that were imposed from above and that had been supported primarily by external funds. Members of the research team reported that studying child immunization policy at the country level had not been easy for a number of reasons, many related to the challenges of studying a global program at the local level, at the same time as retrospectively reconstructing the early history of child survival initiatives in each country. A consistent problem in the four countries, and at all levels, was the absence of an institutional memory as international staff moved on to other countries, in addition to frequent transfers at the national and local level, so that few people were still available who had been part of the initial decisionmaking process. Not only were they not available to answer the researchers' questions; the people who initially committed to adopt UCI and other child survival initiatives at the country level were no longer in place to implement them, thus increasing the gap between international and local realities.

As previously noted, national leaders certainly benefited from the political popularity of universal child immunization and were frequently portrayed in the national media, which was aggressively used to promote immunization campaigns. Researchers found that the media portrayed national and urban activities, focusing on the political leaders and elites, but that less coverage was given to activities and personalities at the local level in peri-urban communities and rural areas, where the real work was being carried out.

The researchers also studied how the global immunization policy was adapted to local conditions. The situations differed in each country. For example, in Indonesia, prior to the international promotion of child survival initiatives, the government had an integrated maternal and child health program (Posyandu) throughout the country and initially tried to integrate Universal Child Immunization into this existing program. In other countries, however, external pressure to reach the internationally set immunization coverage target of 80 percent was so great that other approaches and activities—often less suited to local conditions—were adopted. In Uganda the government health services were just being reestablished after the long years of war, and at first the international child immunization program was seen as helping to organize and focus local health services. Immunization of children was described as the mother's entry into the health system, but the campaign approach promoted by UCI separated immunization and health care. As a result, many mothers did not even understand that immunization was related to health care of their children.

Official evaluation of the universal immunization program at the country level also was often conducted in such a way as to support the goals of the international policy, rather than the reality of local programs. These are only a few of the comparative findings, but they confirm that global objectives and goals were dominant even at the local level.

The research also identified several factors contributing to the child immunization initiative's popular appeal and political success at the global and national level. Of particular significance is the ideological content that fits with the current political climate and meets the demand for greater accountability in organization and government spending, because implementation involves narrowly defined, quantifiable goals, and the limited focus appears to be cost-effective. For example, child immunization is accountable because it focuses on only one measurable program—immunization—which can be targeted and counted. Such methods make it possible to calculate success statistically and establish a direct relationship between money contributed and outcomes achieved. Similarly, the child immunization initiative's reliance on technological intervention rather than changing health behavior offers the reassurance of tangible tasks to be performed with tangible results.

As previously discussed, child survival initiatives have marketing appeal with their focused approach that can be quickly and simply explained, in addition to strong emotional appeal. "Saving infant lives" and "averting deaths" make perfect subjects for promotional materials used in the immunization campaign. These factors have contributed to the success of the immunization initiative at the global level and to the social marketing of other child survival interventions (such as ORS) at the national and local level, but at the same time often create problems and confusion at the local level.

Conclusion

The history of international health policy and its outcomes illuminates several important points about the global policymaking process and its impact at the country level.

First, policies developed at the global level in response to international pressures can be beneficial to local populations, but at the same time often create unanticipated costs for the country. Although external funds are made available to cover initial costs, countries are required to use their limited human and financial resources to implement these global initiatives at the local level.

Second, the international health community often fails to recognize the fragility of health systems and the scarcity of resources in countries. Global health initiatives are frequently promoted without enough regard to the particular local setting in which they are being introduced: for instance, the availability of trained personnel, ability to deliver supplies, ability to finance recurrent costs to operate externally provided capital investments, and follow-up. Nevertheless, as confirmed by the country case studies, national programs are weighted toward global priorities because of the international resources.

Third, the practical implications of new global initiatives and approaches are often not adequately investigated. For example, pilot immunization projects—often more suitable to local conditions—were first conducted in some countries, but it was not clear to the researchers how the lessons learned from such demonstration projects informed the rapid expansion from small-scale pilot projects to national immunization programs and other global child survival initiatives.

Fourth, the frequent shifts and increasingly narrowing focus in international priorities make it difficult for national health systems to respond and absorb them. For example, since the 1980s health priorities have moved from primary health care, to child survival, to child immunization, to the eradication of polio by the year 2000 (Pan American Health Organization 1995; Gounder 1998). Individual agency priorities also undergo rapid change as demonstrated by the shift in UNICEF's role from being the primary promoter of child immunization until 1990 to its current focus on child rights. In fact, in November 1997 an email from a UNICEF staff member stated in bold letters "Immunization is out at UNICEF," meaning that since declaration of the achievement of universal childhood immunization in 1990, UNICEF had moved on to new priorities, leaving the sustainability of universal child immunization to the countries to manage without external assistance. As a result of the shifting priorities at the global level, immunization rates are dropping in many countries (UNICEF 1996, 1998).

* * *

On a personal note, I must confess to a sense of déjà vu as I listened to my colleagues at our team research meetings (held at the Bellagio Center in 1997 and 1999) describing their research findings, as these were the same conclusions I drew twenty years ago when first studying the fit between international health policies and local priorities. I was depressed to realize that although the priorities and actors had changed, we still have not found a way to close the gap between the international and the local. As my colleagues and I discussed how best to distribute the findings of our research to decisionmakers, I wondered if we would be more successful in communicating the lessons learned than I had been earlier. And thus we are left with the question in this era of globalization: How can our research results, in addition to lessons learned from experiences of well-intentioned international initiatives such as child survival, help in contributing to a better fit between the global and the local?

Notes

1. The name of the International Cholera Research Centre was changed to the International Center for Diarrheal Disease Research, Bangladesh (ICDDR-B).
2. The individual case studies were conducted in-country by national researchers—anthropologists and medical doctors with public health training: Charles Rwabukwali conducted the Uganda study; Salwa Gomaa conducted the study in Egypt with support from Jocelyn de Jung; Dileep Mavalankar studied child immunization in India; and Abby Ruddick and Meiwita Iskandar Budiharsana conducted the Indonesian study.
3. Ibid.
4. Funding for the country studies was provided by the Rockefeller Foundation, Ford Foundation, and the University of California Pacific Rim Program.

References

Arora, R. R. 1980. "Morbidity and Mortality in Infants in a Rural Community of Rajasthan," *Journal of Communicable Diseases* 12: 27–33.
Banerji, D. 1988. "Hidden Menace in the Universal Child Immunization Program," *International Journal of Health Services* 18: 293–299.
———. 1990. "Crash of the Immunization Program: Consequences of a Totalitarian Approach," *International Journal of Health Services* 20: 501–510.
Basch, P. 1990. *Textbook of International Health.* Oxford: Oxford University Press.
BASICS (Basic Support for Institutionalizing Child Survival). 1996a. "Accomplishment in Child Survival Research and Programs," B. Sack, Ricardo Rodrigues, and Robert Black. Current Issues in Child Survival Series. Arlington, VA: BASICS.
———. 1996b. "Challenges to Immunization," *Quarterly Technical Newsletter* (3).
———. 1996c. "Monitoring and Evaluation: Tools for Improving Child Health and Survival," *Quarterly Technical Newsletter* (5).
———. 1996d. "Overcoming Remaining Barriers: The Pathway to Survival." Arlington, VA: BASICS.
———. 1997a. "Review of Child Survival Funding: 1990–1995," Deborah A. McFarland, Current Issues in Child Survival Series. Arlington, VA: BASICS.

———. 1997b. "The Recent Evolution of Child Mortality in the Developing World." Arlington, VA: BASICS.

Black, M. 1996. *Children First: The Story of UNICEF, Past and Present*. Oxford: Oxford University Press.

Bland, J., and J. Clements. 1998. "Protecting the World's Children: The Story of WHO's Immunization Programme," *World Health Forum* 19: 162–173.

Bowles, N. R. 1998. "The Task Force for Child Survival and Development. Hope as Energy: An Experiment 1884–1998." Unpublished manuscript. Atlanta, GA: Task Force on Child Survival.

Coreil, J., and J. D. Mull, eds. 1990. *Anthropology and Primary Health Care*. Boulder, CO: Westview Press.

Cutts, F. T., and P. G. Smith. 1994. *Vaccination and World Health*. Chichester, UK: Wiley and Sons.

Dick, B. 1985. "Issues in Immunization in Developing Countries." Evaluation and Planning Centre for Health Care, No. 7, London School of Hygiene and Tropical Medicine.

Dietz, V., and F. Cutts. 1997. "The Use of Mass Campaigns in the Expanded Programme on Immunization: A Review of Reported Advantages and Disadvantages," *International Journal of Health Services* 27(4): 767–790.

Fatt, N., and R. Grenell. 1988. Evaluation of the Campaign for Child Survival. Unpublished manuscript.

Foege, W. F. 1989. "Prospects for Universal Immunization: Strategies for Achievement," *Reviews of Infectious Diseases* 11(3): S659–S662.

Foreman, J. 1991. "Sight First: Lions Conquering Blindness," *Archives of Ophthalmology* 109: 624.

Freed, G. L., W. C. Bordley, and G. H. Defriese. 1993. "Childhood Immunization Programs: An Analysis of Policy Issues," *Millbank Quarterly* 71(1): 65–96.

Goodfield, J. 1991. *A Chance to Live: The Heroic Story of the Global Campaign to Immunize the World's Children*. New York: Macmillan.

Gounder, C. 1998. "The Progress of the Polio Eradication Initiative: What Prospects for Eradicating Measles?" *Health Policy and Planning* 13(3): 212–233.

Grant, J. 1991. "The Children's Vaccine Initiative and Other Promises to Keep," *Journal of Tropical Pediatrics* 37: 272–274.

Greenough, P., and P. Streefland. 1998. "Social Science and Immunization: New Possibilities and Projects." *Items* 52(1): March. New York: Social Science Research Council.

Grossman, M. 1995. "Immunization: Past Successes, Future Challenges," *Infectious Disease Clinics of North America* 9(2): 325–334.

Guerrero, R. 1995. *The Task Force for Child Survival and Development: An Evaluation*. Washington, DC. Unpublished report.

Gupta, A., and J. Ferguson. 1997. "Beyond 'Culture': Space, Identity, and the Politics of Difference." In *Culture, Power, Place: Explorations in Critical Anthropology*, A. Gupta and J. Ferguson, eds. Durham, NC: Duke University Press.

Gwatkins, D. 1980. "How Many Die? A Set of Demographic Estimates of the Annual Number of Infant and Child Deaths in the World," *American Journal of Public Health* 70: 1286–1289.

Halstead, S. B., and F. Hartvelt. 1990. "Children's Vaccine: A Strategy to Provide More and Better Vaccines." Presentation at the Programme for Vaccine Development, World Health Organization, June 24, Geneva.

Heggenhougen, K., and J. Clements. 1987. "Acceptability of Childhood Immunization: Social Science Perspectives." Evaluation and Planning Centre Publication No. 14, London School of Hygiene and Tropical Medicine.

Henderson R. H. 1994. "Vaccination: Successes and Challenges." In *Vaccination and World Health,* F. Cutts and P. Smith, eds. Chichester, UK: Wiley and Sons.

———. 1998. "Keynote Address to the International Conference on Global Disease Elimination and Eradication and Public Health Strategies," February 28, Atlanta.

Jamison, D. T., W. H. Mosley, A. R. Measham, et al. 1993. *Disease Control Priorities in Developing Countries.* Oxford: Oxford University Press.

Jamison, D. T., and H. Saxenian. 1994. "Investing in Immunization: Conclusions from the 1993 World Development Report." In *Vaccination and World Health,* F. T. Cutts and P. G. Smith, eds. Chichester, UK: Wiley and Sons.

Justice, J. 1986. *Policies, Plans, and People: Foreign Aid and Health Development.* Berkeley: University of California Press.

———. 1987. "The Bureaucratic Context of International Health: A Social Scientist's View," *Social Science and Medicine* 25(12): 1301–1306.

———. 1995. "The Cultural and Political Dimensions of International Health Policy." Paper presented at the Social Science and Immunization Research Planning Conference, Dhaka, August 18–24.

Kent, G. 1991. *The Politics of Children's Survival.* New York: Praeger.

Kleinman, A. 1995. "A Critique of Objectivity in International Health." In *Writing at the Margin: Discourse Between Anthropology and Medicine.* Berkeley: University of California Press.

LaFond, A. 1994. "UNICEF," *Health Policy and Planning* 9(3): 343–346.

Langsten, R., and K. Hill. 1995. "Treatment of Childhood Diarrhea in Rural Egypt," *Social Science and Medicine* 40(7): 989–1001.

Lee, K., and G. Walt. 1992. "What Role for WHO in the 1990s?" *Health Policy and Planning* 7(4): 387–390.

McDivitt, J. A., and K. Wilkins. 1991. "Keeping the Promise of the World Summit for Children: One Year Later." Paper presented as part of the panel Report Card to the Nation: FY90/91 Actions Taken by the United States to Benefit Children Internationally, at the 119th Annual Meeting of the American Public Health Association, Atlanta, November 12.

Miller, P., and N. Hirschhorn. 1995. "The Effect of a National Control of Diarrheal Diseases Program on Mortality: The Case of Egypt," *Social Science and Medicine* 40(10): S1–S30.

Mitchell, V. S., N. M. Philipose, and J. P. Sanford, eds. 1993. *The Children's Vaccine Initiative: Achieving the Vision. Institute of Medicine.* Washington, DC: National Academy Press.

Mosley, W. H., and L. C. Chen. 1984. "Child Survival: Strategies for Research," *Population and Development Review,* a supplement to vol. 10.

Muraskin, W. 1995. *The War Against Hepatitis B: A History of the International Task Force on Hepatitis B Immunization.* Philadelphia: University of Pennsylvania Press.

———. 1998. *The Politics of International Health: The Children's Vaccine Initiative and the Struggle to Develop Vaccines for the Third World.* Albany: State University of New York Press.

Murugasampillay, S. 1994. "Who Determines National Health Policies?" In *Vaccination and World Health,* F. T. Cutts and P. G. Smith, eds. Chichester, UK: Wiley and Sons.

Nader, L. 1974. "Up the Anthropologist: Perspectives Gained from Studying Up."

In *Reinventing Anthropology*, D. Hymes, ed. New York: Vintage Books.
Newell, K. 1988. "Selective Primary Health Care: The Counter Revolution," *Social Science and Medicine* 26: 903–906.
Nowels, L. Q. 1991. "Foreign Aid: Budget, Policy, and Reform." CRS Issue Brief, Library of Congress, Congressional Research Service.
Okuonzi, S. A., and J. Macrae. 1995. "Whose Policy Is It Anyway? International and National Influences on Health Policy Development in Uganda," *Health Policy and Planning* 10(2):122–132.
Onta, S. R., S. Sabroe, and E. H. Hansen. 1998. "The Quality of Immunization Data from Routine Primary Health Care Reports: A Case from Nepal," *Health Policy and Planning* 13(2): 131–139.
PAHO (Pan American Health Organization). 1995. "The Impact of the Expanded Programme on Immunization and Polio Eradication Initiative on Health Systems in the Americas." Report of the Taylor Commission, Washington, DC.
Phillips, M. A., R. G. Feachem, and A. Mills. 1987. "Options for Diarrhoea Control: The Cost and Cost-Effectiveness of Selected Interventions for the Prevention of Diarrhoea." EPC Publications No. 13, Evaluation and Planning Centre for Health Care, London School of Hygiene and Tropical Medicine.
Quinley, J. C., and T. D. Baker. 1986. "Lobbying for International Health: The Link Between Good Ideas and Funded Programs: Bread for the World and the Agency for International Development," *American Journal of Public Health* 76(7): 793–796.
Rifkin, S. B., and G. Walt. 1986. "Why Health Improves: Defining the Issues Concerning 'Comprehensive Primary Health Care' and 'Selective Primary Health Care,'" *Social Science and Medicine* 23: 559–566.
Rockefeller Foundation. 1984. "Protecting the World's Children: Vaccines and Immunization." A Bellagio Conference Report, New York.
Skolnick, A. A. 1993. "Rotary Clubs Offer Help in Preschool Immunization," *JAMA* 270(24): 2908–2910.
The Task Force for Child Survival. 1985, 1986. "Protecting the World's Children." Atlanta, GA: Task Force for Child Survival.
———. 1988. *Protecting the World's Children: An Agenda for the 1990s*. Atlanta, GA: Task Force for Child Survival.
The Task Force for Child Survival and Development. 1994. *Proceedings: Achieving Health: New Perspectives on Integrated Services and Their Contributions to Mid-Decade Goals*. New Delhi. Atlanta, GA: Task Force for Child Survival.
Taylor, C. E., F. Cutts, and M. E. Taylor. 1997. "Ethical Dilemmas in Current Planning for Polio-Eradication," *American Journal of Public Health* 87(6): 922–925.
Unger, J., and J. R. Killingsworth. 1986. "Selective Primary Health Care: A Critical Review of Methods and Results," *Social Science and Medicine* 22(10): 1001–1013.
UNICEF. Annual report 1980–1998. *State of the World's Children*. New York, Oxford: Oxford University Press.
———. 1985. "Universal Child Immunization by 1990." *Assignment Children* 69/72.
———. 1989. *Statistics on Children in UNICEF Assisted Countries*. New York: UNICEF.
———. 1990. *Children and Development in the 1990s: A UNICEF Sourcebook on the Occasion of the World Summit for Children*. New York: UNICEF.
———. 1995. *The Bamako Initiative: Rebuilding Health Systems*. New York: UNICEF.
———. 1996. *Evaluation Research: Sustainability of Achievements: Lessons*

Learned from Universal Child Immunization: Report of a Steering Committee. New York: UNICEF.

———. 1998. "Immunization Dropout: A Sign of Trouble." *The Progress of Nations*, ed. UNICEF. New York: UNICEF, p. 19.

U.S. Agency for International Development. Annual report 1985–1998. *Child Survival: Report to Congress.* Washington, DC: USAID.

Walsh, J., and K. Warren. 1979. "Selective Primary Health Care: An Interim Strategy for Disease Control in Developing Countries," *New England Journal of Medicine* 301: 967–974.

Walt, G. 1993. "WHO Under Stress: Implications for Health Policy," *Health Policy* 24: 125–144.

Werner, D., and D. Sanders. 1997. *Questioning the Solution: The Politics of Primary Health Care and Child Survival.* Palo Alto, CA: Health Wrights.

WHO (World Health Organization). 1979. *Formulating Strategies for Health for All by the Year 2000: Guiding Principles and Essential Issues.* Geneva: World Health Organization.

———. 1988. Report of the Expanded Programme in Immunization. Global Advisory Meeting, 9–13 November 1987. Geneva: World Health Organization.

———. 1991a. "Universal Child Immunization: Goal Attained," *World Health Forum* 12: 493.

———. 1991b. *Update: Expanded Programme on Immunization.* Geneva: World Health Organization.

———. 1992. *Programme Report for 1992, Expanded Programme on Immunization.* Geneva: World Health Organization.

———. 1995a. *Integrated Management of the Sick Child.* Geneva: World Health Organization.

———. 1995b. *Geneva and Global Programme for Vaccines and Immunization, Programme Report for 1994.* Geneva: World Health Organization.

———. 1997. *Polio: the Beginning of the End.* Geneva: World Health Organization.

WHO/UNICEF. 1996. *State of the World's Vaccines and Immunization.* Geneva: World Health Organization/UNICEF.

Wiener, B. 1988. "GOBI Versus PHC? Some Dangers of Selective Primary Health Care," *Social Science and Medicine* 26: 963–969.

World Bank. 1993. *World Development Report 1993: Investing in Health.* Oxford: Oxford University Press.

2

Administering the Epidemic: HIV/AIDS Policy, Models of Development, and International Health

Richard Parker

Over the course of nearly two decades now, the HIV/AIDS pandemic has taken shape as a key crisis in international health. Correctly or incorrectly, AIDS has been described as the quintessential epidemic of the late twentieth century, inseparable from a period of increasingly rapid globalization and an era of unprecedented social change. It has been suggested that the spread of HIV infection, wherever it has taken place, has tended to uncover the fault lines of social cleavage—as well as the capacity (or incapacity) of different social, cultural, and political systems to respond to impending disaster in more or less humane and efficacious ways. More broadly, within a global framework, and given its complex dynamics and remarkable diversity (which might be better described as a set of multiple, though often intersecting, epidemics rather than a single pandemic), AIDS has become a kind of test case for the ways in which the international system can respond to a perceived emergency in the area of health.

In this chapter, I examine three of the key paradoxes or contradictions that have emerged over the course of the past fifteen years, as we have struggled to come to terms with the epidemic, and explore some of the implications that they may have for an understanding of international health more broadly. In so doing, I would also like to situate myself in relation to the processes that I will seek to examine, and to make clear that my interpretation is conditioned in a number of complex ways. Perhaps most important, I find that I write in a sense less as an anthropologist (however much my anthropological training may shape my view of the world and the way I interpret its events) or as a professor of public health (however much my commitment to the notion of health as a public good may shape the kinds of work that I have sought to develop) than as someone who has been involved in a variety of capacities in AIDS-related work over the past fifteen years. My perspective is surely shaped by my experience as a researcher, but also by the brief period that I spent in 1989 and 1990 as a staff member at the World Health Organization's Global Programme on AIDS, the even briefer period in 1992 when I served as chief of the Prevention Unit for the Brazilian National AIDS Programme, and, perhaps above all, by my experience from 1992 to the present as executive director and later secretary general and then president of the Brazilian Interdisciplinary AIDS Association (ABIA), a community-based AIDS service and advocacy organization based in Rio de Janeiro. My view is also very much that of a gay man living with the impact of AIDS in a number of different gay communities that have been profoundly affected by the epidemic, someone who has both lived and worked closely with people living with HIV and AIDS, and, perhaps especially important, someone who has lived and worked both in the center and in the periphery, both north and south. In short, my analysis is shaped by a range of social and institutional insertions that have conditioned the ways in which I have interpreted the epidemic and the responses that it has generated. This chapter is fundamentally an attempt to put on paper some of the concerns that this rather eclectic experience has generated, and to open up a dialogue about what I view as a number of the most complex dilemmas that currently confront us as we face the HIV/AIDS pandemic—dilemmas that I consider symptomatic of an even broader set of issues related to contemporary processes of globalization, capitalist development, and international health.

Over the course of the past decade, a number of key paradoxes have emerged in relation to global AIDS policies and politics that have serious consequences for both analysis and action. At least three of these paradoxes, or contradictions, raise especially difficult dilemmas for the future, which I explore precisely because I have no answer with regard to their possible resolution, and because I am convinced that only by understanding how very unlevel the playing field on which we stand is will we somehow be able to find a way forward.

The first paradox can be stated quite simply. Vulnerability to HIV and AIDS has increasingly come to be understood as fundamentally linked to questions of social and economic inequality and injustice. This analysis has forced us to reexamine the dynamics of power, whether at the level of gender and sexual relations, or at the level of global structures and processes. Yet at the same time, institutional responses to the epidemic have become timid and bureaucratic, sometimes adopting progressive rhetoric, but largely implementing programs that are all too appropriate to an era of globalized capitalist development and neoliberal economic policy.

On the one hand, we can point to a growing awareness of the fact that the spread of HIV infection has been fundamentally driven by "structures of oppression" (Parker 1996). Wherever the epidemic has emerged, it has uncovered and acted upon structures of social cleavage and inequality. Whether we are talking about the forms of sexual oppression and discrimination that have been associated with communities of men who have sex with men, sex workers, the marginalization and criminalization of injecting drug users, the relations of gender power that have been associated with HIV infection among women, or the economic injustice that has been associated with the epidemic among the poor (in the so-called developed countries as well as in the underdeveloped world), oppression and inequality have been the most powerful forces shaping the HIV/AIDS epidemic everywhere around the globe (see, for example, Farmer 1992; Farmer, Connors, and Simmons 1996; Jonsen and Stryker 1993; Parker 1996; Singer 1997; Wallace 1988).

This basic understanding, in turn, has pushed us away from our early preoccupation with diverse forms of *risk behavior,* understood in largely individualistic terms, toward a new understanding of *vulnerability* as socially, politically, and economically structured, maintained, and organized, and has made it possible, in recent years, to begin to reconceptualize the fight against AIDS as part of a much broader process of social change that must necessarily take place within the struggle to build a more just social order (Parker 1996; see also Mann, Tarantola, and Netter 1992; Mann and Tarantola 1996). It has helped us understand that without effecting long-term changes in the structure of society, in the relations of power that subject certain populations and communities to increased vulnerability in the face of HIV infection (while simultaneously protecting others), there can be no real hope of ending or even slowing the epidemic. Without overcoming the consistent denial of their basic rights and dignity, gay and bisexual men, sex workers, and injecting drug users will continue to suffer the effects of the epidemic, independent of the degree of behavior change on the part of individuals within these groups (see Altman 1994; de Zalduondo 1991; Parker 1996). Without transforming the unequal relations of power that structure gender in virtually every society, women around the world will continue to be key targets of HIV infection and will be largely unable to negotiate and guarantee their own safety (see Farmer, Connors, and Simmons 1996). Without redressing social and economic injustice that exists within nations and between the developed and the developing world, the poor (both in the north and in the south) will continue to suffer the major impact of an epidemic that has already become all too intimately linked to poverty and misery (see, for example, Farmer 1992; Lurie, Hintzen, and Lowe 1995; Singer 1997; Wallace 1988).

Yet precisely at the same time that this growing understanding of the relations between oppression, exploitation, inequality, and HIV infection have become more apparent to us, it would appear that the global response to the epidemic has simultaneously become more timid and in many ways far more bureaucratic. One needs only to review briefly the history of the three clear phases of the intergovernmental response to the epidemic to see this process at work. Only in 1986 was a Special Programme on AIDS (SPA) created in the World Health Organization (WHO), and only in 1987 did this program take more formal shape as the Global Programme on AIDS (GPA). From 1987 to 1990, what I describe as GPA I grew rapidly to become the single largest program at the WHO. From an initial staff of two, it had grown to a staff of two hundred at headquarters alone by 1990 and commanded the largest budget with the WHO. Its accomplishments, though articulated from the top down rather than the bottom up, were nonetheless quite impressive. By 1989, 159 countries had received WHO support to establish National AIDS Programmes (NAPs). The largest meeting of ministers of health ever held on a single issue had been organized, and for the first time in history the United Nations General Assembly had met to address a global health problem (see Flemming et al. 1988; Mann 1987; Mann and Kay 1991; WHO 1988). As is perhaps best exemplified in WHO/GPA director Jonathan Mann's speech to the United Nations General Assembly in 1987 (Mann 1987), the language of human rights had begun to be incorporated into the field of health. And, at least in principle, through the creation of nongovernmental organization (NGO) liaison offices, a range of novel partnerships (as well as productive conflicts) had begun to emerge between community-based activists and official agencies at various levels (see Altman 1994; Mann, Tarantola, and Netter 1992).

By 1990, however, AIDS had also become a growth industry, and the stakes had clearly become high enough to spark interest even in sectors that had previously resisted any significant involvement. GPA had been charged with breaking the rules of "business as usual" in the field of international health, and power struggles between its leadership and the WHO system had become intolerable. While staff in GPA argued in favor of the need for streamlined administrative procedures in order to confront an epidemic out of control, the office of WHO director-general Hiroshi Nakajima sought to impose additional bureaucratic restraints in order to rein in a program that had increasingly come to be seen as competing with the WHO hierarchy for funding, authority, and influence. After a growing number of bureaucratic dogfights in the late 1980s, when Nakajima's office finally went so far as to deny routine travel authorizations for GPA's founding director, Jonathan Mann, the ongoing power struggle essentially forced Mann's resignation in early 1990.

Following Mann's resignation, Nakajima selected Dr. Michael Merson, previously head of WHO's Diarrheal Disease Programme, to serve as director of GPA, and charged him with the task of restructuring the program and bringing it into conformity with standard WHO operating procedures.

Following this change in leadership, from 1990 to 1995, in what I would describe as GPA II, a fundamental shift began to take place in which the perceived activist excesses of the earlier institutional response to the epidemic would gradually be replaced by a more orderly, more professional, and better coordinated response—aimed less at stimulating action (from the top down) than at "coordinating" efforts emerging locally, and at providing support for the initiatives taking place nationally. This is not to say that GPA II did not have its own important successes and innovations, or to imply that its staff was any less committed to controlling the epidemic, but is to suggest that a new set of constraints had begun to be imposed on GPA by the intergovernmental system. GPA's mission very clearly became one of supporting (technically more than financially) the efforts of National AIDS Programmes,[1] and the relationship between GPA and a range of affected communities became far more ambiguous and unclear. By 1995, following a long process of negotiation culminating in a report to the United Nations Economic and Social Council (ECOSOC),[2] GPA would ultimately give way to the Joint United Nations Programme on AIDS (UNAIDS), which was created by the United Nations General Assembly as the key forum for establishing a global response to the epidemic (Piot 1996; UNAIDS 1995).

In many ways, the shift to UNAIDS after 1995 is a logical outcome of the very same process found in GPA II. By bringing together six UN agencies—the WHO, the United Nations Development Programme (UNDP), the United Nations Children's Fund (UNICEF), the United Nations Population Fund (UNFPA), the United Nations Educational, Scientific, and Cultural Organization (UNESCO), and the World Bank—in part of a more unified structure, UNAIDS has offered the hope of increased "coordination" in responding to the epidemic (predicated on the conviction that fighting the epidemic can be more effectively carried out once different agencies stop fighting among themselves). Yet, if anything, UNAIDS also symbolizes a new configuration in which AIDS has been reframed as *not simply a health issue,* but as *a broader question of development.* Nowhere is this more evident than in the involvement of the World Bank as perhaps the key player within this new configuration. More or less quietly, over the course of the 1990s, the bank has emerged as the major funder of HIV/AIDS prevention work in the developing world (see Mann and Tarantola 1996; World Bank 1997, 1998). Today it is the Bank, rather than the WHO, that issues the most important statements and reports on the status of the epidemic and the policies that should be pursued to control it; one needs only to think of the example of *Confronting AIDS,* the World Bank's recent analysis and policy statement (World Bank 1997), which not only constituted the major international statement about the epidemic in 1997, but which also recently served to frame the discussion at a major

NIH-sponsored workshop on how the National Institutes of Health (NIH) in the United States could most effectively invest in and support HIV/AIDS research and practice internationally.

In short, much the same institutional constellation that gave us the politics of international debt in the 1970s, and structural adjustment in the 1980s, today leads the global fight against an epidemic that its own previous policies did so much to structure. That there is indeed more than a little irony in all of this goes without saying, particularly for those of us who have been involved in AIDS-related work long enough to remember that the red ribbon—today worn proudly not only by entertainers from Hollywood but also by politicians, government bureaucrats, and even World Bank economists—was in fact created not simply as a symbol of sympathy or even solidarity, but of the need to cut red tape, to do away with the status quo, with the mentality of business as usual, in seeking to build a more militant response to the epidemic.

The second paradox that I explore is very much linked to the first: it is what I see as the basically false or unnecessary choice that has been posed with increasing force in recent years—at least for the so-called developing world—between primary prevention on the one hand, and treatment and care on the other. This choice has been articulated, above all, by representatives of what we might describe as the "development establishment" (again, multilateral agencies such as the World Bank, or bilateral agencies such as the United States Agency for International Development [USAID] or the Overseas Development Agency [ODA]), but has been imposed (much like "policy-based lending") primarily on the policymakers and public health systems of the developing countries—independent of the public policies that those countries might prefer to establish as a result of their own internal policy debates concerning the prevention and control of AIDS. The result of this imposition increasingly would seem to be the abandonment of what we might describe as "inclusive" or "inclusionary" strategies in response to HIV and AIDS and the adoption of "exclusive" or "exclusionary" approaches—approaches whereby the interests of people already living with HIV and AIDS, at least in the poorer countries, have been placed consistently at the bottom of the list of priorities in seeking to respond to the epidemic.

This choice between prevention on the one hand, and care and treatment on the other, is fundamentally linked, I believe, to the reconceptualization of AIDS as first and foremost a question of economic development, subject to a relatively crude calculus of costs and benefits, that is not only devoid of any real ethical reflection, but is largely determined (or overdetermined) by the unquestioned assumptions of the late-twentieth-century world capitalist system (and by the model of dependent development that of course structured vulnerability to HIV in the first place).[3] Within this framework, primary prevention is understood as cost-effective—convincingly presented as the means to reduce the loss of "disability-adjusted life years" (World Bank 1993), enabling governments to achieve the biggest bang for their buck, the best return for their investment in light of limited health budgets.[4] Indeed, though for political reasons it would never be stated so crudely, the often repeated assertion that AIDS is an exceptionally expensive condition to care for and treat can hardly help but lead to the conclusion that the more rapidly those people living with HIV in the developing world become sick and die, the more "cost-effective" the response to the epidemic would be.[5]

It is striking, however, how very different this 1990s conception is from the articulation of a more *inclusive* approach during the 1980s. Based both on the changing precepts of what has been described as the "new" public health, as well as on the relative "exceptionalism" that characterized many early policy responses to the epidemic,[6] during the late 1980s, again with WHO/GPA as its leading voice, a powerful awareness of the interconnection between the infected and the uninfected was constructed. Emphasis was placed on the need to break down divisions between "us" and "them," between the HIV+ and the HIV− (Mann 1987; Panos Institute 1990; Sabatier 1988). The public health logic behind this approach was the fundamental need to bring people infected with HIV into structures of social, psychological, and medical support—to avoid driving the epidemic underground, where it would continue to spread silently and efficiently (Mann 1987). What was strategically quite brilliant about this was that the argument against discrimination and for the protection of the human rights of those living with HIV, as well as of those vulnerable to HIV infection, could be made not *just* because it is ethically correct (though clearly it is) but also because it is sound public health policy. It was clearly this underlying connection between concepts of human rights and health that was the most powerful mark of GPA director Jonathan Mann's 1987 address to the UN General Assembly previously mentioned (Mann 1987).

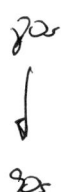

Over the course of the 1990s, however, as the response to the international pandemic evolved—and as a development framework replaced notions of health and well-being as the key to interpreting and analyzing the epidemic and its "handling"—this relatively inclusive approach was increasingly replaced by a very different framework, which in its crudest expression had been little more than a calculation of economic cost and benefits. I want to stress that this conception of "development" was by no means the only conception that might have emerged—on the contrary, in my opinion it was itself the outcome of a complex ideological and political struggle between competing notions of development that can perhaps be most usefully (though perhaps oversimplistically) symbolized through the UNDP on the one hand and the World Bank on the other. While admitting that the opposition, in practice, has been complex and nuanced, it is still possible, I think, to draw a distinction between a broader conception of *human* development, more closely associated with UNDP (and with the AIDS program at UNDP), and a more restricted focus on *economic* development, traditionally championed by the bank and the International Monetary Fund.[7]

Indeed, in the early and mid-1990s, the international discussion of AIDS policy was marked by often heated debates involving such diverse conceptions between differing notions of health and human development, linked to institutional power struggles among agencies such as the WHO, UNDP, and World Bank (as well as the diverse approaches of otherwise allied governments in countries such as the United States, Great Britain, Australia, the Netherlands, and Denmark). Gradually, however, out of these various struggles AIDS has been reframed as a question of economic development, just as the World Bank has emerged as the major funder of international AIDS control programs (through large-scale project loans to countries like Brazil and India [see World Bank 1998]). In turn, as this has happened globally no less than in the industrialized democracies, it has been argued that exceptionalism in response to the epidemic must give way to normalization. Yet in the so-called developed countries, this has meant one thing—in the poor countries of the developing world, subject to decisions made in the international intergovernmental system, emanating from Washington, Brussels, and Geneva, it has meant something quite different: an almost exclusive emphasis on primary prevention and vaccine research at the expense of investment in treatment and care (World Bank 1997). Recent media/academic debates about the ethics of clinical trials in developing countries—subject, it would seem, to a different set of ethical rules because of the unpleasant realities that their limited economies impose upon their possibilities for investing in health—are but one example of this trend, with the need for such research justified by the imperative of containing infection due to the unacceptably high cost of HIV/AIDS treatment (see Lurie et al. 1995). (That very different economic constraints impinge upon the economies of some developing nations [Haiti or Cameroon, for example] than on those of others [Brazil or Thailand, for example] is largely ignored within such formulations, as the differences that characterize such vastly incomparable contexts are rarely acknowledged—a strange leveling of differences that would of course be unthinkable were the comparison being made between the health care systems of the United States and the United Kingdom or Australia.)

When viewed from the south rather than from the north, however, such debates take on rather different dimensions, and the choices they articulate may be redefined in a number of important ways. To illustrate this just briefly, we can take an example from the Brazilian case—which is obviously not typical, but which is illustrative precisely because it is atypical (and which has the virtue of being relatively well known to me, because I have worked on AIDS in Brazil for more than fifteen years at the time of writing). In 1991, the Brazilian National AIDS Programme had taken the rather unusual step of making AZT available through the free distribution of medications provided to all Brazilian citizens (independent of socioeconomic status) (see Parker 1997). This was by no means a humanitarian gesture; according to the director of the NAP, it was intended to remedy serious problems of underreporting in the epidemiological surveillance system. Due to widespread discrimination, many physicians (particularly private physicians) tended to comply with their patients' wishes in disobeying case reporting laws—from their point of view, patients had little or nothing to gain from such reporting and, potentially, a good deal to lose due to stigma and discrimination if confidentiality was violated.

Because of strong demand for AZT, at least one major pharmaceutical producer had decided to violate patent laws, and to produce AZT locally at a significantly reduced price. The NAP then jumped at the chance to purchase bulk quantities and made AZT available free of charge—but only to officially reported cases, thus providing a payback or incentive for all the risks entailed in case reporting. Epidemiologically, this policy certainly had the desired effect of reducing underreporting, though it of course drew a good deal of international criticism both for patent violation and for economic inefficiency. Following the reform of the Brazilian government and the reorganization of the National AIDS Programme in 1992, when for a brief time I served as chief of the Prevention Unit for the Brazilian National AIDS Programme, the World Bank expressed interest in providing a loan for AIDS prevention and control. Throughout the long process of negotiation, the continued policy of antiretroviral distribution would become a major point of contention, classified as it was by the bank as economically irrational and unsustainable. In spite of opposition from the bank, the Brazilian Ministry of Health maintained the program, seeking to improve the logistics of distribution, but agreed to the bank's stipulation that none of the U.S.$160 million loan finally agreed upon would be devoted to treatment or care (Parker 1995).

Although the Brazilian policy has continued to draw international criticism, it has nonetheless been defended not only by AIDS activists but also by progressive public health officials. Indeed, the latter have ingeniously elaborated their own economic arguments, focusing on the reduced hospital costs and the increased economic productivity of HIV-infected citizens who receive access to treatment and care that significantly extends their working lives and reduces the burden that they would otherwise place on health care services. Because the jury is still out on the long-term consequences of recent advances in treatment therapies, all predictions (whether those of development economists or those of progressive public health officials) are of course exercises in futurology, based more often than not on ideological convictions (whether neoliberal or socialist) that may or may not be borne out over time. Yet it is hard to deny the assertion, made by more than a few policymakers and activists (in Brazil and elsewhere), that public policy must ultimately stem from discussion and debate concerning the nature of a good society—and that decisions about what constitutes the public good can be contested from various points of view. From the perspective of health workers fighting in the front lines against the epidemic even in very poor nations, the assumption that developing countries cannot afford to provide care and treatment for people living with HIV and AIDS (and that the development establishment and the pharmaceutical industry have no global responsibilities in this regard) may seem just as indefensible as the assertion that the United States (or other similarly well-to-do nations) cannot afford to care for the elderly. What any society can afford, whether in military spending or health care services, is ultimately a political question in large part about the allocation of resources—and northern assumptions about the availability of resources in the south may be as questionable as the kinds of structural adjustment policies that have been imposed by international development agencies on the countries of the developing world over the course of recent decades.

Finally, the third paradox I examine is in some ways tied to the first two, yet at another level provides a distinct dilemma. Stated simply: Many of the most effective responses to the epidemic (both in the developed and the developing worlds) have emerged at the local level as a result of what might be described as a *politics of identity*. Yet the very effectiveness of local-level identity politics has made it difficult to build a broader coalition to address HIV/AIDS as a global issue, and the kinds of social movements that have emerged around other (similarly global) issues (such as the environment or reproductive health and rights) have largely failed to emerge in response to AIDS. This, in turn, has left undisputed control over the "administration" of the epidemic in the hands of an international system that has already proved itself unable to address the underlying factors that shape the epidemic (and this, of course, is where the third paradox relates to the first two in a number of problematic ways).

In setting after setting, in spite of the often distracting noise produced by agencies such as the WHO, UNAIDS, or the World Bank, it has become apparent that *local-level responses* to the epidemic have in general been the most powerful. These responses have for the most part emerged from society itself, from community-level organizing, rather than from a more controlled process of planning and programming (see, for example, Altman 1994, 1995; Daniel and Parker 1993; Dowsett 1996; Mann and Tarantola 1996; Parker et al. 1995). The quintessential (and also overused) example is the response to AIDS on the part of gay communities in the United States, and in particular in San Francisco, where the greatest documentation probably exists. Although this story has of course become more complex (as debates over "relapse" and seroconversion rates among young gay men attest [see, for example, Davies 1993; de Wit 1996; Dowsett 1996; Stall and Ekstrand 1989; Stall et al. 1992]), the fact remains that massive behavioral and cultural responses took place in the gay community, which in large part preceded any kind of formal programming (see Kirp and Bayer 1992). At different points in time and clearly shaped by a range of different factors, similar changes have taken place in other sexual communities (see, for example, Coxon 1992; Davies et al. 1993; Dowsett 1996). We can point to the relatively effective control of the epidemic in Australia, for example, and recount the history of the gay community response in Sydney and other major urban centers (see, for example, Dowsett 1996; Kippax et al. 1993; on Australian national AIDS policy, see also Ballard 1992; Manderson 1994). Or we can look at the largely out-of-control epidemic in Brazil (Daniel and Parker 1993; Parker 1997), where my colleagues and I monitored the behavioral response to HIV/AIDS among men who have sex with men from 1990 to 1993 to 1995, and where we found that the greatest change had already taken place by 1993, when the first formal interventions for homosexual and bisexual men in Brazil were initiated (Parker and Terto Jr. 1998).

These changes are clearly not limited to a single community, such as gay or bisexual men. Exactly the same kind of community-based response has been documented cross-culturally among female and male sex workers in Western Europe and North America, as well as in different African, Latin American, and Asian sites (see, for example, Aggleton 1998; Gillies and Parker 1994; Miller, Turner, and Moses 1990). Perhaps more surprisingly, it has also been documented among injecting drug users in at least some sites. Against the grain of what some might describe as common-sense expectation, injecting drug users in sites as distant as São Paulo and Santos in Brazil, and New York City in the United States, have demonstrated greater ability than was ever expected to organize around their shared identity and to develop local-level responses to the epidemic (see, for example, Bastos 1995; Des Jarlais and Friedman 1996; Friedman et al. 1987; Friedman, de Jong, and Wodak 1993). More broadly, as the impact of HIV infection on women has increasingly been felt not only in Africa but throughout the world, organizing around women's issues, within the context of HIV/AIDS, has become one of the most powerful contemporary responses to AIDS, and feminist and women's health organizations have in many places become important leaders in the fight against the epidemic.

Clearly, these responses have not been absolute. They have not turned back the tide of the epidemic. They have not accounted for many populations that fall through the cracks of social and cultural identities (such as the female partners of male injecting drug users, or many men who have sex with men without adopting a gay identity). But, north and south, in the so-called developing world as much as in the developed world, they have nonetheless offered the most powerful response to AIDS that has thus far been seen (Parker 1996).

At the same time, by the very nature of their focus on local-level identities, such responses have for the most part not been particularly well suited to the organization of a more global social movement (whether *global* here is taken to mean broad-based within a particular society or nation-state, or global at the level of international and transnational responses to AIDS). Although a good deal of time and money has been spent seeking to organize the international response to AIDS (see Mann and Tarantola 1996; Abaogye-Kwarteng, Manderson, and Msiska 1997), local-level responses have for the most part failed to take shape within a broader vision of political organizing—what we might think of as a *politics of solidarity* as opposed to a *politics of identity* (see Parker 1994, 1996, 1999; see also Altman 1994; Minkler 1997; Rorty 1989). Any number of structures have been elaborated, such as the International Council of AIDS Service Organizations (ICASO), but for the most part with a relatively limited impact that hardly goes beyond offering opinions about the speakers for the next International AIDS Conference. Perhaps the most effective of these organizations, both locally and increasingly globally as well, has been the Global Network of People Living with HIV. This effectiveness has in large part been based on the powerful construction of seropositivity as itself the basis for a politics of identity, and GNP, for all its recent accomplishments, has not been able to stimulate a broader political response outside this context. The kinds of interconnections that seem to link environmentalists in Bangkok and Boston (see Rich 1994), or reproductive rights advocates in Lima and London (see Petchesky and Judd 1998), have largely failed to emerge in the case of HIV/AIDS—in spite of (though some might say because of) the very concerted efforts that have been made to stimulate such interaction.

Admittedly, there may be understandable reasons for these disparities. The very interconnectedness of the environment and global warming, or that a certain essentialization of women's bodies and reproductive biology is perceived to link reproductive health and reproductive rights issues globally simply fail to be present in health issues like HIV, in which vulnerability to infection seems to be distributed so differentially (mapping, of course, socioeconomic inequalities) that making common cause becomes difficult if not impossible. Theoretically, however, the area of treatment activism may ultimately prove to offer greater possibilities for coalition building globally, again because of a certain essentialism that may take shape through the perceived commonality of the experience of the virus itself. Thus far, however, this has been the case only to a very limited degree, and the record of first-world treatment activists in relation to questions of treatment access for people living with HIV in the rest of the world, until now at least, gives little reason for great optimism.

Unfortunately, the end result of these various developments has been that effective control—not over the epidemic, but over the responsibility for responding to it—has been concentrated in the formal structures of the international system (and its national, state, and local counterparts). From 1986 to 1995, undisputed control was held by the WHO (at times in competition with other UN agencies), which hired community activists as consultants, funded NGO partnerships, and in a variety of ways sought to nurture the "community-based response"—but without ever sacrificing its own relative control, and in large part legitimizing the overriding hegemony exercised by National AIDS Programmes around the world. From 1995 to the present, with the creation of UNAIDS, these tendencies have become even more glaring, as NGO representatives have become part of the governing bodies of UNAIDS (though without any structures for actually defining representativeness), as the principles of human rights have become integrated into programmatic documents, and as coordination and horizontal collaboration (between countries in the south) have become the order of the day—yet for the most part without any sense of popular support or sustainability as part of a broader social movement. The world system has increasingly learned how to "administer" the epidemic, but has certainly not made much progress in doing away with it.

The obstacles that these paradoxes present, if my assessment of them is at all correct, are clearly immense. Yet we would ignore them, I believe, at our own peril, since in many ways they structure the playing field on which we today find ourselves at work, at least in the specific case of HIV/AIDS. Perhaps even more troubling, they suggest a number of broader tendencies in the general field of international health. HIV and AIDS are part and parcel of a much broader social and economic configuration in which the processes of globalization, unequal capitalist development, and the politics of international health are intertwined in multiple ways that ultimately seem to increase the sum total of human suffering in the world today rather than alleviate it. As we find ourselves moving from one century into the next, history may well judge us on the extent to which we are able to analyze these interconnections critically, and, ultimately, to dismantle them, as part of a broader struggle for solidarity and social justice.

Notes

1. It is important to point out that this kind of role is typical of other Special Programmes at the WHO, which are often focused heavily on research and technical

support and which generally have a much less "proactive" approach than that which had been pursued by GPA initially.

2. ECOSOC is a body composed of fifty-four governmental representatives, in large part drawn from diplomatic and foreign services, that has a constitutional mandate to coordinate the UN system of international agencies, including the World Bank and the International Monetary Fund. It has a key role in developing recommendations for eventual UN General Assembly approval (see Gordenker et al. 1995).

3. The relationship between economic dependency and unequal development in Africa, Asia, and Latin America has of course been the subject of a vast literature that is far too extensive to review here—though such a review, in my opinion, will ultimately be crucial for a fuller understanding of the political and economic context of HIV/AIDS in the developing world. For a key conceptual framework of dependency theory, see in particular Cardoso and Faletto (1979). For a discussion of HIV/AIDS within the context of political economy, dependency, and the world capitalist system, see Baer, Singer, and Susser (1997), Farmer (1992), and Lurie, Hintzen, and Lowe (1995).

4. Introduced by the World Bank in the *World Development Report 1993: Investing in Health* (World Bank 1993), the concept of disability-adjusted life years (or DALYs) includes both the disability and the mortality effects of disease and uses age weights to discount the importance of infant and elderly deaths in order to calculate the global burden of different diseases. The World Bank calculates that, in 1990, poor health resulted in the loss of 265.2 DALYs per thousand persons per year in developing countries. Of this total, infectious disease accounted for 24.5 percent of total lost DALYs. HIV accounted for 0.8 percent. By 2020, it is estimated that the total burden of disease will have dropped to 186.2 lost DALYs, and the burden due to infectious disease will have dropped to 13.7 percent of this total, but that the burden directly linked to HIV will have climbed to 2.6 percent (World Bank 1997).

5. This is of course an exaggeration of far more cautious declarations on the part of different agencies, but nonetheless takes an especially frequent line of argument to its logical conclusion. That said, it is important to emphasize that AIDS policy discourses have been neither monolithic nor unchanging in this regard. A good example of this is USAID, which has increasingly incorporated a concern with care for people living with HIV into its agenda—a shift that is especially evident, for example, in comparing the approaches of the USAID-supported AIDS-CAP Project in the early 1990s with the round of contracts awarded by USAID for AIDS-related work in the late 1990s. UNAIDS has also adopted at least a rhetoric of concern for care and treatment issues. In this regard, the World Bank would seem to be by far the most articulate agency in championing prevention at the expense (no pun intended) of treatment and care programs in developing countries (see in particular World Bank 1997).

6. On the concept of "exceptionalism" in relation to the policy response to HIV and AIDS, see in particular Kirp and Bayer (1992).

7. At a discursive level, many of these differences are crystalized in the Human Development Index and the World Development Reports. See also the analysis of "development" as a discursive field in Escobar (1995).

References

Abaogye-Kwarteng, T., L. Manderson, and R. Msiska. 1997. "Reviews and Strategic Planning for HIV/AIDS Prevention and Care: Anthropology and the Expanded Response to AIDS," *AIDS and Anthropology Bulletin* 9(2): 1, 8–10.

Aggleton, Peter, ed. 1998. *Men Who Sell Sex: International Perspectives on Male Prostitution and AIDS*. London: UCL Press.
Altman, Dennis. 1994. *Power and Community: Organizational and Cultural Responses to AIDS*. London: Taylor and Francis.
———. 1995. "Overview of Community Responses." *Development* 2: 8–15.
Baer, Hans A., Merrill Singer, and Ida Susser. 1997. "AIDS: A Disease of the Global System." In *Medical Anthropology and the World System*. Westport, CT, and London: Bergin and Garvey.
Ballard, John. 1992. "Australia: Participation and Innovation in a Federal System." In *AIDS in the Industrialized Democracies: Passions, Politics, and Policies*, David Kirp and Ronald Bayer, eds. New Brunswick, NJ: Rutgers University Press.
Bastos, Francisco Inácio. 1955. *Ruína e Reconstrução: AIDS e Drogas na Cena Contemporânea*. Rio de Janeiro: ABIA/IMS-UERJ/Relume-Dumará Editores.
Cardoso, Fernando Henrique, and Enzo Faletto. 1979. *Dependency and Development in Latin America*. Berkeley: University of California Press.
Coxon, Anthony P. M. 1992. *Homosexual Response Study: A Report to the Steering Committee of the World Health Organization/Global Programme on AIDS/Social and Behavioural Studies Unit*. Geneva: World Health Organization.
Daniel, Herbert, and Richard Parker. 1993. *Sexuality, Politics and AIDS in Brazil: In Another World?* London: Falmer Press.
Davies, P. M. 1993. "Safer Sex Maintenance Among Gay Men: Are We Moving in the Right Direction?" *AIDS* 7(2): 279–280.
Davies, P. M., et al., eds. 1993. *Sex, Gay Men and AIDS*. London: Falmer Press.
de Wit, John B. F. 1996. "The Epidemic of HIV Among Young Homosexual Men," *AIDS* 10(suppl. 3): S21–S25.
de Zalduondo, Barbara O. 1991. "Prostitution Viewed Cross-Culturally: Toward Recontextualizing Sex Work in AIDS Research," *Journal of Sex Research* 28: 223–248.
Des Jarlais, Don, and Samuel R. Friedman. 1996. "Risk Reduction Among Injecting Drug Users." In *AIDS in the World II*, Jonathan Mann and Daniel Tarantola, eds. Oxford: Oxford University Press.
Dowsett, Gary W. 1996. *Practicing Desire: Homosexual Sex in the Era of AIDS*. Stanford: Stanford University Press.
Escobar, Arturo. 1995. *Encountering Development: The Making and Unmaking of the Third World*. Princeton, NJ: Princeton University Press.
Farmer, Paul. 1992. *AIDS and Accusation: Haiti and the Geography of Blame*. Berkeley and Los Angeles: University of California Press.
Farmer, Paul, Margaret Connors, and Janie Simmons, eds. 1996. *Women, Poverty and AIDS: Sex, Drugs and Structural Violence*. Monroe, ME: Common Courage Press.
Flemming, Alan, et al., eds. 1988. *The Global Impact of AIDS*. New York: Alan R. Liss.
Friedman, S. R., W. de Jong, and A. Wodak. 1993. "Community Development as a Response to HIV Among Drug Injectors," *AIDS* 7(suppl. 1): S263–S269.
Friedman, Samuel R., et al. 1987. "AIDS and Self-Organization Among Intravenous Drug Users," *International Journal of the Addictions* 22: 201–219.
Gillies, Pamela A., and Richard G. Parker. 1994. "Cross-Cultural Perspectives on Sexual Behaviour and Prostitution," *Health Transition Review* 4(suppl.): 257–271.
Gordenker, Leon, Roger A. Coate, Christer Jönsson, and Peter Söderholm. 1995. *International Cooperation in Response to AIDS*. London and New York: Pinter.

Jonsen, Albert R., and Jeff Stryker. 1993. *The Social Impact of AIDS in the United States*. Washington, DC: National Academy Press.
Kippax, Susan, et al. 1993. *Sustaining Safe Sex: Gay Communities Respond to AIDS*. London: Falmer.
Kirp, David, and Ronald Bayer, eds. 1992. *AIDS in the Industrialized Democracies: Passions, Politics, and Policies*. New Brunswick, NJ: Rutgers University Press.
Lurie, Peter, Percy Hintzen, and Robert A. Lowe. 1995. "Socioeconomic Obstacles to HIV Prevention and Treatment in Developing Countries: The Roles of the International Monetary Fund and the World Bank," *AIDS* 9: 539–546.
Manderson, Lenore. 1994. "Drugs, Sex and Social Science: Social Science Research and Health Policy in Australia," *Social Science and Medicine* 39(9): 1275–1286.
Mann, Jonathan. 1987. Statement to the UN General Assembly, October 20, New York.
Mann, Jonathan, and Daniel Tarantola, eds. 1996. *AIDS in the World II*. Oxford: Oxford University Press.
Mann, Jonathan, Daniel J. M. Tarantola, and Thomas Netter, eds. 1992. *AIDS in the World*. Cambridge, MA, and London: Harvard University Press.
Mann, Jonathan M., and Kathleen Kay. 1991. "Confronting the Pandemic: The World Health Organization's Global Programme on AIDS, 1986–1989," *AIDS* 5(suppl. 2): S221–S229.
Miller, Heather G., Charles F. Turner, and Lincoln E. Moses, eds. 1990. *AIDS: The Second Decade*. Washington, DC: National Academy Press.
Minkler, Meredith, ed. 1997. *Community Organizing and Community Building for Health*. New Brunswick, NJ, and London: Rutgers University Press.
Panos Institute. 1990. *The Third Epidemic: Repercussions of the Fear of AIDS*. London: Panos Institute.
Parker, Richard. 1994. *A Construção da Solidariedade: AIDS, Sexualidade e Política no Brasil*. Rio de Janeiro: ABIA/IMS-UERJ/Relume-Dumará Editores.
———. 1995. *Historic Overview of Brazil's AIDS Programs and Review of World Bank AIDS Project*. Arlington, VA: Family Health International/AIDSCAP Project.
———. 1996. "Empowerment, Community Mobilization, and Social Change in the Face of HIV/AIDS," *AIDS* 10(suppl. 3): S27–S31.
———. 1999. *Beneath the Equator: Cultures of Desire, Male Homosexuality, and Emerging Gay Communities in Brazil*. New York and London: Routledge.
———, ed. 1997. *Políticas, Instituições e AIDS: Enfrentando a Epidemia no Brasil*. Rio de Janeiro: Jorge Zahar Editor/ABIA.
Parker, Richard, et al. 1995. "AIDS Prevention and Gay Community Mobilization in Brazil," *Development* 2: 49–53.
Parker, Richard, and Veriano Terto Jr., eds. 1998. *Entre Homens: AIDS e Homossexualidade no Brasil*. Rio de Janeiro: ABIA.
Petchesky, Rosalind P., and Karen Judd, eds. 1998. *Negotiating Reproductive Rights: Women's Perspectives Across Countries and Cultures*. London: Zed Books.
Piot, Peter. 1996. "Why UNAID?" In *AIDS in the World II*, J. Mann and D. Tarantola, eds. Oxford: Oxford University Press.
Rich, Bruce. 1994. *Mortgaging the Earth: The World Bank, Environmental Impoverishment, and the Crisis of Development*. Boston: Beacon Press.
Rorty, Richard. 1989. *Contingency, Irony and Solidarity*. Cambridge, England: Cambridge University Press.

Sabatier, Renée. 1988. *Blaming Others: Prejudice, Race and Worldwide AIDS.* London: Panos Institute.

Singer, Merrill, ed. 1997. *The Political Economy of AIDS.* Amityville, NY: Baywood.

Stall, Ron, and Maria Ekstrand. 1989. "Implications of Relapse from Safe Sex," *Focus: A Guide to AIDS Research and Counseling* 4 (February): 3.

Stall, Ron, et al. 1992. "Maintenance of HIV Risk Reduction Among Gay-Identified Men." In *AIDS in the World,* Jonathan Mann, Daniel J. M. Tarantola, and Thomas Netter, eds. Cambridge, MA: Harvard University Press.

UNAIDS (Joint United Nations Programme on HIV/AIDS). 1995. "Strategic Plan, 1996–2000." Background document for the second meeting of the Programme Coordinating Board. Geneva, November 13–15 (UNAID/PCB[2]/95.3, October 31).

Wallace, R. 1988. "A Synergism of Plagues: 'Planned Shrinkage,' Contagious Housing Destruction and AIDS in the Bronx," *Environmental Research* 47: 1–33.

WHO (World Health Organization). 1988. *AIDS Prevention and Control: Invited Presentation and Papers from the World Summit of Ministers of Health on Programmes for AIDS Prevention.* Geneva: WHO; Oxford: Pergamon Press.

World Bank. 1993. *World Development Report, 1993: Investing in Health.* Oxford: Oxford University Press.

———. 1997. *Confronting AIDS: Public Priorities in a Global Epidemic.* Oxford: Oxford University Press.

———. 1998. "World Bank HIV/AIDS Interventions: Ex-ante and Ex-post Evaluation," World Bank Discussion Paper No. 389. Washington, DC: World Bank.

3

Local Identity, Globalization, and Health in Cuba and the Dominican Republic

Linda M. Whiteford

Recently, I saw a photograph of a young Fidel Castro, beardless and in New York in the 1950s. It gave me pause and a chance to unravel a conceptual knot in the writing of this chapter. The central concept of this chapter is that history, politics, and economics intersect with cultural experiences to commodify health, and that the creation of local identities both reflect and augment that commodification process. To demonstrate this, I draw on my own research in the Dominican Republic and Cuba to show how local identities can impede or facilitate community-based health promotion campaigns to control, for example, dengue fever.

These local identities are associated with idioms, phrases, and even slogans that capture and reinforce lived experiences. In earlier work I have written about two of these idioms—*mala unión* in the Dominican Republic and *sembrando el futuro* from Cuba (Whiteford 1998a, 1998b). As I analyzed these idioms and the local identities they express in writing this chapter, I realized that the idioms of hope that *sembrando el futuro* held for Cubans in the 1980s may no longer be true, and that I, because of my own constructed identity, did not want to write that. I wanted the Fidel of promise still to be real. My own reluctance to acknowledge the waning of that promise made writing about Cuba and its social suffering at the end of the twentieth century difficult. I suspect that the idioms of hope that once brightened local identities of Cubans may have been replaced by more darkly colored sentiments similar to those expressed by Dominicans who spoke of powerlessness and lack of faith in their political authorities, or the *mala unión* between Dominicans and their government.

But this chapter no more speaks of the Cuban experiences in the last decade of the twentieth century than it refers to the young Fidel Castro in

New York in the 1950s. Instead it situates itself in the decade of the 1980s during a period of severe economic crisis yet, still, of possibilities.

The process of health commodification in the Dominican Republic and Cuba demonstrates how ideological seeds sown in national and global politics are transformed into local identities. Cuba is offered as a limited contrast with my more extensive experience and data from the Dominican Republic, to suggest the comparative utility of the analysis of globalization, the commodification of health, and local identities.

Cuba and the Dominican Republic can be seen as exemplifying how political history and global forces shape local rights, responsibilities, and obligations associated with individual, community, and national activities. These local responses reflect an ongoing process of negotiated cultural identities. In the arena of health, global forces, national responses, and local identities transform health experiences into forms of commodification, one consequence of which may be an increase in social suffering. Investigating these forms of commodification provides insight into the process of globalization, culturally negotiated identities, and the underpinning of the moral scarcity of health.

My use of the term *globalization* is based on Michael Kearney's definition of the "social, economic, cultural and demographic processes that take place within nations but also transcend them, such that attention limited to local processes, identities and units of analysis yields incomplete understandings of the local" (Kearney 1995:548). Conversely, exclusive attention to global processes blinds us to the national and local context particularly significant in understanding the nexus between local identity, social suffering, and health.

The commodification of experience, in this case of health, is the conceptualization of a particular type of occurrence in terms of its social and symbolic significance, as well as the economic and cultural conditions of contemporary global capitalism. Globalization, therefore, results in the capitalization of health. The analysis of contemporary health experiences in this context then takes on added significance as a reflection of the dispersion, decentering, interpretation, and general complexity of globalization (J. Fisher 1993; W. F. Fisher 1995, 1997; Ferguson 1996; Escobar 1995).

Mala unión and *sembrando el futuro*, idioms of hope and despair, were responses to ideological and economic strategies designed to combat global financial threats. In the 1980s, Dominicans used the phrase *mala unión* to refer to a "bad partnership" between ordinary citizens and their government (Whiteford et al. 1991; Whiteford 1997, 1998a, 1998b). The symbolic capital of such a phrase translates as a powerful deterrent to community-based activities like mosquito control, even though Dominicans suffer from a variety of debilitating, painful, and potentially fatal mosquito-borne diseases such as malaria and dengue fever (Salazar 1993;

Whiteford 1993, 1997), diseases that could be controlled through cooperative government-community response programs. In contrast, during the same period in Cuba, health was a central focus of postrevolutionary reforms, symbolized by the phrase *sembrando el futuro,* or sowing the seeds for the future, suggesting a relationship between current acts and future rewards.

Mala unión and *sembrando el futuro* are evocative phrases symbolizing identities imbued with differential expectations, reflecting distinctive social relations between citizens and their government, created from perceptions of material realities and social promises. The commodification of health, expressed in both symbolic and material forms, occurs in both contexts. In the Dominican Republic the commodification is played out in the loss of primary health care, the unequal distribution of human and fiscal resources, the increase in infectious disease, at the same time that the Dominican government continued to pay a relatively large percentage of its gross domestic product for the declining health of its people.

In Cuba, health was a symbolic public success both at home and abroad. Its success was also commodified for international distribution. And, as the following data show, health commodification for Cuba translated into more than symbolic successes.

On any summer day the fast beat and driving sound of merengue can be heard from New York to Paris, and all across the Caribbean. The music so loved in the Dominican Republic is part of the global transformation of music, images, and dance that fly across space with apparent disregard for geopolitical and cultural boundaries, erasing cultural histories and mixing local identities, shrinking the global world. But even in a world that appears to be shrinking, cultural identities powerfully root people in time and place. These identities, often changing and yet somehow enduring, shape how people feel about themselves, how they perceive their surroundings, and how they imagine their future.

In the arena of international policy, local identities are often overlooked as too amorphous, too changing, too ambiguous, and too great a complication in already complex processes. Yet local identities embody culturally constructed expectations that shape the ways transported music, for instance, is enjoyed, images understood, and dance interpreted. When music created in Africa is heard in the Andes, it is transformed by the listeners' Andean experiences. And so it is with all things, including health. Whereas health may be commodified by global economic and political forces, transformed through international health policies and programs, and interpreted by history and proximity, it is internalized in local idioms and identities.

Global processes are played out in the cultural, historical, and political contexts in which they occur, and they have distinct consequences for the presentation and experience of health. Far too frequently international health policy planners attempt to standardize their programs in form and function, regardless of the historical/economic particularities of the country in which they will be applied. Sometimes health planners refer to this as the assumption that all countries are playing on the same level playing field, that is, that a health care program developed and administered from a central source such as the World Health Organization (WHO) can and will be applied in a standardized way, whether in Uganda or Bolivia.

In this chapter and others in this volume, we challenge that assumption and question the very efficacy of centralized health programs designed without attention to local identities and context, be they for the control of cholera, dengue fever, AIDS, or tuberculosis. Here I present some ideas about how local, national, and transnational histories shape local identities, citizens' perceptions of their rights and obligations, their expectations and exasperation, and their abilities to improve their own and others' health. My underlying argument is that local identities embody the perceived relations between sectors of the population and the officials charged with protecting the health of the community. These local identities, then, shape how health care programs are received and sustained. That is, the cultural construction of local identities, including citizens' rights and responsibilities for health, emerges from national historical and political experiences. Community willingness to participate, for instance, in community-based interventions such as those described in this chapter reflect constructed local identities. And, as this chapter demonstrates, those very identities unlevel the playing field. In short, there *is* no level playing field, and health programs developed and administered without cognizance of that at best will fail to maximize their effectiveness and, at worst, will contribute to the very suffering they seek to alleviate. The fallacy of the level playing field has implications beyond program ineffectiveness. Inattention to the disjuncture between globalizing discourses and localized social realities may actually increase the social suffering of the community and thereby multiply its losses. The following examples of local idioms and identities in Cuba and the Dominican Republic in the 1980s shows how they reflect distinctive realities and their consequences in the control of dengue fever.

Dengue Fever: A Vector-Borne Disease

The Pan American Health Organization (PAHO), the Americas' sister to the World Health Organization (WHO), declared war on *Aedes aegypti,* the mosquito vector of dengue fever (DF), in 1947. The program was ambitious, its aim no less than the eradication of *Aedes aegypti* from the Western

Hemisphere by "complete and thorough coverage of the infested areas with frequent treatment cycles" (Gubler and Kuno 1997:444). Opinions vary concerning the efficaciousness of the eradication campaigns (Gubler and Kuno 1997; Coreil et al. 1997), but there is no disagreement that dengue today is one of the most prevalent emerging diseases in the world, and that the public health consequences of dengue hemorrhagic fever (DHF) are no longer limited to the tropical countries of Asia, but now must be faced in the tropical areas of the Americas as well.

Since 1980 both the Dominican Republic and Cuba have experienced dengue fever epidemics, yet the countries' ability to respond to the epidemics has been fundamentally different. An analysis of these responses provides an opportunity to analyze how local identities shape what strategies were available to the Dominican and Cuban governments in their attempts to control dengue epidemics. During the period of the epidemics (between 1980 and 1990), both Cuba and the Dominican Republic were governed by strong-willed, independent, and isolated men—the last caudillos—Castro in Cuba and Balaguer in the Dominican Republic. Each had been in power for a prolonged period of time during which they came to be well known by the people they governed. Balaguer, almost blind and in his eighties, was supported by the United States. Castro, in power at that time for more than twenty years, relied on support from the Soviet Union. In both cases, the population on each island knew their caudillo—they had years of experience in dealing with him, his policies, and his programs; Cubans and Dominicans created local identities reflecting those experiences.

Vector-borne diseases are not new to the islands. Yellow fever, malaria, and dengue-like illnesses have been described in the Caribbean since 1635 (Gubler and Kuno 1997:5). According to Gubler and Kuno, as early as 1779 and 1780 there were reports of major epidemics of a dengue-like illness in Asia, Africa, and North America. Even earlier descriptions of a disease similar to dengue are found in a Chinese encyclopedia of disease symptoms and remedies first published during the Chin Dynasty (AD 265–420) (Nobuchi 1979, cited in Gubler and Kuno 1997:4). In 1635 an outbreak of a dengue-like disease occurred in the French West Indies, and later, in 1699, in Panama. The symptoms described during the Panama epidemic closely mirror those found in patients with classical dengue: acute pain in the joints and bones (giving rise to the name "bone-break fever," as dengue fever was sometimes known), rash, fever, headache, nausea, vomiting, pain behind the eyes, and prolonged exhaustion (Gubler and Kuno 1997:4). For most individuals, dengue fever is not fatal. However, since 1780 a new, more severe, and sometimes fatal hemorrhagic disease, dengue hemorrhagic fever, has been reported. DF and DHF now have reached a worldwide pandemic stage. Again according to Gubler and Kuno:

Epidemic DF/DHF has become one of the most important emergent global public health problems in tropical countries in the waning years of the twentieth century. In 1977, DF/DHF was the most important arbovirus disease of humans occurring in all major tropical areas of the world, with over 2.5 billion persons at risk of infections. Each year, an estimated 50 to 100 million cases of dengue fever and several hundred thousand cases of DHF occur. (1997:17)

Dengue is one of the leading causes of pediatric mortality and morbidity in the tropics (Halstead 1980) and is caused by a virus being injected by the mosquito into the human host. There are four antigenically related, but distinct, dengue virus serotypes (DEN-1, DEN-2, DEN-3, and DEN-4). Repeated infections can lead to conditions such as dengue hemorrhagic fever or dengue shock syndrome (DSS), particularly dangerous for children and the elderly. Even when people recover from DF/DHF, they are often in a weakened state for a prolonged period. Clearly, successful public health DF/DHF interventions need to be understood.

Dengue fever has much in common with yellow fever, although many people are more aware of the latter, perhaps because of its place in history books and its association with the construction of the Panama Canal. Both dengue fever and yellow fever are flavivirus infections in primates. They both have a zoonotic forest cycle and are present in urban and periurban settings. DF/DHF's principal urban and periurban vector in the Americas is the *Aedes aegypti* mosquito that breeds in domestic environments such as household containers (flowerpots, water-storage receptacles) and common trash like discarded old tires. Although today there is a yellow fever vaccine, there is no vaccine available for dengue fever, and therefore control of DF/DHF is dependent upon breaking its cycle of transmission.

Dengue Fever in Cuba

A number of dengue epidemics swept through the Caribbean during and immediately following World War II. Although between 1946 and 1963 there was no recorded evidence of epidemics (Gubler and Kuno 1997:13), by the 1980s the picture radically changed. Vector control spraying campaigns were active in the Americas until the 1970s, when concern about the long-term effects of the chemical agents ended the eradication campaigns, and in a few years the mosquitoes reinvaded the countries from which they had been banished in the previous decades. In addition, increased international travel allowed humans to transport various serotypes of the virus from one part of the world to another, spreading and then maintaining disease transmission. In short, the environmental conditions favored a resurgence of the *Aedes aegypti* mosquito at the same time that previous control activities failed (Kendall 1998).

According to Gubler and Kuno, the changing epidemiology of dengue in the Americas that took place in the decades of the 1970s and 1980s mirrors what was observed in Southeast Asia in the 1950s and 1960s (Gubler and Kuno 1997).

> The reinvasion of Central and South America by *Ae. aegypti* in the 1970s and 1980s, combined with the increased movement of people and with them dengue viruses, resulted in most countries evolving from nonendemicity (no viruses present) or hypoendemicity (one virus present) to hyperendemicity (multiple virus serotypes cocirculating). This resulted in increased frequency of epidemic activity and the emergence of DHF as a major public health problem. (Gubler and Kuno 1997:15)

The environment was right and the mosquito was ready. In 1977 a dengue epidemic occurred in Jamaica and Cuba, and the following year another epidemic was identified in Puerto Rico and Venezuela. Within four years, the reinfestation was extensive. DF was found throughout the Caribbean, Mexico, Texas, Central America, and northern South America. These were the less dangerous classic dengue fever, DEN-1 serotype. But in 1981 a new and more deadly strain of DF (DEN-2) was identified in Cuba and resulted in the first dengue hemorrhagic fever epidemic in the Americas. The DEN-2 serotype found in Cuba may have been introduced from Southeast Asia, most likely from Vietnam (Gubler and Kuno 1997: 14) and resulted in a major epidemic with thousands of cases of severe hemorrhagic bleeding. It is estimated that 10,000 cases of DHF and dengue shock syndrome occurred in Cuba during a three-month period in 1981 (Kouri et al. 1986).

And yet, with more than 10,000 clinically diagnosed cases, and more than 116,000 people hospitalized, only 158 died. How did Cuba succeed in limiting mortality? What can we learn from an analysis of the successful Cuban campaign? The Cuban government's response to the 1981 DHF epidemic was massive and military in its execution. The military public health model was not rare; previous public health campaigns to eradicate yellow fever used a military model (used by Soper in the 1930s), a vertical, top-down program aimed at source reduction. In the 1981 epidemic the Cuban government mobilized fifteen thousand health workers to conduct a house-to-house source reduction campaign during which disposal containers were treated with insecticides, malathion was sprayed from planes, portable blowers were used to fog inside dwellings, sanitary laws affecting disposal of containers were enforced, and health education intensified (Gessa and Gonzalez 1986; Kouri et al. 1986; Gubler and Kuno 1997). Massive resources were deployed, in both economic and human terms. Close to U.S.$43 million was spent on the campaign, mostly on insecticides (Gubler and Kuno 1997), but human resources throughout the island were also mobilized, from top public health officials to individual householders and community members. Much of the actual work of inspection of premises and removal of breeding grounds was conducted by community members who were organized into brigades, trained, supervised, and transformed into "vector controllers" (Gessa and Gonzalez 1986).

In May 1981 when the first cases were diagnosed, and between May and October when the Cuban epidemic ended, a total of 344,203 cases were reported. Two-thirds of the deaths reported occurred among children under the age of fifteen (101 cases); at the height of the epidemic on July 6 there were more than eleven thousand cases. In addition to environmental surveillance and insecticides, the Cuban government established mobile field hospitals and a liberal hospitalization policy, allowing more than 116,151 people (33.7 percent of all reported cases) to be admitted and treated (Kouri et al. 1986:26). Without doubt this policy reduced both morbidity and mortality rates significantly. As Kouri notes:

> This policy appears to have played a significant role in reducing fatalities; in other epidemics elsewhere, where the index of hospitalization was typically much lower, patients were hospitalized when they were already in shock, and the indexes of mortality and lethality were higher. (1986, 26)

The Cuban case is remarkable not only for its low mortality rates, but also for the high level of sustainability the campaign engendered. The Cuban campaign against dengue fever and its *Aedes aegypti* vector enjoyed powerful governmental support, extensive personnel assigned to the campaign (15 provincial directors, 60 entomologists, 27 general supervisors, 729 team leaders, 3,801 inspectors, and 1,947 vector controllers), and a mass media health education campaign that built upon previous governmental activities to develop community-based prevention programs. The sustainability of these efforts draws extensively on the Cuban commitment to community-based primary care, and the successful experiences of health-based community participation programs.

The almost two thousand women vector control brigade members were responsible for many of the activities designed to reduce *Aedes aegypti* breeding places—a crucial element in any long-term reduction plan and one that needs broad community support to be effective. During the epidemic the government instituted a number of laws designed to reduce breeding places, such as banning the use of water-bearing containers in cemeteries, requiring that all water storage containers be covered with lids, and prohibiting the use of vehicle tires or tubes for animal feeding or as drinking troughs. Another common breeding place for *Aedes aegypti* is bromeliads; following the Cuban epidemic, planting bromeliads was banned. Vector controllers were authorized to fine people not in compliance with these regulations designed to reduce breeding sites (Kouri et al. 1986).[1]

Dengue Fever in the Dominican Republic

Dengue fever is so common in the Dominican Republic that people accept it—along with the summer rains, heat, and humidity—as part of island life. For much of the Dominican population, life is lived outdoors, where evening breezes diminish the heat of the day. As the sun sets, people gather to recount the day and relax. Electrical power, often interrupted and always unreliable, makes houses hot and uncomfortable. Few houses without their own power supply have air conditioning, and most houses have no screens on the windows. In addition, the electrical power shortages mean that almost everyone stores water in buckets, tubs, and fifty-five-gallon drums for times when there is no running water (Whiteford 1997). The water storage containers and the lush foliage create perfect breeding receptacles in which *Aedes aegypti* flourishes.

Surveys conducted in the late 1970s showed that approximately 70 percent of children younger than ten years in some poor, urban neighborhoods of Santo Domingo had antibodies to dengue fever, and that dengue was endemic in the area (Tidwell et al. 1990). By 1988 approximately 40 percent of the blood samples from febrile children in Santo Domingo showed a positive screen for dengue fever, both DHF and DSS (Tidwell et al. 1990). These data underlie the grave concern that Tidwell et al. expressed in 1990 concerning the likely possibility of a serious dengue epidemic: "In view of the high population densities of *Aedes aegypti,* the endemicity of all four dengue serotypes, and the continuing use of essential water storage containers, it is probable that Santo Domingo will experience a serious epidemic of dengue hemorrhagic fever" (1990:521). How did this situation of endemicity come to pass, and given the extant data and documentation of the dengue problem, could the Dominican Republic undertake programs similar to those successfully employed in Cuba to control the vector and avoid an epidemic?

Between 1950 and 1960, the population of Santo Domingo increased sixfold; simultaneously, the percentage of the population living in urban centers doubled. The majority of that increase was due to rural migration to the capital city of Santo Domingo, resulting in 25 percent of the Dominican population living in 3.2 percent of the country's geographic area (Beestra 1984). By 1989 Santo Domingo had a population of 2.25 million inhabitants (Tadeu and Rauner 1989).

However, the increase in urban population crowding into the capital was not matched by an increase in the ability of the government to provide services for them. As shown in Table 3.1. Piped water and electricity, always in short supply, became even more difficult to secure, and as those necessities became harder to access legally, people became more adept at securing them through alternative means. One response to the capricious

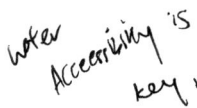

Table 3.1 Access to Public Health Services (percentage)

	Cuba (1994)	Dominican Republic (1990)
Access to improved water		
Urban	96	82
Rural	85	45
Access to sanitation		
Urban	71	95
Rural	51	75

Source: Health Statistics Report, Center for International Health Information, December 1996.

provision of water was the Dominicans' constant concern with getting it and storing it. Another was the wide variety of ways people managed to obtain water: They tapped into city water pipes; they stood in line for hours to get water from public distribution points; they borrowed it from friends; they used communal standpipes. Wherever and whenever water was running, people collected and stored it.

In 1988–1990 I had the opportunity to study dengue fever in the Dominican Republic. The objectives of our research[2] were to conduct an ethnographic study of dengue fever, describe the household ecology of *Aedes aegypti,* identify constraints to community-participation activities, and propose means to overcome those constraints.

Integrated ethnographic methods were used to design and conduct a community study and small-scale survey to learn about people's knowledge of and behavior toward dengue fever. A walking survey and map of the community were drawn, and key informant interviews, structured observations of households, and in-depth interviews were conducted with a limited sample of men and women. In addition, school-based essay competitions provided access to families in the community.

Based on the qualitative data acquired through ethnographic techniques, a survey was constructed to elicit information concerning water-handling behavior, distribution of household tasks, the ethnoecology of dengue fever, knowledge about dengue fever and its causes, means of prevention, and perception of relative severity. The survey was administered to a random sample of one hundred adults living in the study neighborhood and was augmented by historical and ethnographic information. One individual per household was surveyed. Fifty-six males and forty-four females responded to the sixty-four-item interview schedule (Whiteford 1997).[3]

Following the ethnographic and survey components of the research, nine households were selected for structured direct observations. Day-long observations were designed to validate information provided during the survey concerning allocation of tasks, duration of tasks, and behavior related to dengue fever. During the household observations, the project field director took special note of the physical and social environment of each household. Nine individuals were selected as key informants based on their knowledge of the history and population of the neighborhood. In addition, demographic and epidemiological data provided a national context in which to examine individual interviews and other qualitative data.

The Dominicans exposed to years of dengue eradication and control activities, including health education messages, understood the transmission cycle of dengue fever and the role of the mosquito in that process. However, they were unwilling to participate in the community-based prevention activities critical to control dengue transmission. Those activities did not necessitate large expenditures of time or money, but did require a community-based response. Water storage receptacles needed to be kept covered, refuse removed, and trash collected and disposed of. Dominicans explained the community's lack of willingness to engage in simple activities designed to control a potentially deadly disease as a result of the local identity of *mala unión,* lack of political will, lack of a viable partnership between the community and the government.

Idioms of Hope and Despair

Mala unión in the Dominican Republic and *sembrando el futuro* in Cuba are local idioms that reflect people's willingness to engage in community-based participatory activities. In the case of dengue fever, these activities are the control and prevention programs so necessary to the interruption of the cycle of transmission. The epidemiologic and ethnographic data from the Dominican Republic and Cuba contextualize these local identities from two Caribbean island countries so similar and dissimilar to each other. When Dominicans talk about *mala unión,* they evoke images of a partnership gone bad, of a relationship of trust soured. The identity is weighted with disappointment, failed expectations, and expectations of failure. It is a burden of knowledge borne from the past, carried into the future. *Mala unión* permeates Dominicans' explanations of past failures, and it predicts future outcomes. It surrounds their social suffering, explaining unemployment, power shortages, lack of teachers, powerlessness, and disease. While the Dominican idiom of *mala unión* looks backward as if at a failed marriage, the Cuban phrase *sembrando el futuro* is one of hope and expectation. The crop is planted for the future.

The Cuban phrase exemplifies a local identity defined by reciprocally achieved results in which participants and the government clearly have identified rights, responsibilities, and limitations. This identity includes a strong governmental role and equally strong community role, a cultural construction of health care surety played out against a backdrop of economic hardship and political risk. Whereas the Cuban images look forward, the Dominican images suggest a local identity of failed expectations, loss of faith in health care rights, and community and governmental withdrawal from health obligations.

The Dominican Republic and Cuba share similar colonial histories: indigenous, diasporan, and colonial populations and physical environments. However, following the overthrow of Batista and Trujillo (the Cuban and Dominican leaders who controlled the islands during the middle third of this century), the political directions of the two islands diverged. As their political histories parted ways, in each country emerged the idioms of hope and despair grounded in individual political and economic realities and reflecting citizens' relations with their government and among themselves. The two countries exemplify distinctive national geopolitical and ideological identities and concomitant divergent global, political, and economic processes influencing the commodification of health.

In order to understand how health becomes commodified in local identities, national ideologies, and global pressures, I discuss some of the economic forces that prevailed upon the Dominican Republic and Cuba between 1980 and 1992, describe how responses to those pressures are expressed in changed health conditions, and analyze how accumulated symbolic and material capital are the result of both the process of globalization and its intersection with constructed identity.

Triggered by increases in world oil prices, the global recession of the late 1970s forced the Dominican Republic into a debt crisis from which every effort to extricate itself saddled it with crippling economic agreements. The International Monetary Fund imposed perilous structural adjustments on the Dominican economy as part of lending agreements, while simultaneously U.S. trade policies dealt a serious blow to Dominican sugar exports with the development of the U.S. Economic Recovery Act. In the early 1980s international economic policies resulted in the loss of Dominican revenue from sugar exports, a reduction of gross domestic product (GDP) that resulted in a severe decrease in government expenditures on health. Even when the percentage of the GDP dedicated to health increased in the mid-1980s, little was available for discretionary costs. Most was committed to the maintenance of the administrative and infrastructural fixed costs.

The economic crisis attacked the Dominican quality of health from several directions. For instance, loss of personal income led to increasingly crowded living conditions, deteriorating sanitation, declining nutritional status, and increased exposure to infectious disease. Simultaneously, as more women entered the workforce to supplement the decreased incomes of male wage earners, childcare became more problematic as it was more dispersed and less adequate. Meanwhile, at the very moment of increased health risk and need for services, the economic crisis forced the Dominican government to withdraw support from its already ailing primary health system (Whiteford 1990).

In Cuba the thirty-year-old U.S. trade embargo not only continued, but also was strengthened (Santana 1992:1). The U.S. government continued its attempt to isolate Cuba economically through world trade by imposing sanctions against countries trading with Cuba. Of equal, if not greater, significance was the loss of the Soviet Union as both a trading partner and provider. Previous to 1989, the Soviet Union and its trading system had provided Cuba with food, medical supplies, and fuel; without this trade, the Cuban population suffered deficiencies in all three. Food shortages became so common in Cuba in the early 1990s that one could determine if a shop had food by the presence of a line of people waiting outside: "No line, no food." Bread, always a staple in the Cuban diet, became expensive and difficult to obtain; bakeries were unable to make enough because of the shortages in raw materials (Deere 1991:62).

Although almost all babies are born in hospitals in both the Dominican Republic and Cuba, and official statistics for each country suggest that most women receive prenatal care (Ubell 1983:438; Benjamin and Haendel 1991:4; Whiteford 1990), there is less similarity between the two countries than it first appears. Besides sharing an economic crisis, Cuba and the Dominican Republic share history, geography, and proximity to the United States. In terms of local identities, one of the greatest differences between the two islands is that Cuba transferred its vision of *sembrando el futuro* by creating an islandwide primary health care network and a community-based health care system, whereas the Dominican Republic allowed to lie fallow its rural primary care system and turned its resources instead to urban-based hospitals and clinics. Because of its emphasis on community and preventive health, the Cuban public health system appears to be withstanding the current economic challenges by relying on the accumulation of both symbolic and medical capital, whereas the Dominican commodification of health remains costly for its poor results.

In the 1960s and 1970s, Cuba developed a system of community health centers, family health providers, public health education, potable water, and collection of human and solid wastes, each dependent on the central government and on the goodwill and participation of the community. Had the economic crisis not occurred, and had development continued according to Cuba's Public Health Plan, by 1995 Cuba would have been the first country to have comprehensive family practice coverage for 100 percent of its people (Nelson 1991). The economic crisis made that an impossible goal to achieve by 1995. Nevertheless, Cuba's health accomplishments are significant. In 1991 Cuba had thirty-eight thousand physicians and a physician-to-population ratio of 1:534, compared to the 1:2,320 physician-to-population ratio in the Dominican Republic, making total coverage a realistic possibility (Nelson 1991). In addition, by 1992 Cuba had achieved a life expectancy rate within two years of that for the United States, and an infant mortality rate within one point of that in the United States, and had reduced low birth weights to within two percentage points of the United States' figure (*New York Times* 1994). Although the Cuban trends in infant mortality, birth weights, and deaths from infectious disease—each relatively sensitive indicators of changes in health status—show recent small increases in the number of low birth weight babies born and number of deaths from infectious disease, the overall infant mortality rate continues to drop (Figure 3.1).

In light of the economic restructuring that Cuba has endured, one must ask, How were they able to do so much? In the early 1960s, Cuba set four national health goals: "(1) increased emphasis on preventive medicine, (2) improvements of sanitation and related areas, (3) raising of nutritional levels for the disadvantaged social groups, and (4) education of the public regarding health matters" (Diaz-Briquets 1983:105–106). To accomplish those goals, the government provided free access to medical care; increased the number of trained health workers; increased the number of medical facilities in rural areas; increased chemical treatment of water; eradicated malaria; began food rationing to allocate food to those most in need; and began aggressive early intervention strategies to treat both problem pregnancies and diarrheal diseases (Diaz-Briquets 1983: 107–112).

In so doing, Cuba made equity and access a central focus of both its policy and practice. It accumulated symbolic and medical capital that

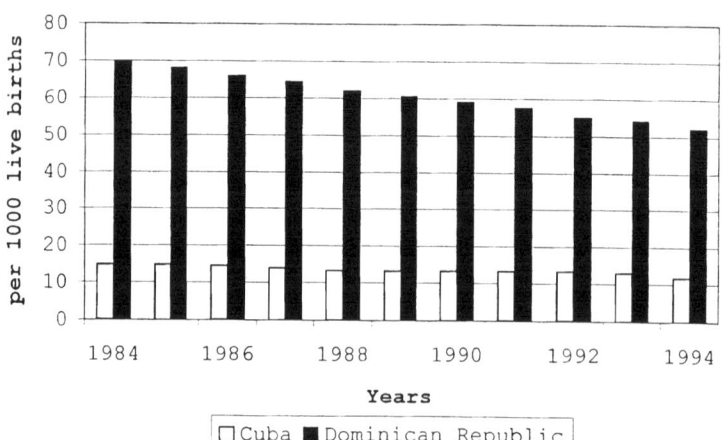

Figure 3.1 Infant Mortality Rates, 1984–1994

Source: *New York Times*, 1994.

serves the people during the economic crisis. Both Dominicans and Cubans face conditions that challenge their survival—shortages of food, housing, and medical supplies. However, Dominicans also struggle with the problems of little health education, restricted access to health care, inadequate services within the health system, a centralized, urban-based medical infrastructure, the lack of access to clean water and waste disposal, and the lack of political will to improve health.

Global and transnational economic pressures on the Dominican Republic resulted in increased external flows of capital and labor. Labor migration and remittances became increasingly significant as a survival strategy for Dominicans. More than seven hundred thousand Dominicans have emigrated since the 1970s, most of them during the decade of the 1980s, and especially since 1985 (PAHO 1996b). In the Dominican Republic, global pressures in the form of international lending institutions and their conditions for loan repayments, coupled with high unemployment, labor strife, and high levels of emigration, transformed health policies and, in so doing, commodified health away from the public good. During the financial crisis of the 1980s, provision of clean water and health policies directed toward improved sanitation and prevention were put aside as the commodification of health moved away from traditional public health themes and toward the provision of more centralized and curative practices. For many Dominicans, this turn away from community-based health programs was seen as a reflection of the global market in which one had to have money to purchase health at a time when the government was reducing the accumulated medical capital and restricting equity and access to public health programs. "The connection between income and health depends not only on current flows but on the stock of capital—including medical capital as well as safe water supplies and sanitation—accumulated from the past" (Musgrove 1987:421). As Musgrove points out, medical capital—like savings in a bank—continues to accumulate and reward the investor after the initial investment is made. Even with international pressures and high out-migration of labor, had the Dominican government maintained that initial commitment to public betterment through public health, that medical capital might well have changed local identities so antithetical to cooperation.

For the Dominican Republic the issue of accumulated capital is particularly critical because there was little medical capital previously accumulated, and what little there was does not serve to reverse community sentiment of *mala unión*. Cuba, on the other hand, showed real gains in accumulated and symbolic capital, particularly in the areas of public health, equity and access, and community identity.

These global pressures commodify Dominican health in "quick fix" immunization campaigns while ignoring the long-term health needs of communities. This loss of support for communities further erodes the belief of Dominicans in their government, and even in their own abilities to participate in the alleviation of shared problems. *Mala unión* expands to permeate not only relations between the national government and individuals, but also between individuals, defeating community-based solutions.

The Dominican local identity of *mala unión* abrogates necessary government-community collaboration. Because the Dominican Republic, unlike Cuba, chose not to make prevention, health education, equity, and access to health care a major thrust of its public policy, Dominican health identity is one of failed campaign promises, hospitals without doctors, pharmacies without medicine, and rural health outposts without patients. In contrast to the constructed identity that places Dominicans in a *mala unión* with their government, the Cuban local identity of *sembrando el futuro* is one of promises fulfilled now and for the future.

Analysis and Conclusion

How do we measure the well-being of people in the 1980s living in these two countries? Standard health indicators such as maternal mortality, infant and child mortality, and total fertility rates suggest that health is more precarious in the Dominican Republic than in Cuba. By the mid-1990s, international agencies estimated 95 maternal deaths per 100,000 live births in Cuba, whereas in the Dominican Republic the rate was slightly higher at 110 (www.cihi.com, 1998). Infant mortality rates are more telling, reflecting the greater coverage of primary care doctors and family physicians in Cuba. Cuba's infant mortality rate was ten per one thousand live births, whereas in the Dominican Republic it was estimated that thirty-eight infants would die for every one thousand born live (www.cihi.com, 1998). Likewise, the death rate for children under the age of five was considerably higher in the Dominican Republic than in Cuba (fifty-two deaths per one thousand live births in the Dominican Republic as compared to thirteen in Cuba).

Other health indicators suggest that health coverage in Cuba is more equally distributed across the island than it is in the Dominican Republic. Measures of oral rehydration therapy (ORT) access rates in Cuba show 100 percent coverage, whereas in the Dominican Republic only 13 percent of the children have access. The use rate for ORT in Cuba is a remarkably high 80 percent, whereas in the Dominican Republic, only 29 percent of the population say that they use ORT (see Table 3.2).

A higher proportion of infants die in the Dominican Republic than in Cuba, perhaps a reflection of Cuba's emphasis on prevention and level of physician coverage. Access to sanitation, potable water, and education are

Table 3.2 Access to Health Services in Cuba and the Dominican Republic

	Cuba	Dominican Republic
Oral rehydration therapy (%)		
ORS access rate	100[a]	13[b]
ORT use rate[a]	80	29
HIV prevalence		
Adults (per 100,000)[b]	21	987

Source: Health Statistics Report, Center for International Health Information, December 1996.
Notes: a. 1991
b. 1989

also indicators of quality of life. If we consider only sanitation and access to "improved" (not necessarily potable) water—items that would improve the likelihood of survivability—96 percent of the urban households in Cuba have access to improved water, and 82 percent of the households in the urban areas of the Dominican Republic do (www.cihi.com, 1998). Both countries are undergoing serious economic crises, affecting the population's access to basic commodities, continuous electrical power, and basic sanitation. There is no doubt that social suffering exists in both countries in the form of a shortage of employment opportunities and the pressures of the global market—and, in Cuba, a lack of political freedom. The many similarities between the two countries, however, mask the importance of local identities. These local identities and the idioms that express them should be understood to mediate the unfolding of health programs and their local applications.

I have used the idioms *mala unión* and *sembrando el futuro* to suggest how two distinctive local identities could facilitate or impede health programs. These images are only two of the multiple identities that people have, only two of the many that people use at different times and in different contexts. Each identity is important in relation to the other identities in the community and serves to highlight the need to listen to the voices in the community, to learn their categories, and to fit health-program aims and objectives to local needs and identities—not to force local realities into global outcomes. The playing field will be more level only when its dimensions come from the users on the ground and in the communities. Until then, the idea of a level playing field is a fallacy.

In 1996 Kleinman and Kleinman wrote: "Existential processes of pain, death and mourning are metamorphosed by . . . historically shaped rationalities and technologies, which again all-too-regularly are inattentive to how the transformations they induce contribute to the suffering they seek to remedy" (1996:xii). Attention to local realities, constructed histories, and power differentials between funding agencies and recipient countries can smooth out the craters and mountains on the playing field so that all players have equal opportunities to decrease social suffering and to improve their lives. Jean J. Schensul, past president of the Society for Applied Anthropology, suggested that applied anthropologists use their skills to level the playing field by equalizing the imbalance of power between funders and field sites, centralized programs and their field applications, globalized policies and in-country cultural contexts (personal communication, 1998). Attention to local identities and local realities can ground the social analyst in the application of programs shaped by politics and economics, thereby mediating the process of social transformation to reduce social suffering.

Even the semisacred cows of international health and development programs should be critically appraised to see how their local fit occurs. The three key concepts often employed in health and development projects, "empowerment," "participation," and "community" (Fisher 1997), may needlessly reify what Kleinman and Kleinman refer to as "routinized misery" because they are treated as processes whose outcomes are predetermined by funders (1996:xiii). That is, although community empowerment and participation are the cornerstones for many health and development programs (both in the United States and abroad), they are envisioned as processes for which planners have predetermined definitions (via funders) of acceptable outcomes. The process itself is rarely the outcome, and consequently the desired intervention outcome (increased immunizations, for instance) does nothing to alleviate the routinized social suffering of unemployment, lack of water and housing, and unequal social relations. In an era of globalization of international health programs, local realities—though often given lip service—are denied because they do not fit into predetermined categories. Local realities and identities are locally constructed, shaped by history and context, and often not globally generalizable. One consequence of this is the denial of the local because programs must fit into predetermined funding categories and their outcomes measured in units that are globally comparable—measures that may be locally inappropriate, meaningless, or even detrimental. Yet, as the Cuban and Dominican Republic examples show, local identities facilitate or prohibit types of interventions; those identities give contour to the playing field and define the rules of the game.

Perhaps it is time to throw out the idea of a "level playing field," for without attention to local identities as well as national infrastructures, the globalization of health will only result in the globalization of social suffering. As Farmer (1996) and others have suggested, health policy and social policy are inseparable, and the discussion of social suffering brings a moral perspective to social analysis. It forces the social analyst to embed issues in a defined moral, political, and cultural space, reducing escapes into cultural relativity or global abstractions.

The Kleinmans suggest that routinized misery results from the lack of the level playing field, where local needs are not given weight and meaning comparable to the internationally generated agendas of funding sources. They draw our attention to the fact that even with the "miracles of modern medicine and public health measures, it is not nearly so apparent that the social suffering . . . is reduced" (1996:vii). We need to ask why this is the case. Could it be that we have too narrowly defined our roles as applied social scientists by confining our research foci to particular categories of physical health, thereby ignoring how suffering itself becomes reified as a process of social mediation and transformation (Kleinman and Kleinman 1996:xvii)? In an earlier work (Whiteford 1997) I suggested that dengue fever control projects in the Dominican Republic failed due to their inability to recognize and transform a local identity of powerlessness, that community participation failed because of historical circumstances. Now I wonder if even that explanation was too narrowly conceived, and in this chapter I have tried to expand my understanding of the social suffering embedded in the concept of *mala unión,* and explore the idea of local identities as keys to our understanding of the ways in which people interact with national health care systems. Social suffering "results from what political, economic, and institutional power does to people, and reciprocally, from how these forms of power themselves influence responses to social problems" (Kleinman and Kleinman 1996:xi). Although the Kleinmans include health as a possible indicator of social suffering, their concept is much wider than just health. They incorporate perspectives from economics, politics, social medicine, anthropology, and critical literature applied to levels of analysis stemming from the intersubjective connections of experience to localized social realities and global processes. Using the examples of the Dominican Republic and Cuba, I am suggesting that unexamined local identities become barriers to care, thereby increasing the social and physical suffering of people we work with and for. In a time of increasing globalization and commodification of health, it is time to understand how local realities transform people's lives and their abilities to live them well.

Notes

This chapter is the result of fieldwork conducted under the auspices of Rockefeller grant 8908–45878 (co P-I, Jeannine Coreil, Diego Salazar, project director), Johns Hopkins University, and the University of South Florida. I want to thank Lenore Manderson, Alpa Patel, and Dinorah Martinez for their editorial and technical assistance in bringing this chapter to light, and Kim Hopper for insightful commentary on an earlier version.

1. Fifteen years after the 1981 dengue fever epidemic, Cuba again experienced a reemergence of dengue. The 1998 epidemic was detected through an active

surveillance system. Early detection through active surveillance and ongoing detection through passive surveillance allowed for a rapid response to the threat. It appears that the vector control activities instituted following the 1981 epidemic made it possible to limit the transmission to one of 169 municipalities known to have *Aedes aegypti* mosquitoes, and that one municipality where dengue was found (Santiago) had a breakdown in vector control activities (wysiwyg:://106/http://www/cdc.gov/ncidod/EID/vol4no1/kouri.htm).

2. The research was funded by a grant from the Rockefeller Foundation and the International Center for Community-Based Health Research at Johns Hopkins University School of Hygiene and Public Health.

3. For more detailed information about research design and methodology, see Coreil and Whiteford 1997; Whiteford 1997.

References

Beestra, Teresa. 1984. "Dinamic Regional y el Proceso de Urbanizacion en la Republica Dominicana," *Estudios Sociales* 17(57): 21.
Benjamin, Medea, and Mark Haendel. 1991. "A Health Revolution?" *Links: Health and Development Report* 8(3): 3–6.
Ceara, M. 1987. *Nacional Sobre la Situación de la Niñez y la Mujer Dominicana.* Santo Domingo: UNICEF.
Coreil, Jeanine, Linda M. Whiteford, and Diego Salazar. 1997. "The Household Ecology of Disease Transmission." In *Anthropology and Infectious Disease*, Peter Brown and Marcia Inhorn, eds. Amsterdam, NY: Greenwood Press.
Deere, Carmen O. 1991. "Cuba's Struggle for Self-Sufficiency," *Monthly Review* (July/Aug.): 55–73.
Diaz-Briquets, Sergio. 1983. *The Health Revolution in Cuba.* Austin: University of Texas Press.
Eberstadt, Nicholas. 1986. "Did Fidel Fudge the Figures? Literacy and Health: The Cuban Model," *Caribbean Review* 15(2): 4–7, 37–38.
Escobar, A. 1995. *Encountering Development: The Making and Unmaking of the Third World.* Princeton, NJ: Princeton University Press.
Farmer, Paul. 1996. "On Suffering and Structural Violence: A View from Belo," *Daedalus* 125(1): 261–283.
Ferguson, A., and F. Ox-Salzberger. 1996. *An Essay on the History of Civil Society.* Cambridge, England: Cambridge University Press.
Fisher, J. 1993. *The Road from Rio: Sustainable Development and the Nongovernmental Movement in the Third World.* New York: Praeger.
Fisher, W. F. 1995. *Toward a Sustainable Development: Struggling over India's Narmada River.* Armonk, NY: Sharpe.
———. 1997. "Doing Good? The Politics and Antipolitics of NGO Practices," *Annual Reviews in Anthropology* 26: 439–486.
Gessa, Armada Jose A., and Rafael Figueredo Gonzalez. 1986. "Application of Environmental Management Principles in the Program for Eradication of Aedes (Stegomyia) Aegypti (Linneus, 1762) in the Republic of Cuba, 1984," *PAHO Bulletin* 20(2): 186–193.
Gubler, Duane G., and G. Kuno. 1997. *Dengue and Dengue Hemorrhagic Fever.* New York: CAB International.
Halstead, Scott B. 1980. "Dengue Haemorrhagic Fever: A Public Health Problem and a Field for Research," *Bulletin of the World Health Organization* 58: 1–21.

Instituto de Estudios de Poblacion y Desarrollo. 1986. *Poblacion y Salud en la Republica Dominican.* Dominican Republic: PROFAMILIA.

Kearney, Michael. 1995. "The Local and the Global: The Anthropology of Globalization and Transnationalism," *Annual Reviews in Anthropology* 24: 547–565.

Kendall, Carl. 1998. "The Role of Formal Qualitative Research in Negotiating Community Acceptance: The Case of Dengue Control in El Progreso, Honduras," *Human Organization* 56(2): 217–221.

Kleinman, A., and J. Kleinman. 1996. "The Appeal of Experience, the Dismay of Image: Culture Appropriations of Suffering in Our Time," *Daedalus* 125(1): 1–23.

Kleinman, Arthur, Veena Das, and Margaret Lock, eds. 1997. *Social Suffering.* Berkeley: University of California Press.

Kouri, Gustavo, Maria G. Guzman, and Jose Bravo. 1986. "Hemorrhagic Dengue in Cuba: History of an Epidemic," *PAHO Bulletin* 20(1): 24–30.

Musgrove, P. 1987. "The Economic Crisis and Its Impact on Health and Health Care in Latin America and the Caribbean," *International Journal of Health Services* 17: 411–441.

Nelson, Harry. 1991. "Overmedicated? An Excess of Success May Ail Cuba's Top Flight Health Care System," *Los Angeles Times,* July 22.

New York Times. 1994. "Health Care in Cuba Falls on Tough Times," October 30, 6y.

Nobuchi, H. 1979. "The Symptoms of a Dengue-like Illness Recorded in a Chinese Medical Encyclopedia" (in Japanese), *Kanpo no Rinsho* 26: 422–425.

PAHO (Pan American Health Organization). 1996a. http://www.paho.org/english/cuba.htm.

———. 1996b. http://www.paho.org.english/dominicanrepublic.htm.

Ramirez, N., I. Duarte, and C. Gomez. 1987. "Sintesis del Estudio: Población, Producción de Alimentos y Nutrición en la Republica Dominicana," *Población y Desarrollo* (Octubre-Diciembre): 1–4.

Salazar, Diego. 1993. "Folk Models and Household Ecology of Dengue Fever in an Urban Community of the Dominican Republic." Unpublished Ph.D. diss., University of South Florida.

Santana, Sarah. 1992. "Cuba: Trends and Conditions in Health, Food and Nutrition." Paper presented at the Annual Latin American Studies Association Meeting, Los Angeles, September.

Tadeu, Americo, and Julie Rauner. 1989. "Dominican Republic's Attractive Beaches and Investment Incentives Lure Tourism Industry," *Business America* 110(22): 14–15.

Tidwell, M. A., D. C. Williams, T. Carvalho Tidwell, C. J. Pena, T. A. Gwinn, D. A. Focks, A. Zaglul, and M. Mercedes. 1990. "Baseline Data on *Aedes Aegypti* Populations in Santo Domingo, Dominican Republic," *Journal of the American Mosquito Control Association* 6: 514–522.

Ubell, Robert N. 1983. "Twenty-five Years of Cuban Health Care," *New England Journal of Medicine* 309(23): 1468–1472.

Whiteford, L. M. 1990. "A Question of Adequacy: Primary Health Care in the Dominican Republic," *Social Science and Medicine* 30: 221–226.

———. 1992. "Contemporary Health Care and the Colonial and Neo-Colonial Experience: The Case of the Dominican Republic," *Social Science and Medicine* 35(10): 1215–1223.

———. 1993. "Child and Maternal Health and International Economic Policies," *Social Science and Medicine* 37(11): 1391–1400.

———. 1997. "The Ethnoecology of Dengue Fever," *Medical Anthropology Quarterly* 11(2): 202–223.

———. 1998a. "Children's Health as Accumulated Capital: Structural Adjustment in the Dominican Republic and Cuba." In *Small Wars: The Cultural Politics of Childhood,* Nancy Scheper-Huges and Carolyn Sargent, eds. Berkeley: University of California Press.

———. 1998b. "Sembrando el Futuro: Globalization and the Commodification of Health." In *Crossing Currents: Continuity and Change in Latin America,* Michael B. Whiteford and Scott Whiteford, eds. Upper Saddle River, NJ: Prentice Hall.

Whiteford, L. M., and J. Coreil. 1991. "The Household Ecology of Dengue Fever." Unpublished monograph, Johns Hopkins University.

Whiteford, Linda, Jeannine Coreil, and Deigo Salazar. 1991. "Household Ecology of Dengue Fever." Unpublished monograph prepared for the Rockefeller Foundation, Johns Hopkins University.

4

Health Care from the Perspectives of Minahasa Villagers, Indonesia

Peter van Eeuwijk

If the dream of postmodernism[1] and cosmopolitanism were to come true, world citizens would live in one big global village characterized by heterogeneity and cultural fragmentation. As Geertz (1995:140) states, "'modernity' may not exist as a unitary thing"; the interpretation of a particular culture as a monolithic body based on consensus, and on shared common values and modes of behavior, is untenable in a globalized world. We live in a paradoxical state in which global processes of transformation create uniformity and transnationalism on the one hand, but on the other, these processes lead to a strengthening of cultural differences within and between societies. The more people are interconnected, the greater the plurality of senses of belonging and modes of existence (Geertz 1996:24).[2] The popular slogan "think globally, act locally"[3] puts into words the active protection of cultural difference as well as the carefully orchestrated transformation of "traditional" cultures. As Kearney's (1995) definition[4] implies, present-day local processes and identities cannot be understood without understanding the ongoing global processes and their impact on local conditions. Conversely, local culture-specific circumstances always shape global processes. In this sense, the construction of cultural identity may function as a prerequisite for security, peace and well-being,[5] but not as a shield against global influences. The simple oppositions of "the global versus the local" or "the universal versus the particular" are alleged contradictions that postmodernism overcomes with the concept of "glocalization"[6] (Featherstone and Lash 1995:4), that is, global localization as "a global outlook adapted to local conditions" (Robertson 1995:28). For instance, worldwide local knowledge undergoes a process of hybridization[7] resulting in "blurring distinctions between scientific and other knowledge on socio-cultural grounds" (Sillitoe 1998:205). The dichotomous thinking in "either-or" terms—that is, "the modern scientific perspective versus the traditional local view"—has to be abandoned in social sciences. Local and global realities are not mutually exclusive anymore,[8] and ideas and ideologies defy the conventional boundaries of time and space (it can happen anywhere, anytime). Therefore, global phenomena are re-created against backdrops of local realities. For instance, lay knowledge of health and illness is, perhaps everywhere, a rich mélange of fragmented, loosely coherent, and popularized concepts that may originate from the professional (e.g., biomedical and/or Ayurvedic traditions) and the folk health sector (e.g., local healers and/or complementary medicine). The spread and exchange of new ideas and notions do not result in increased uniformity of knowledge, but rather lead to a multitude of variations and combinations of knowledge. In this sense, indigenous knowledge systems show their adaptability to new incentives "from outside." "Indeed globalization has generated a whole new diversified pattern of responses at national, regional and local levels" (Long 1996:39).

Global processes in medicine have a long history. In the wake of imperialism, the industrial revolution, free enterprise, and scientific progress, worldwide so-called cosmopolitan Western medicine began to influence medical reality. Nonbiomedical professional regional and local medical traditions were overlaid and at times displaced or marginalized by biomedicine and its institutions.[9] Biomedicine postulated health as an alienable commodity, which could be sold and bought, its profit reinvested; cosmopolitan biomedicine is therefore clearly linked to a particular political economy, namely, the capitalist world order.[10]

Medicalization,[11] as a worldwide process that invents new needs and creates new expectations, unilaterally defines health as a global supervalue. Physical wellness and fitness as well as bodily beauty and emotional "feel good" factors enter the medical market: to stay well becomes a moral condition or even imperative; to be ill would be immoral. Accordingly, well-being could be construed as an achievement of globalization, sickness the everyday reality of localization. It is a fallacy of the level playing field that health is attainable. Biomedicine gives people an ideal image of what a healthy and happy life consists of, but in reality individual and socio-economic circumstances—living in poor urban slums in third world megacities, for instance—do not allow people to stay well.

By constructing and defining international guidelines, the World Health Organization (WHO) as a multilateral body has had a strong global impact on medical reality.[12] For instance, the universality of the Declaration of Alma-Ata (1978) and its idealistic target "Health for All by the Year 2000" made these documents a global charter. Thus, primary health care (PHC) has become an important option in many pluralistic medical systems.

Furthermore, in developing PHC programs, traditional practitioners, traditional birth attendants, and local herbalists at times have been incorporated into health projects, as so-called locally rooted agents of medical change by national and international health authorities, to bridge the gap between global concepts and local settings. In many cases global agendas and national policies have led to a decontextualization of local medical knowledge and/or to an etic construction of what is "traditional."[13]

Generally speaking, worldwide local health care systems are pluralistic and do not consist of mutually exclusive and unadaptable structures. It is therefore extraordinary that international health planners and national health providers frequently try to overrun the already existing medical structures rather than make use of these given pluralistic forms and respect local cognitive systems of health and illness. Biomedicine, through its claim to universality, considers itself to be entitled to judge what is right and what is wrong in local health care. From a provider's view, this process leads to worldwide uniformity in medicine, whereas from the user's view, it will lead to a global decline in medical variety.

Globalization in the Indonesian Context

Indonesia's constitutional frame is shaped by "Unity in Diversity" *(Bhinneka Tunggal Ika)* and the state philosophy of Five Principles *(Pancasila)*.[14] The country has experienced the processes of globalization in a multilayered and sometimes ambiguous way. The rulers in Jakarta, the majority Javanese, consider the country's great ethnic diversity "a component of the national culture" (Schefold 1998:276)[15] that has to submit to a nation-building state ideology and to serve so-called pan-Indonesian vested interests such as the exploitation of raw materials, the promotion of tourism, and the provision of a cheap workforce to global industry. On one hand, global processes and relationships encompassing local, regional, and even national boundaries have strengthened detribalization and moves toward cultural uniformity in the Indonesian Archipelago, which encompasses 13,667 islands and about 583 language groups. It has finally led to the creation of a national identity—One Land, One Nation, One Language. On the other hand, transnational networks for the first time have offered sociopolitical bodies and various ethnic groups the opportunity to express and promote their interests and concerns on an international platform, and to ask for global support.[16]

Indonesians' views of globalization and its processes have been strongly influenced by one of the world's top social forecasters and futurists, the American John Naisbitt, a political scientist and entrepreneur. In Southeast Asia, his ten "Megatrends 2000" were considered as "gateways to the twenty-first century" and "a new world view" based on "the Asian model."[17] Naisbitt (1996:246) prophetically concluded:

> Combined with science and technology, Asians could present the world with a new model, one that takes modernization and combines it with the virtues of Eastern and Western values, one that reconciles freedom and order, individualism with communitarian concerns. . . . In giving new meaning to modernization, Asians will give birth to a model for the new civilization.

These statements were enthusiastically embraced by Southeast Asian national decisionmakers and top leaders in, for example, Malaysia, Thailand, and Indonesia. As a consequence, they were convinced to join the forces of global transformation believed to be an "Asianization of Asia" and not a "Westernization of the Pacific Rim," which combined "Asian virtues" and Western high technology.

In Indonesia, Naisbitt's "Megatrends" became the official guidelines for the state economic policy, and he was appointed chief consultant of the government. His catchy slogans—"The more universal we become, the more tribal we act" (Naisbitt 1994:26), "The bigger the system, the more efficient must be the parts" (Naisbitt 1996:4)—entered national and regional newspapers ("The worldwide success of the Indonesian economy begins with every individual clove farmer in the district of Kombi"), speeches of officials of the ruling party Golkar ("You are Minahasa, you are Indonesian, you are Asian—you will take part in prosperity, if you vote for Golkar!"), and students' howls of protest ("We are the fuel for political change, and the Indonesian society is its engine"). Even in remote villages, the ten Megatrends were cited, mostly in a very fragmentary form, by village heads at birthday parties, by religious leaders in their prayers, and by secretaries of local rotating saving and credit associations *(arisan)* during their weekly meetings. Regional and provincial leaders held workshops on Naisbitt's Megatrends, where their subordinates were informed of what *globalisasi* consists of. Thus, Indonesians' notions of globalization were deeply influenced by Naisbitt's writings. At the village level, this kind of opinion forming resulted mostly in a very simplified impression and images of globalization, which were usually condensed into availability of Coca-Cola drinks, Pizza Hut fast food, fashionable Nike sneakers, trendy Marlboro cigarettes, and the top disco hits of pop star Michael Jackson.[18]

After decades of self-imposed economic and political isolation, Indonesia opened its doors in the 1980s especially to multinational enterprises. In the economic field, globalization was warmly welcomed by the top national decisionmakers, and a policy of deregulation and liberalization led in the late 1980s and the 1990s to a certain level of national prosperity.

Consequently, Indonesia became a newly industrialized country.[19] The Suharto family, the national government in Jakarta, and certain leaders of conglomerates took increasing profit from globalized world markets as well as from prospering economies in neighboring Southeast and East Asian countries. In the sociopolitical field, conversely, the Indonesian government tried, as in previous years, to tightly control intruding global influences such as free access to mass media, unlimited electronic mailing, and the import of "Western signs of decadence" such as pornography and recreational drugs. In discourse of these factors, globalization was represented by the Indonesian rulers as a threat to their well-established order of power. The then government of Indonesia under President Suharto declared spheres that it considered particularly sensitive—for instance, human rights, freedom of speech, free access to information versus censorship, democratization of political parties, the armed forces, and the civil administration as well as legal claims of ethnic minority groups and environmental care—as Western and therefore not culture-specific Indonesian issues. This point of view was articulated in certain catch-phrases—"The Indonesian culture does not know such issues such as Human Rights," "Democracy is an imported Western product and does not match our cultural identity and political heritage"—and clearly manifested the rejection of emerging global concerns in politics while justifying and maintaining the power of the national rulers.[20] In consequence, most Indonesians perceived *globalisasi* as a purely economic process of transformation, whereas political, social, and ecological issues with regard to globalization were not admitted as issues to be addressed officially and were not incorporated into the same discourse.

The vast majority of Indonesian citizens began to discuss the pros and cons of *globalisasi* only after the resignation of President Suharto in May 1998 and the subsequent abolition of the government's New Order *(Orde Baru)* policy.[21] The economic and financial collapse in Indonesia—at the same time a far-reaching political, social, and ecological crisis—is considered to be an outcome of national incompetence and corruption as well as globalization. Today, in the so-called *era reformasi* (the era of reformation), nearly every Indonesian sees himself or herself as a victim of global processes that went wrong in Indonesia.[22] Although globalization has led to a more pragmatic political behavior of the ruling class, in the last few years Indonesians have had to pay a very high price to achieve their "reformation." Reformation is regarded now as a very bitter and sometimes traumatic experience for both rural and urban people all over Indonesia, as even the most established health and education systems collapsed within a few months of the end of the "New Order." The paradox in Indonesia is the perceived role of globalization in the overthrow of a corrupt regime and increased political freedom, at the cost of mass impoverishment.

Indonesia: The Concept of National Development and the Process of Globalization

In 1966 the New Order period, under the then newly appointed president General Suharto, formally commenced, after the nightmare of the alleged attempted Communist overthrow of the Sukarno government (in September 1965). The main task of the New Order policy was development *(pembangunan)*, with prosperity and modernity of the Indonesian people defined as the two general aims (Cribb and Brown 1995). Several campaigns—for instance, the Green Revolution *(Revolusi Hijau)* in agriculture, transmigration *(transmigrasi)* to the Outer Islands, and family planning *(keluarga berencana)*—were powerful transregional instruments to achieve these, for the most part, idealistic targets, and they served as substitutes for politics. This Period of National Development *(Era Pembangunan Nasional)* "gave a generation of Indonesians a sense of participation in their country's future which the political system refused them" (Cribb and Brown 1995:119). Participation in development *(partisipasi dalam pembangunan)* linked with catchy slogans—for instance, *modernisasi* (modernization) through *industrialisasi* (industrialization) and *teknologi* (technology)—became a prominent ideological vehicle of progress.

The figures reflecting the achievements of development in Indonesia during the subsequent thirty years illustrate quantitatively the more or less successful implementation of concrete development steps. True "stories of success" embody the national systems of health and education,[23] and Indonesia's economic progress in the 1980s and early 1990s resulted, in spite of great social and regional differences, in an increase of average wages per worker from U.S.$743 (1980) up to $1,128 (1993) (Sunanda 1996:10).[24]

If we look at the local level, we become aware of the villagers' positive tenor in respect to national and regional development and its achievements, but much less so at a village level. Each of the three Minahasa villages that were my research sites had a primary school *(sekolah dasar)*, a local health post *(posyandu)*, a community hall *(balai desa)*, and church buildings *(gedung gereja)*. The respective school enrollment rate had reached nearly 100 percent by 1993; voluntary village health workers *(kader kesehatan)* provide basic preventive and curative services in each of the villages. People enjoy these local achievements, but at the same time they still feel backward *(terkebelakang)*, left behind *(tertinggal)*, not really advanced *(kurang maju,)* and isolated *(terpencil)*. A Minahasa village head came to the following conclusion (in the year 1987): "As long as we don't have a permanent connection to the outside world, we feel like an isolated tribe *[suku terasing]*." His notion, and those of his fellow community members, of "global relations" between his neatly arranged small world and the "world behind the hills" consists of an all-weather street (for vehicle traffic), means of communication (radio and television with satellite dish), and "doing business with the others" (trade and commerce).

This kind of backwardness is "promoted" by the government in two antagonistic ways. On one hand, the alleged intellectual backwardness of villagers (*"Orang kampung kurang berpendidikan dan masih bodoh"* ["The villagers have not enough formal schooling and are still stupid"]) serves as an excuse for state planners and administrators to neglect rural areas. Even village heads in my research sites told me (in 1997!): "People are not yet ready to receive modern life" (*"Orang kampung belum siap untuk menerima hidup modern"*). On the other hand, government officials in low and middle levels of administration instrumentalize poverty and backwardness for very pragmatic reasons: the poorer a village, a district, or a regency is, the more development funds are channeled to it. It is a miraculous fact that many village heads are still keen to declare their already well-developed villages as backward villages *(desa tertinggal)* by manipulating figures in order to receive financial and material aid from higher authorities or from abroad.

In the opinion of villagers, the era of development in Indonesia has not, since the 1980s, met their primary expectations: that is, better access to services and more information to their village from the "outside," and the successful expansion of markets for the various commodities they were producing, for example, agricultural and forest products. As we shall see, these are essential elements of the villagers' view of globalization. Village inhabitants observe from newspapers the fashionable and sophisticated world of the country's capital, Jakarta, on faraway Java, with its trendy and busy people, its glittering saloon cars, and its towering skyscrapers. They do not at all feel jealous of the emerging urban middle and upper class, nor are they frustrated with their own living conditions. On the contrary, they are very proud of what their country has already achieved—and it is only a matter of time until this new dimension of *modernisasi* representing Jakarta will reach their village. Therefore, globalization ideally embodies a postmodern or postdevelopment dimension; it consists of a dynamic, all-embracing movement that makes it possible for locals to profit from global links and connections and to join these networks as active "players."

From a local view, the development period of the 1980s and early 1990s was a static "thing," in which they perceived their role as passive objects to which progress was brought. Their initial hope to become actors in "participation in development" only reached the degree of consumption and utilization of services provided by the government and Christian churches. Nevertheless, all adult villagers of the three Minahasa communities with whom I spoke in 1998 frankly acknowledge that their lives have changed for the better over the last thirty years.

Global Influence on Local Reality

The three Minahasa villages of Makalisung (760 inhabitants; ethnic and language group: Tondano), Pinenek (490 inhabitants; Tonsea), and Liandok (420 inhabitants; Tonsawang) are located on the Minahasa Peninsula at the northeastern tip of North Sulawesi (Island of Sulawesi, the former Celebes). Their population is predominantly Christian, that is, Protestants, Roman Catholics, and members of American-based free churches, and consists largely of ethnic Minahasa.

Makalisung lies on the hilly and fertile Minahasa east coast. During the 1970s, this village changed completely from extensive coffee and coconut cultivation (including copra production) to highly intensive clove cultivation. In the 1970s and 1980s, this "clove fever" resulted in amazing material prosperity and financial wealth in this area (from *daerah minus* to *daerah dolar* [from poor to rich region]). The "hanging gold" (i.e., clove) became the only cash crop, and the cultivation of core foods such as cassava, taro, corn, rice (on dry fields [*ladang*]), sago, and vegetables ceased. As in urban areas, daily food was bought in shops, social relations were "capitalized," and traditional mutual support systems were quickly abolished. By the appropriation of prestige items, villagers gained more *gengsi* (high status, class, and respect), but seldom their practical use. Refrigerators and freezers were used as bookshelves and Sony TVs as flower stands (because there was no electricity until 1991), and in the village reassembled Toyota Jeeps served as garden arbors or chicken coops (because there was no road). After only ten years, however, this almost affluent village society collapsed, when the Suharto family monopolized the entire clove trade in Indonesia (1991–1992) and, as its consequence, clove prices hit rock bottom. Only a few households had sufficient savings to buy rice and fish once a day.

The national economic crisis also hit this village very hard, and in 1997 and 1998, the inhabitants of Makalisung began to know hunger and poverty again—indeed, a very bitter experience! For the past five years, the young village head, a university dropout, has strictly followed an "antiglobal" strategy to improve the villagers' life: back to subsistence agriculture, away from monoculture and cash crop cultivation, back to interhousehold payment in kind, back to traditional mutual assistance bodies, back to solidarity structures in the community, and back to an ordinary peasant lifestyle.

Pinenek is located in a swampy, sandy, very hot area near the Molucca Sea. Since colonial times, this poor, isolated, and backward village has depended completely on coconut cultivation and copra production. The coconut palm is called "the tree of life" because of its multiple uses. Although copra prices fluctuate, copra selling ensures a small but permanent monetary income for the villagers. For food production (e.g., cassava, corn, rice, and some vegetables), most Pinenek households make use of "slash and burn" techniques in a faraway (and theoretically protected) primary forest area. Until 1994 Pinenek had no permanent road connection, and in the rainy season the village was completely cut off for weeks from the outside world. Three families related to each other by kinship dominate the community, for example, in economic matters (big landowners, in possession of all copra grate kilns), in political and religious affairs (filling all important governmental and church offices), in information (owner of the one and only TV set, including parabola antenna), and in transport (owners of the only two cars—copra jeeps used for goods and passenger traffic). This constellation has led to more or less permanent dependence of the villagers on these dominating "clans" that consider the village of Pinenek—their "hunting ground"—a rich source of human and natural assets. These three families hold a protective shield over the community, deflecting external harmful influences. On the other hand, the families in power keep the majority of the villagers isolated and ignorant to ensure eager, good, and cheap labor at their disposal.

Liandok lies like a tiny oasis in the midst of primary forest in a mountainous region. The community is characterized by its natural surroundings, and the rain forest is still the favorite environment of its residents; hunting prey and gathering wild fruits and wood products (e.g., resin, rattan, and lianas) remain an important weekly activity. Only in the last decade have villagers turned from settled hunters and gatherers to part-time gardeners (e.g., cassava, sweet potatoes, taro, corn, and sago) and cash crop cultivators. Life changed when in 1986 a first development project implemented by the Ministry of Agriculture introduced irrigated rice cultivation (on *sawah* fields), a technique that was unknown to them until then. In spite of an abundance of fresh water and land, most villagers are still reluctant to go into muddy *sawah* water and to work there for hours. "This is work for Javanese people, but not for Tonsawang!" they say with contempt. In 1989 vanilla plants were successfully introduced as the main cash crop. Every household had dozens of vanilla plants in its "slash and burn" plantations or around the houses. Once per year the dried black vanilla sticks were carried down to the valley and sold to intermediaries, with the cash so generated used for clothes, tools, and batteries. In 1997 a semipermanent road was constructed, and in 1998 electricity entered Liandok. These development steps brought short-term wealth; soon they had a detrimental effect on the villagers' prosperity. The surrounding primary forest area immediately became a target of several logging companies and of a foreign gold-mining company; regional overproduction of vanilla led to a very dramatic drop in prices; an unknown plant virus brought into Liandok in 1997–1998 destroyed the entire vanilla cultivation; and new settlers ignore and despise the local *adat* traditions (manner, customs, and law). For decades the village chief and his council of elders watched over the villagers' compliance with the *adat* law. Until the 1990s, Liandok remained a traditional and neatly organized village. In 1993 the son of the former village chief, a forestry engineer who lived for ten years in the provincial capital, took over his father's office. He is still trying to find a balance between existing local traditions and emerging global influences.

In these three villages, the economic sector especially has had a strong global influence, although primarily for the export or cash crop system. Villagers speak of *globalisasi* when they discuss clove, copra, or vanilla prices, a tendency that points to a sense of dependence on somebody invisible and unknown, far away from the village, manipulating prices. Besides this perceived global economic impact, which, villagers sense, cannot be prevented, one element of global culture can be heard in every village: "Western" music. Disco music, heavy metal songs, rap melodies, and Asian and African ethno pop music are booming almost twenty-four hours a day, even in remote places such as Liandok. Every household has a cassette recorder run on ordinary batteries or on old truck accumulators, and music cassettes are bought in shops outside the village. It is very prestigious to play, incessantly, American Christmas songs as early as November, and with plastic Christmas trees (made in the People's Republic of China) decorated with snow down (made in Brazil), silver tinsel (made in Thailand), and colorful flash light garlands (made in South Korea), religion has also been subject to globalization. Yet to my surprise, villagers do not at all perceive Christianity as a global phenomenon. "It is our faith, not others'!" they argue.

Makalisung, Pinenek, and Liandok are far from being interconnected with global or even national information networks. Current newspapers and journals are not available in the villages. TV sets are the only actual channel to regional, national, and worldwide news, the evening newscast from Jakarta providing villagers with access to virtual reality. For example, in Pinenek dozens of villagers attentively watched coverage of the Rwanda genocide, and an airplane crash in Colombia, the commentary on the English soccer league, or the weather forecast for New York, London, and Paris, often lead to the enthusiastic remark, *"Itulah globalisasi!"* ["That is what comes from globalization!"]. In Makalisung, where three private TV sets were exclusively used for watching videocassettes (mostly "brutalos," [illegal] American soft pornos or Indian love stories) and in Liandok (without electricity or generators, hence without TV sets), "news from the world" arrives weeks and months after a main event has happened (for instance, the news about the outbreak of the Iraq War in 1991 was heard in Liandok two months after it was over). Therefore, on a local level, topics of conversation of current interest still consist of village affairs and events in neighboring villages or nearby cities.

If Makalisung and Liandok could be generally categorized as partial victims of global economic processes, Pinenek still profits from (indirect) global links because of its copra production. Nevertheless, in every village we find some "global players" who turn their connections to profit. For instance, the manager of the local state cooperative (Koperasi Unit Desa [KUD]) in Makalisung has successfully linked rich Chinese traders in Singapore, powerful representatives of the KUD organization from Java, leaders of the (then) ruling Golkar party from Jakarta, and members of the executive board of the Protestant Minahasa Church (Gereja Masehi Injili Minahasa [GMIM]) in the provincial center. His private as well as his official business runs well; even in the difficult times of the East Asian economic crisis, his international relations did not let him down. However, very rarely does he spend his money on community affairs. The village head of Pinenek, a dynamic and impetuous man, based his network on relatives and influential friends inside the Golkar party and the government of the province North Sulawesi and in Jakarta. Through his personal links in Jakarta, he managed in 1995 to convince a Canadian development agency to invest in a river control project in his village, and in 1997 he convinced managers of an Australian gold-mining company to invest money in prospect sites. Both he and other villagers gained from these projects. The heavy loss of land and buildings due to river erosion was stopped, and many villagers were well paid for their work in this project. The foreign mining company paid substantial compensation to numerous landowners in Pinenek.

During the past years, health conditions in the three Minahasa villages have not changed a lot. Sixty percent of all households still experience at least one illness episode per month. Acute respiratory infections, skin diseases and infections, gastrointestinal diseases, tuberculosis, and external injuries are widespread, and malaria remains the main source of sickness. It causes 62 percent of all illness cases in the villages, and especially the insidious but usually underestimated *Malaria tropica* takes a heavy toll on human lives, particularly babies and children under five years. Four to five times a year every villager suffers from regular malaria attacks. Some cases of leprosy and filiariasis are still found in the three communities. Household sanitation, hygiene, and waste disposal as well as access to safe water are still poor. People use "natural" toilets behind bushes and palm trees, where stray pigs compete to dispose of and "recycle" these deposits; it is therefore advisable always to take a large stick with you on ablution trips. Brooks and rivers still serve as main sources of water for household purposes, and their banks are used as the washing places for clothes, kitchen utensils, and human bodies. In periods of extended drought, water becomes the most restricting factor for a healthy life. For instance, in the course of the three extremely dry years 1987, 1991, and 1997, we had to dig deep holes in riverbanks to gain some glasses of muddy water, and even these at times were shared with thirsty and thus obtrusive pigs, dogs, and cows.

Because of their remote location, the three villages were integrated relatively late into already existing primary health care (PHC) networks (Makalisung, 1983–1984; Pinenek, 1985–1986; Liandok, 1987–1988). Biomedical services other than PHC are available only outside the villages, usually at distant district health centers *(puskesmas)*. State or church PHC teams visit the villages irregularly and during the rainy season not at all, and for the most part, the health-seeking behavior of the villagers involves regular attendance at traditional healers and frequent use of herbal plants and modern drugs. After the roads were built, the three communities immediately expected better and regular professional medical services in their villages. Their hopes were not realized. Because of improved transportation from and to rural areas, PHC providers expected the patients to come to their health centers and polyclinics. Nevertheless, the new roads led to new medical options: retailers of modern drugs extended their networks to the villages and offered a variety of new modern drugs now sold in local shops and kiosks; conversely, patients from Makalisung, Pinenek, and Liandok left their villages to see traditional healers in other regions or to see doctors with private clinics in Manado, the provincial center, thus bypassing the official PHC services. This unexpected change in health-seeking behavior is a manifestation of how villagers' "globalized" thinking led to their use of new realities.

Nevertheless, the locals get a proper and consistent idea of what should be done in their communities to improve health care. Most villagers would like a biomedical professional of the same ethnic group to be based in their village, so that curative care could be provided night and day. A married nurse, for instance, could ideally run a local health center *(puskesmas pembantu)*, monitored and regularly supervised by a health district center *(puskesmas)* and its head *(dokter puskesmas)*. This kind of service would allow villages better access to more effective and stronger pharmaceuticals than those sold over the counter in local kiosks and small shops. A medical reference system—guidelines to medications, a small diagnostic encyclopedia—would complete the provision of a curative service. Many villagers stress that the quality of care has improved in "their" local health center, and this contrasts with their largely negative experiences in distant district health centers. Villagers still also hope for the implementation of conventional preventive programs such as safe water, hygiene, sanitation, and clean housing, not merely as promises by state health planners before each national election. Many villagers would like to improve preventive programs for young children and pregnant women—and for the elderly and the disabled. Rapid demographic change has taken place all over Indonesia. In Minahasa, in rural areas as well as in towns, the health transition (for example, communicable as well as noncommunicable diseases are found in the same community) requires new ideas and solutions. Community-based home nursing could be one option. Many older people are already afraid to grow old and become sick, infirm, and dependent without the help and support of their children or grandchildren.

The Local Perception of *Globalisasi*

Entering Minahasa villages, people "from outside" are very frequently welcomed with colorful posters, spanning over the main street at the village's entrance arch, postulating "Let's welcome the era of globalization!" (*"Mari kita menyongsong era globalisasi!"*). With amazing ease villagers on the way to their remote gardens, with their hoes on their shoulders, try to stress their open-mindedness by saying, "Of course, we are ready to participate in globalization!" Village heads, parish elders, and treasurers of the state Family Welfare Organization (*Pembinaan Kesejahteraan Keluarga,* or PKK) place particular emphasis on the readiness of their respective bodies by repeatedly saying the magic word *globalisasi* in their mostly long-winded speeches. It is nearly impossible to deliver a formal speech without several references to "globalization." Analyzing these statements of local authorities, we recognize straightaway that the actual impact of globalization on community members and its concrete consequences, as well as the dimensions of space and time, are omitted or are acknowledged only in a very vague manner. The inflationary use of the term *globalisasi* should not obscure the fact that the local perspective of the amorphous world "behind the forest hills" has not yet changed a lot.

The term *globalisasi* is one of numerous foreign words that have entered the villagers' vocabulary in a relatively short period. During my first stays in Minahasa villages in the late 1980s, no one ever used this term. It was only in 1990, after the spread of Naisbitt and Aburdene's *Megatrends 2000* in Southeast Asia, and especially in Indonesia, that the term became common even in the everyday discourse of peasant farmers. In Minahasa villages, the word *globalisasi* was, like *liberalisasi* (in the late 1980s) and many other *"-sasi"* suffixes in the Indonesian language, adopted from mass media (e.g., TV or regional newspapers like *Manado Post* or *Cahaya Siang*) and supralocal formal norm setters such as district heads *(camat)* or officials of the ruling political party, Golkar. Villagers subsequently popularized the term. From a local perspective, the term itself remained an "empty shell" until its initial semantic hollowness was filled, step by step, with popular interpretations of globalization. More than three quarters of those with whom I spoke in the three villages had established a link between globalization and modernity, wealth, prosperity, and well-being, thus generally emphasizing a better life. People think of more or less vague characteristic features or signs of globalization, but not of the causes or occasions for it. This felt gap results in a certain conceptual vagueness.[25]

As previously discussed, the term "globalization" was brought from outside into the communities, and the primary carriers of its meaning were people from outside, too. As social phenomena, the initially "empty shell" called *globalisasi*, and therefore its future content, "are constructions produced historically through human activity" (Berger and Luckmann 1989: 106). On the local level, the constructors of meaning are, to a great extent, people who act in the overlapping area of "the inner" and "the outer world," as, for instance, village heads (*kepala desa;* through external administrative duties), cash crop peasants (through trade), shopkeepers (*pemilik toko;* through commerce), officials of political parties (through information), and, where there are roads, bus drivers (*sopir oplet;* through exchange of information). They are the prominent bearers of knowledge "from outside," and they construct the local version of globalization by combining the micro and the macro level of information and notions. According to their professional activities, economic, infrastructural, technical, or political issues may characterize the term *globalisasi*.

Villagers' perceptions of globalization comprise rather heterogeneous ideas of a better life in the near future. The future will be less laborious and more harmonious, and the children will be healthier and wealthier than the present generation. Core elements of their understanding of globalization include hope and patience, not fear or concern. *Globalisasi* is not valued as good or bad, but considered to be something dynamic *(yang bergerak)* and sophisticated *(canggih)* that will, in some way, have an impact on their lives.

Locals understand globalization as a thing moving in from outside, like a vehicle *(kendaraan)* that will stop one day in their village. It is therefore essential for every villager to be ready and prepared to join this process. Those individuals who want to participate have to get onto the vehicle *(naik kendaraan)* called "globalization." If you miss this "mystery train," you will stay a backward peasant and be caught in your traditions. *Globalisasi* consists of something in motion that one day enters the village *(tiba-tiba masuk desa),* stops *(berhenti)* at the "global train station" or "bus stop," picks up those passengers who are already waiting with a ticket or "boarding card" *(karcis untuk naik),* and continues its ride to a new destination *(melanjutkan jalan).*[26] This brief outline of the local concept of "globalization" is based on the assumption that it will be the "outside world" *(dunia di luar)* that will come to the village and connect it with different, already existing global trajectories. Inconsistent and sometimes contradictory notions of many villagers remain. On one hand, they consider globalization a great challenge, which offers them the opportunity to play an active role in structuring their own future. On the other hand, they have adopted a more or less passive "wait-and-see" attitude, until the externally started process has reached their safe shelter. One young man, in one very remote Minahasa village, expressed the widespread metaphor of globalization as a vehicle toward progress in the following words: "Look, we have globalization when the doctor of the district health center *(puskesmas)* in his white dress can reach our village with his white Suzuki Samurai Jeep for his monthly medical visit, and can still return to his center in the evening of the same day!"

The Local Health Care System and Globalization

Following Kleinman's model of the internal structure of local health care systems, medical pluralism in the three Minahasa villages comprises the professional, the popular, and the folk health sector (Kleinman 1980: 49–60). Health-seeking behavior of sick villagers shows a rich variety of complementary and mutually nonexclusive patterns of resort. According to locals, cosmopolitan "modern medicine" is only one of several medical options that are available ideally to sick persons. However, their real health-seeking behavior clearly demonstrates that therapy choice at the village level is limited to a more or less popular-folk curative field. What people say they would do if sick is different from what they really do. From this realistic approach, cosmopolitan biomedicine is far from being synonymous with "global medicine." The local healer *(dukun, tonaas)* may well decorate his or her chest with a stethoscope and proudly wave the blood-pressure cuff, but medical knowledge is still local, not global.

According to villagers' experience, the professional health sector and its services are not yet satisfactory, although some global health programs, such as the expanded program on immunization (EPI), the under-five-weighing and nutrition program *(Upaya Peningkatan Gizi Keluarga* [UPGK]), the village or community health worker (VHW/CHW, *kader kesehatan*) program, and the malaria control program, have been adopted by government and private health providers and are already known to the majority of villagers. The WHO's slogan "Health for All by the Year 2000" decorates the T-shirts worn by elderly trained traditional birth attendants (TBAs), and the official health chart *(kartu menuju sehat,* "road to health" chart) given to mothers with children under the age of five has become an elementary and symbolic document for the provision of preventive health activities.

The first visible and concrete forerunners of globalized health care at the local level had already arrived in Minahasa villages in the 1980s:

modern drugs *(obat modern)* and injections *(suntikan)*. All kinds of pharmaceuticals—whether a doctor's prescription is requested or not, and including drugs long banned in North America and Western Europe—are readily available, sold over the counter of small local kiosks *(warung)* and shops *(toko)* by lay sellers. The frequent use of pharmaceuticals has already had an impact on villagers' health-seeking behavior. For example, in many cases local shopkeepers and lay sellers of modern drugs become the main consultants and new decisionmakers in health-related matters and thus partly replace the patient's social reference groups such as the household. Modern drugs have become an important curative option for many villagers for common ailments and symptoms, for instance, malaria fever and headache.[27] The application of injections by nurses *(perawat, mantri)* and physicians *(dokter)* on their visits to villages and in *puskesmas* has become a core element in biomedical health care.[28] It is an interesting and important detail that villagers of the three Minahasa communities consider the diagnostic and therapeutic procedures of medical professionals as rituals in which the application of drugs and injections—from the user's view—is a normative, irreversible, and formal action and should therefore be an integral part of every biomedical intervention. Not to give medicaments means that "the healing ritual" of nurses and physicians is not complete and therefore not successful. From this local perspective, it is possible to speak of a "local ritual with global ingredients."

Global elements such as time, money, transport, and information play an increasingly important role in illness behavior. System factors such as the Five A's (accessibility, acceptability, availability, accommodation, and affordability [Coreil et al. 1994]) gain importance even on the micro level, such as within the household. The people of the three Minahasa villages are certainly aware of the decisive influence of these pragmatic or "modern" issues on their health decisionmaking. Therefore, biomedical health programs and services need to be "globalized" in such a sense that global elements such as money, time, and distance are integral parts of a medical framework in less-developed areas. The villagers' unspoken critique of conventional primary health care asks for a more transparent, user-oriented, and quality-of-care-oriented health care framed by both local and global perceptions and experiences.

But how can the process of globalization in health care have a decisive impact on the three local health sectors, other than through tablets, pills, and syringes? The key word is "medicalization," a process affecting all areas of life. Medicalization is not the outcome of globalization, but paves the way for it. This process strives to gain social control and economic dominance in local health care systems. Its platform is the professional health sector whose areas overlap with the popular and the folk health sector and is the ideal "entrance gate" for medicalizing local health care. For instance, self-medication with pharmaceuticals—without professional overview—has already been practiced for several years. But there are more subtle things. Pregnancy is defined as a state of sickness—and antenatal care is provided; conception is defined as a medical action—and medical contraception, family planning, and reproductive methods are offered; aging is defined as a critical period in one's life—medical interventions for elderly people are provided. From a villager's perspective it is difficult to recognize the direction of this medicalizing process. If medicalization, acting as a pioneer of globalization, means more available, accessible, affordable, and reliable health care in his or her village, it is most welcome. However, if medicalization aims to displace other medical options and impose its global values on the villagers, *globalisasi* means a step back for them.

Conclusion

If globalization refers to the availability and provision of telecommunications and information, trade and commerce, a road network, and reliable health services, it would meet the basic demands and expectations of the majority of Minahasa villagers. Nevertheless, it is not as simple as it looks: global factors clash with cultural factors; quantitative aspirations and technical feasibility clash with quality of life and psychological resistance. The example of Indonesian development policy of the previous thirty years has clearly shown that progress is a highly sensitive process of awareness building and consciousness-raising. Many material achievements in Indonesia were, in a technical sense, very successful. But they were not sustainable in the end because the "target population" could not participate, and the steps toward progress were not adjusted to daily life circumstances.

In this Indonesian discourse of progress, the Minahasa villagers' perception of *globalisasi* connects their own notions of low-risk, step-by-step development with external methods and support. This idealistic view would at least share the same playing field with moderate regional development planners. Those players who introduce new techniques and ideas from "the outside world" to the villages should act with a great sense of responsibility and sensibility. This is very true for the health sector, too, even more for global or cosmopolitan biomedicine. For instance, the use of pharmaceuticals and the application of injections should not be left to other laymen or paramedics in the villages, but have to be at least supervised by those professionals who are ex officio responsible for this task. Ideal health-seeking behavior of villagers has shown that they are willing to increase their use of biomedical services on condition that biomedical interventions are safe and that professional service is reliable. In the case of the three Minahasa villages, however, this has failed to be the case!

"Traditional" concepts of health and illness are not major barriers to the use of global professional medical practices. Conversely, "modern" thinking does not exclusively lead to a therapy choice in the professional health sector. Worldwide medical pluralism makes health and illness behavior a multilayered phenomenon where different cultural, system, and user factors play an important role. Global behavioral determinants such as time, money, distance, and quality of care have an increasingly strong influence on health- and illness-related behavior. Health professionals have to become more aware of the meaning of these aforementioned criteria. In a globalized world where "traditional" is more an etic construction for "the other," "the alien," and "the old-fashioned," the social sciences have a responsibility to take part in the "game of transformation" not as a neutral referee, but as an active field player.

Notes

I am much indebted to Lenore Manderson for revising and commenting on this chapter. During a visit to Brisbane in 1998, she strongly encouraged me to turn my attention to local perspectives of global processes. Brigit Obrist van Eeuwijk and John Litaridis have supported me to improve the quality of this chapter.

1. Giddens (1991:2–3) speaks of "high" or "late" modernity instead of postmodernism, because we experience the direct consequences of modernity, for example, through reorganization of time and space and disembedding mechanisms in social relations. On this issue see also Giddens (1990). On Giddens's theory of modernization and Robertson's contra-concept, see, for instance, Waters (1995: 38–53).

2. Geertz (1996:71) concludes: "Je mehr die Dinge zusammenruecken, desto mehr bleiben sie getrennt" [The more things move together, the more they are divided].

3. This catch phrase is frequently used in the discourse of, for instance, politics, ecology, and economy. Environmentalists investigating global warming, politicians shaping the European Union and introducing the "Euro" currency, and activists of nongovernmental organizations (NGOs) claiming human right violations underline their actions with this slogan.

4. "Globalization . . . refers to social, economic, cultural, and demographic processes that take place within nations but also transcend them, such that attention limited to local processes, identities, and units of analysis yields incomplete understandings of the local" (Kearney 1995:548).

5. I am well aware that the construction of cultural identity can be misinterpreted and/or deliberately misused for certain claims of power. Ex-Yugoslavia (e.g., Bosnia-Herzegovina and Kosovo) and Rwanda are tragic cases in point. On the other hand, identity building can reinforce cultural differentiation, which also leads to a clash of interests, as experienced in East Timor and Irian Jaya (Indonesia) as well as in Chiapas (Mexico).

6. Featherstone and Lash (1995:4) describe Robertson's term of "glocalization" as "a global creation of locality."

7. Nederveen Pieterse (1995:45) views "globalization as a process of hybridization which gives rise to a global mélange." For a critical discussion of the

interlocking of global and local culture leading to difference as well as to similarity, see Nederveen Pieterse (1994).

8. Beck (1997:90) argues: "Das Lokale und Globale . . . schliessen sich nicht aus. Im Gegenteil: Das Lokale muss als Aspekt des Globalen verstanden werden" [The local and the global . . . do not exclude each other. On the contrary: the local must be seen as an aspect of the global].

9. The connection between dominance and power of biomedicine in medical systems is well described, for example, by Lindenbaum and Lock (1993). On legal aspects in medical pluralism, see, for instance, Stepan (1983). Boomgard and colleagues (1996) give an accurate historical analysis of colonial power, political economy, and biomedical supremacy on Java in the Netherlands Indies (Indonesia). For an excellent description of colonial medical reality and state power in British Malaya, see Manderson (1996).

10. On these issues in critical medical anthropology, see, for example, Turshen (1977), Singer (1990), and Scheper-Hughes (1992).

11. Lock (1988:44) defines "medicalization" as follows: "[T]he medical community attempts to create a 'market' for its services by redefining certain events, behaviors, and problems as disease."

12. Keane (1998) has classified "world health" into four ideal images; accordingly, the dominant perspective of the WHO considers the nation-state the principal agent of world health.

13. For critical comments see, for example, Stone (1986), Jordan (1989), and Pigg (1995).

14. These inseparable and interrelated "Five Principles" are (1) Belief in the One and Only God, (2) Just and Civilized Humanity, (3) The Unity of Indonesia, (4) Democracy Guided by the Inner Wisdom in the Unanimity Arising Out of Deliberations Among Representatives, and (5) Social Justice for the Whole of the People of Indonesia.

15. The entire volume (1998, 154 [2]) of *Bijdragen tot de Taal-, Land- en Volkenkunde* is dedicated to the topic "Globalization, Localization and Indonesia" (edited by J. M. Nas).

16. On Indonesian indigenous people and their worldwide links, see Persoon (1998); on environmental protection and nongovernmental organizations (NGOs) in Indonesia, see Colombijn (1998). The case of U.S.-based PT Freeport Indonesia (copper and gold mining) in Irian Jaya (e.g., human rights violations and environmental destruction) has won worldwide attention because several national and international NGOs took the Indonesian government and the company to court and launched a wide "bad image" campaign against Freeport.

17. The ten Megatrends 2000 comprise (1) the booming global economy of the 1990s; (2) a renaissance in the arts; (3) the emergence of free-market socialism; (4) global lifestyles and cultural nationalism; (5) the privatization of the welfare state; (6) the rise of the Pacific Rim; (7) the decade of women in leadership; (8) the age of biology; (9) the religious revival of the new millennium; and (10) the triumph of the individual. See Naisbitt and Aburdene (1990:xi).

18. The lifestyle of Minahasa people was by no means always American oriented. Before Independence (1945), villagers gained prestige via their ability to adopt Dutch cultural values (e.g., dances, songs, clothes, language, food, and church activities). During the Japanese occupation (1942–1945), a Japanese-like lifestyle (e.g., discipline, clothes) was held in high esteem. After independence, national Indonesian values covered the emerging prestigious American lifestyle, whereas the latter influenced people's trendy behavior in the 1960s (e.g., music,

clothes). In the 1970s and 1980s, the possession and use of Japanese goods (e.g., radios, TVs, cameras, telephones, cars) was highly esteemed. The 1990s saw again the rise and (very often) the imitation of an American lifestyle, strongly influenced by Javanese, mostly urban values (e.g., *dangdut* disco music, Javanese fast food, trendy *batik* ties, hand phones in protective covers made of *ikat* textile). Schouten (1998:231–233) has explored these changes by examining first names of different Minahasa generations.

19. In my fieldwork villages, this fact was brought home by the national TV evening news *(Dunia dalam Berita)*. The villagers could regularly watch the highlights of pretentious opening ceremonies of crucial production plants and listen to the inaugural address of proud (former) President Suharto. Prestigious symbols of new industrialized Indonesia are, for instance, petrochemical plants, a national automotive and aircraft industry, and glass, plastic, and cement manufacturing plants. These industries emphasize the newly gained independence of Indonesia from foreign import products, and they stress the high level of existing professional know-how.

20. The (democratic) constitution of the Republic of Indonesia is strongly inspired by the age-old Indonesian cultural concepts of *gotong royong* (mutual assistance), *musyawarah* (deliberation), and *mufakat* (consensus). Indonesian rulers consider Western-style democracy such as voting by ballot and, as its result, majority-minority proportions to be unjust, discriminatory, easily manipulated, and inappropriate to Indonesian sociopolitical culture. Mythologies such as the Javanese myth of *Ratu Adil* (the Just Prince or Princess) are used as a means to legitimize and maintain the present rulers' supremacy. In this context, criticism of the Indonesian government's respect for democracy and human rights are interpreted as "anti-Indonesian," imported ideas that challenge local culture and history. For a critical discourse on culture, democracy, human rights, and political freedom in Indonesia, see, for instance, Retboll (1998) and Amnesty International (1994).

21. Generally, the government's New Order policy (1966–1998) was marked by depoliticization of public life, anti-Communism and nonalignment, state secularism, industrialization and diversification of raw material exploitation, planned economy, state paternalism, the rulers' oligarchic behavior, and cronyism, as well as a high degree of organization (of the society) with distinct social structuring (from above to below). See Vatikiotis (1993), Cribb and Brown (1995), and on the "New Order" period in Minahasa, Schouten (1998).

22. In early 1997, the financial crisis, the subsequent drop in production in Indonesia, a sharp increase in living costs, and inflation led to the dismissal without notice of hundreds of thousands of workers. These mostly young women worked in factories (to a great extent on Java), which produced cheap export goods such as toys, T-shirts, or computer bodies. The working conditions were bad, with poor pay, few benefits, and no union representation. Most Javanese people consider themselves direct victims of global economic processes.

23. For example, life expectancy at birth (both sexes) is sixty-five years (1997), the infant mortality rate (per one thousand live births) is 49 (1997), and the adult literacy rate is 83.8 percent (1995). See WHO (1998).

24. The present economic and financial crisis in Indonesia will lead to a very sharp decline of these wages and the per capita income in 1998.

25. For instance, I have tried to explain (to some peasants) the long way of complex connections between global stock market decisions made in New York and the very low price of clove and copra the peasants finally get from their local cooperative or Chinese intermediate traders. It was a difficult task—and without fully convincing those affected by this misery! Somehow the peasants instinctively felt

that there are always winners ("the others") and losers ("we") in this playing field. See Backhaus (1996) with his attempt to demonstrate the complex relationship between global consumer markets and local Balinese seaweed, sea salt, and shrimp producers.

26. Some villagers put in concrete terms the destination to be reached: the next bigger city! I conclude from it that they consider cities as already globalized spots or at least as the place from where this process will start or be launched.

27. See van der Geest (1987) and Nichter and Vuckovic (1994), and Chapter 6 on Uganda and Chapter 5 on Vietnam.

28. See, for example, van Staa and Hardon (1996) and Hardon and van Staa (1997).

References

Amnesty International, ed. 1994. *Indonesien und Osttimor: Kein Paradies fuer Menschenrechte.* Bonn: Amnesty International.
Backhaus, N. 1996. *Globalisierung, Entwicklung und Traditionelle Gesellschaft: Chancen und Einschraenkungen bei der Nutzung von Meeresressourcen auf Bali/Indonesien.* Muenster: Lit Verlag.
Beck, U. 1997. *Was Ist Globalisierung? Irrtuemer des Globalismus—Antworten auf Globalisierung.* Frankfurt am Main: Suhrkamp.
Berger, P., and T. Luckmann. 1989. *The Social Construction of Reality: A Treatise in the Sociology of Knowledge.* New York: Anchor Books.
Boomgard, P., R. Sciortino, and I. Smyth, eds. 1996. *Health Care in Java: Past and Present.* Leiden: KITLV Press.
Colombijn, F. 1998. "Global and Local Perspectives on Indonesia's Environmental Problems and the Role of NGOs," *Bijdragen tot de Taal-, Land- en Volkenkunde* 154(2): 305–334.
Coreil, J., A. Augustin, N. A. Halsey, and E. Holt. 1994. "Social and Psychological Costs of Preventive Child Health Services in Haiti," *Social Science and Medicine* 38(2): 231–238.
Cribb, R, and C. Brown. 1995. *Modern Indonesia: A History Since 1945.* London and New York: Longman.
Featherstone, M., and S. Lash. 1995. "Globalization, Modernity and the Spatialization of Social Theory: An Introduction." In *Global Modernities,* M. Featherstone, S. Lash, and R. Robertson, eds. London: Sage.
Geertz, C. 1995. *After the Fact: Two Countries, Four Decades, One Anthropologist.* Cambridge, MA: Harvard University Press.
———. 1996. *Welt in Stuecken: Kultur und Politik am Ende des 20. Jahrhunderts.* Wien: Passagen-Verlag.
Giddens, A. 1990. *The Consequences of Modernity.* Cambridge: Polity Press.
———. 1991. *Modernity and Self-Identity: Self and Society in the Late Modern Age.* Cambridge: Polity Press.
Hardon, A., and A. van Staa. 1997. "Suntik, Ya? Investigating Popular Demand for Injections in Indonesia and Uganda," *Essential Drug Monitor* (WHO) 23: 15–16.
Jordan, B. 1989. "Cosmopolitical Obstetrics: Some Insights from the Training of Traditional Midwives," *Social Science and Medicine* 28(9): 925–944.
Keane, C. 1998. "Globality and Constructions of World Health," *Medical Anthropology Quarterly* 12(2): 226–240.

Kearney, M. 1995. "The Local and the Global: The Anthropology of Globalization and Transnationalism," *Annual Reviews in Anthropology* 24: 547–565.

Kleinman, A. 1980. *Patients and Healers in the Context of Culture: An Exploration of the Borderland Between Anthropology, Medicine, and Psychiatry.* Berkeley: University of California Press.

Lindenbaum, S., and M. Lock, eds. 1993. *Knowledge, Power, and Practice: The Anthropology of Medicine and Everyday Life.* Berkeley: University of California Press.

Lock, M. 1988. "New Japanese Mythologies: Faltering Discipline and the Ailing Housewife," *American Ethnologist* 15(1): 43–61.

Long, N. 1996. "Globalization and Localization: New Challenges to Rural Research." In *The Future of Anthropological Knowledge,* H. L. Moore, ed. London: Routledge.

Manderson, L. 1996. *Sickness and the State: Health and Illness in Colonial Malaya, 1870–1940.* Cambridge, England: Cambridge University Press.

Naisbitt, J. 1994. *Global Paradox: The Bigger the World Economy, the More Powerful Its Smallest Players.* London: Nicholas Brealey.

———. 1996. *Megatrends Asia: The Eight Asian Megatrends That Are Changing the World.* London: Nicholas Brealey.

Naisbitt, J., and P. Aburdene. 1990. *Megatrends 2000: Ten New Directions for the 1990s.* New York: von Books.

Nederveen Pieterse, J. P. 1994. "Globalisation as Hybridisation," *International Sociology* 9(2): 161–184.

———. 1995. "Globalization as Hybridization." In *Global Modernities,* M. Featherstone, S. Lash, and R. Robertson, eds. London: Sage.

Nichter, M., and N. Vuckovic. 1994. "Agenda for an Anthropology of Pharmaceutical Practice," *Social Science and Medicine* 39(11): 1509–1525.

Persoon, G. 1998. "Isolated Groups or Indigenous People: Indonesia and the International Discourse," *Bijdragen tot de Taal-, Land- en Volkenkunde* 154(2): 281–304.

Pigg, S. L. 1995. "Acronyms and Effacement: Traditional Medical Practitioners (TMP) in International Health Development," *Social Science and Medicine* 41(1): 47–68.

Retboll, T., ed. 1998. *East Timor: Occupation and Resistance.* Copenhagen: IWGIA.

Robertson, R. 1995. "Globalization: Time-Space and Homogeneity-Heterogeneity." In *Global Modernities,* M. Featherstone, S. Lash, and R. Robertson, eds. London: Sage.

Schefold, R. 1998. "The Domestication of Culture. Nation-Building and Ethnic Diversity in Indonesia," *Bijdragen tot de Taal-, Land- en Volkenkunde* 154(2): 259–280.

Scheper-Hughes, N. 1992. *Death Without Weeping: The Violence of Everyday Life in Brazil.* Berkeley: University of California Press.

Schouten, M. J. C. 1998. *Leadership and Social Mobility in a Southeast Asian Society: Minahasa, 1677–1983.* Leiden: KITLV Press.

Sillitoe, P. 1998. "What, Know Natives? Local Knowledge in Development," *Social Anthropology* 6(2): 203–220.

Singer, M. 1990. "Reinventing Medical Anthropology: Toward a Critical Realignment," *Social Science and Medicine* 30(2): 179–187.

Stepan, J. 1983. "Patterns of Legislation Concerning Traditional Medicine." In *Traditional Medicine and Health Care Coverage: A Reader for Health Administrators and Practitioners,* R. H. Bannerman, J. Burton, and C. Wen-Chieh, eds. Geneva: World Health Organization.

Stone, L. 1986. "Primary Health Care for Whom? Village Perspectives from Nepal," *Social Science and Medicine* 22(3): 293–302.
Sunanda, S. 1996. *Growth Centres in South East Asia in the Era of Globalization.* Geneva: UNCTAD.
Turshen, M. 1977. "The Political Ecology of Disease," *Review of Radical Political Economics* 9: 45–60.
van der Geest, S. 1987. "Pharmaceuticals in the Third World: The Local Perspective," *Social Science and Medicine* 25(3): 273–276.
van Staa, A., and A. Hardon. 1996. *Injection Practices in the Developing World. A Comparative Review of Field Studies in Uganda and Indonesia.* Geneva: World Health Organization.
Vatikiotis, M. R. J. 1993. *Indonesian Politics Under Suharto: Order, Development and Pressure for Change.* London: Routledge.
Waters, M. 1995. *Globalization.* London: Routledge.
WHO (World Health Organization). 1998. *The World Health Report 1998: Life in the Twenty-first Century: A Vision for All.* Geneva: WHO.

PART 2

The Global Pharmacy

5

The King's Law Stops at the Village Gate: Local and Global Pharmacy Regulation in Vietnam

David Craig

I am chatting with two women at a pharmacy counter, a glass case loaded with stacks of different-colored capsules in foil slides, on the cluttered footpath of a Hanoi street. Both women are here to buy antibiotics: one mother's child has a cough, the other a sore throat. There are no prices displayed in the drug cabinet, nor is any written product information available. The seller seems eager to make a sale, pushing extra strips into one woman's hand, and making claims for the drug's foreign origins ("It's from France, so it's fast"). His finger taps one of many promotional stickers on the front of his drug cabinet, one advertising a brand of Cefotaxime Sodium, a third-generation cephalosporin, an antibiotic of last resort in Australia, where it is reserved for acute cases, including meningitis. The sticker, ingenuous, says the drug is "an antibiotic with the ability to kill strong germs."

One mother has just bought a slide of Ampicillin, which, like most antibiotics, is readily available over the counter. She already knew the brand and the price and the dosage, and the fact that this particular brand and antibiotic type was the one that her youngest child's body was already "familiar" with, and that therefore would give fastest relief.

"I know the right dose, I know it already," she said. "You have to know the right dose, and the child has to be familiar with the medicine."

"That's right," her friend said, "you have to know clearly. If it's not compatible, it hardly works, could even kill. My little girl always has Am-pi,[1] foreign Am-pi. If she takes inside [Vietnamese] Am-pi, it's not compatible."

"She's not familiar with it," her friend said.

The pharmacy from which she has bought the drugs is one of dozens side by side along one of the many streets of private pharmacies that have sprung up during the last ten years of free market reforms (*doi moi*) and deregulation in Vietnam. Despite the array of choice, both women regularly return to this same shop front, where they are certain they can get the particular brands with which they are familiar, and where they are known by the sales staff and thus get a preferential price—and, they hope, quality drugs, not fakes. The sales staff there are not trained pharmacists, and the women have not much trust in commercially driven advice. Rather, they base purchases on knowledge gleaned from doctors and reputed drug authorities whom they consulted the first few times their child got this kind of illness. In this way, they have memorized, in a mnemonic way not far removed from the way they learned traditional remedies, the name, broad indications, and dosage for a dozen different kinds of antibiotics.

In this risky, deregulated environment of fakes, drug-seller prescribing, and uncertain medical qualifications, women take on the responsibility for regulating their own families' drug consumption. In broader terms, the "rational use of drugs" in Vietnam might be said to be primarily regulated "bottom up," by family caregivers who base their decisions on a patterned array of everyday cultural beliefs and practices, and on a formidable experience of getting the best from freewheeling traders of all kinds. This regulation is fairly exacting, with careful attention paid both to notions of correctness of dose, and "other," less biomedically rational concerns with "compatibility" and "familiarity," the "regulating" and "harmonizing" of bodies, power, and spaces (Craig 1997). It is patterned yet idiosyncratic, by no means always safe or biomedically effective. Obviously, most of this local regulation happens well beyond the institutional and ideological reach of global and even national approaches to "rational" drug use.

This chapter describes some of the contest between the local and the global for regulatory dominance in the everyday consumption of drugs. Here, I describe the basic scope and parameters of this contest: the uneasy passage that globalizing regulatory modes have had into national policy in Vietnam, the blunting of reform through the resistance of existing national regulatory modes, the ways in which the global "King's law" fails to get past the local "village gate."[2] I underscore the differences and similarities between a globalizing consumer-oriented regulation, and the local regulatory practices of mothers in Vietnamese households. Finally, I raise the current possibility of a convergence between local and global kinds of regulation, and map some of the obstacles in its way.

Level Playing Fields?
Rationality, Subjectivity, and Government

Like the industry it pursues, the regulation of pharmacy has become a global business. The field is highly contested, fought over by competing interests (nation-states, health care professionals, multinational pharmacy companies, consumers) (see Chapter 6). Vast sums of money are at stake, and there are clear cases of market failure to deliver socially optimal outcomes. The battle lines have traditionally been drawn between governments, UN multilaterals, NGOs, and consumers on one side, and the industry on the other (Chetley 1990; Silverman et al. 1992; World Health Organization Action Programme on Essential Drugs 1995; Zwi and Mills 1995).

But the phenomenon of globalization in pharmacy regulation enfolds within itself some intriguing contradictions, which this simple conflict model tends to obscure, and which I want to pursue here. First, consumers and regulators are by no means easy allies. The flat universality of drug rationalities (the notion that there is one correct, rational way for drugs to be taken anywhere in the world) is usually at considerable odds with lumpy local cultural formations. And, though numerous studies of cultural "idiosyncrasies" of drug use exist (Van der Geest and Whyte 1988; Hardon 1992; Craig 1997), in general international drug regulators have been at a practical loss as to what should be done with them. They are often dismissed as "descriptive," as useful in understanding problem cases and irrationality, as pointing generally toward needs for education and regulation. The notion that local practice might in itself be seen as regulatory, and as a point to begin from when working toward rational drug use, has not in general attracted project funding or practical support from major international players.

Second, modes of regulation being promoted globally are at considerable odds with national and local political and medical regulatory forms. Gradually, international drug regulatory modes are shifting, like broader regulatory frameworks, toward more market-oriented positions, which seek to incorporate the self-regulatory powers of consumers and enhance these through greater surveillance and dissemination of product information. This regulatory approach, as we will see, carries a number of crucial assumptions about the position of the people it regulates, its regulatory subjects. In particular, it aims to regulate consumers in a way that is deeply at odds with traditional, authoritarian modes of regulation, of the kind found in both socialist Vietnam and hierarchical medical practice.

Globalization, however, is about flattening out barriers. Between markets and consumers, local, national, and global regulators, a new rapprochement may be possible, based on the rescoping of regulation to capture more of the range of slippery local subjectivity. Its eventuality, however, would depend on continuing shifts in the nature of local subjectivity and government. It would require a certain surrender of personal and national sovereignty, the creation of a level playing field of subjectivity and nationality. In Vietnam, the terrains for resistance here are considerable.

The King's Law?
Emerging Modes of Regulation and Government

In the last twenty years, modes of government in many "developed" countries have been refocused around a broad consensus that an effective market is central to economic welfare. The economic, social, and environmental optimization of the market has emerged as the state's major role, along with the broad-based marshaling of the regulatory potential of all the players involved. The changing, mobile market had to be "managed" through "responsive regulation" and "consumer empowerment," if it was to provide optimal outcomes (Ayres and Braithwaite 1992).

The period, however, is widely remembered for its move away from regulation. In the sociology of health and illness, deregulation has occupied the imagination of analysts to the extent that the current era is characterized as "postmodern, deregulated and risky" (Turner 1997:xvii). The post-1980s Vietnamese drug marketplace certainly demonstrates all the elements of a globally decentered, risky environment, having become a place where individuals need to become "self-regulating and self-forming" (Turner 1997:xxi). But in fact, globally, the 1980s witnessed little net reduction in regulatory frameworks (Ayres and Braithwaite 1992). Rather, a different kind of regulation emerged, attuned to governing the activities of private sector agencies and private individuals in what were previously public sector domains (Boston et al. 1991). These modes of government have been generous in their definition of "regulation," and far reaching in the aspects of local subjectivity they can appropriate. In these modes, "sound policy analysis is about understanding private regulation—by industry associations, by firms, by peers, and by individual consciences—and how it is interdependent with state regulation" (Ayres and Braithwaite 1992:3).

Following Foucault, it is possible to see this development and incorporation of self-regulatory mechanisms as representing a fundamental shift in the practice and discourse of "governmentality": a shift, that is, away from the concept of the state as the central and sovereign lawmaker and enforcer, toward modes of government that rely on rational and organizational forms at some remove from the state (Rose and Miller 1992). These modes depend on the subjects actively participating, taking responsibility for their own actions, becoming self-regulating; they set out to equip the subjects for this role by providing a choice of services and the crucial information to allow them to make informed, rational decisions. By factoring in mobility and choice, devolving responsibility, and increasing surveillance through research, these modes produce cost-efficient subjects who can self-manage, yet whose deviances from norms can be followed closely and targeted specifically (Gordon 1987, 1991; Lupton 1995).

Globalizing Governmental Modes

The export of these modes of regulation to developing countries is now proceeding quickly, especially under the influence of multilateral structural adjustment and decentralization programs (Akin 1987; Mills and Zwi 1995), and the World Bank's highly influential *Investing in Health: World Development Report 1993* (World Bank 1993).

To the extent that traveling governmental modes are localized, Rose and Miller suggest, local actors and issues "are assembled into mobile and loosely affiliated networks," and "particular and local issues . . . become tied to much larger ones" (1992:184). Traveling governmental modes thus open up local spaces and practices for redefinition in terms of global rationalities, by itinerant experts and consultants, and decentralized programs. This redefinition casts a new layer of extralocal governance across local and national boundaries, increasing the leverage of in-country programs through international legitimation. International governmental modes thus contest local authority, promoting its recasting in the terms of a global regime and hierarchy of authority. In this way, transnational governmental bodies, including UN agencies and aid and development organizations, are now reproducing neoliberal governmental modes on a global level, even within nation-states like Vietnam whose own governmental modes are not liberal at all (Escobar 1988; Hoggett 1991; Wunsch 1991; Atkinson and Coleman 1992; UNDP 1995).

The net effect, however, has often been the creation of contradictory subject positions for locals. At local and household levels, traveling governmental modes may or may not mediate real power, shape real practice, or subject real people: even in a globalized Vietnam, perhaps, "the king's law stops at the village gate" (cf. Popkin 1979:111). The success of traveling governmental modes depends on their ability to construct local practice, to distance it from local contingency. Rationalities don't arrive on any kind of cognitive or cultural tabula rasa: in the disparate localities to which governmental rationalities travel, they are variously revalued, reworked, hybridized, according to local interests and priorities. The more subtle governmental modes of self-determination, financial transparency, and education fall down in the local absence of the myriad invisible supporting elements of "civil society."

Emerging Global Governmental Modes in Pharmacy

Pharmaceutical consumers first entered the discourse of pharmacy as the unruly subjects of biomedical discipline. The problem of "achieving patient compliance" was viewed largely from the top down, in simple behavioral terms. Noncompliance in these terms becomes "a form of deviance requiring explanation" (Conrad 1985:30), and compliance the ideological expression of medical dominance (Trostle 1988). Compliance across all populations and drug regimens is low. Conrad's (1985) review of compliance literature has most studies showing that at least one-third of patients are noncompliant, whereas Sackett and Snow (1979) suggest around 50 percent.

Recent approaches to compliance have, however, begun to argue the need for "systematic efforts to incorporate the patient's perspective"(Maloney and Paul 1993:287; Roter 1995). Emerging discourses locate medical subjects as "consumers," with responsibility for making their own choices, within a framework of consumers' access to product information, and their legally established rights, protection, and redress. Above all, information—rational, informative, disseminated—is the mainspring of the new pharmaceutical governmentality (Davis 1997:137). The rationale, as elsewhere, is cost-effectiveness. The catch is that these approaches depend on shifting responsibility to the subjects, who thus become "ambulatory (self-)managers" of pharmaceuticals in the community, bearing a heavy weight of responsibility (Smith and Basara 1995:64).

Ironically, "relationship-centered medicine" thus promises to present planners with even better techniques of intervention and surveillance than old-style medical dominance and clinical methods, insofar as it is "a more effective method of establishing interpersonal rapport, gathering data, making diagnoses, educating and counselling patients and motivating patients to comply with medical recommendations than the biomedical model of medicine" (Roter 1995:39).

The Globalization of National Drug Policies

Global drug regulation has by no means fully embraced these new modes of governing pharmacy. In general, biomedical authority still casts "rational drug use" in simple compliance terms. There are, however, slowly emerging shifts in this position, and here I want to chart their tentative emergence into the wider world of global drug regulation.

The global governing of pharmacy comprises a number of international projects, supported by some powerful international health organizations: the International Federation of Pharmaceutical Manufacturing Associations (IFPMA); the World Health Organization (WHO); regulatory bodies in the European Union, the United States, and Japan;[3] the World Bank and other regional development banks; and multi- and bilateral donors. International networks of NGOs and drug consumer activists have had a voice.[4] In general, the drugs themselves have always traveled much more quickly and subtly than the regulatory (and clinical) rationalities and organizations that should accompany them. Although pharmaceutical companies have proved adept in adapting to local conditions, progress on international and national drug regulation has been highly uneven in recent years, despite being given unprecedented attention at all levels (Chowdhury 1995; Murray 1995; Boyd 1997; Tan 1997).

National Drug Policies (NDPs) have emerged as a central mechanism in a global regulatory push, promoted by the WHO, the European Union, and some bilateral donors (notably Sweden, Japan, and Australia). Essential Drugs Policies (EDPs) and later NDPs were formulated in some 130 countries, including Vietnam (twice). Both aimed principally to rationalize supply through generating essential drugs lists for import and public sector procurement, and quality control.

Local Subjects of Global Regulation

The WHO "Guidelines for Developing National Drug Policies" (World Health Organization 1988a) were revised in 1995, reflecting growing experience, but also the contradictory influence of new regulatory approaches to markets, subjects, and information (World Health Organization Action Programme on Essential Drugs 1995). The fine-tuning of regulatory mechanisms has seen an emerging emphasis on consumers, information, and rational drug use (cf. Davis 1997:137).[5] In the original 1988 WHO NDP guidelines, consumers invariably appeared last in any list of policy areas. In 1995 revisions, however, consumers (i.e., "patients") are given greater prominence, usually listed above the (private) drug industry, which now fills the place of limit and frontier. Rational Drug Use, with monitoring and evaluation, is now one of the essential policy components. Wide dissemination of drug information is now described as vital to rational use, and to regulating market efficiency through enhancing competition. In line with wider trends, the new frame relies on shifting responsibility to local subjects themselves, who thus become informed decisionmakers. So in the interstices of global regulation, the first signs of a global pharmaceutical subject are beginning to emerge. One senses a hope within the discourse that this "autonomous consumer," capable of being educated and forming pressure groups, might yet perform all the regulatory functions that governments have not been able to.

The Localization of NDPs

In the world of globalization with the threat from free market systems, the Vietnamese are facing a much more difficult war—a war against invisible threats. The weapons for this war are not physical armaments; instead, Vietnam must develop new invisible weapons through new ways of thinking. The main weapons to fight this war are policies, strategies, and implementation plans developed through the wisdom of group leadership. The leadership has already envisaged such an effort in the process of developing Vietnam's "National Drug Policy (Lalvani et al. 1997).

Despite the WHO exhortations to create NDPs that reflect local and national situations (see, e.g., Brudon 1997:67), international and global policy directions tend to dominate national drug policies, especially in developing countries.

Vietnam's National Drug Policy (VNDP) came about with high levels of instigation from Swedish International Development Assistance (SIDA), guidance from a high-powered international consultative group, and with leverage from the World Bank. The VNDP document, particularly in earlier drafts, reads as a hybrid of international drug regulatory framing concepts and local line ministry activities, interspersed with references to other Asian countries' policies, and reminders that Vietnam itself has actively, if not always successfully, regulated pharmacy.

As Vietnam's NDP process demonstrates, the particular modes of national and local government continue to play crucial roles in mediating between global regulation and local subjects. In Vietnam, existing official modes of governmentality—whether characterized as "bureaucratic socialism," "rump Stalinism," or "Confucian face—empty space"—tend to filter out or radically reformulate civil society notions such as popular participation, consumer rights, and tripartism. In the current order, new modes of governmentality must be applied to local subjects via the often hollow "formalism" of party politics (Porter 1991)—the hierarchical structures of line ministries, with their bureaucratic cultures and didactic styles of correct, top-down information. At the same time, within these bureaucracies they face the likelihood of being captured and deflected by the plural, personal fiefdoms and factions, networks, patron-client relations, and interest groups competing over scarce resources and influence (Fforde and Porter 1994).

Despite a growing pragmatism, the state remains badly positioned to cope with governing a market and legally empowering consumers. There has been ongoing reluctance to embrace officially the private business, and entrepreneurship, despite its legal status. At central levels, many top positions in line ministries continue to be occupied by older cadres from old schools. Their image of how the government should operate is dominated particularly by vertical programs through bureaucratic hierarchies, ministries, and the military, and whose policy reactions (and implementation of programs) are often restricted to short-lived clampdowns on the worst market symptoms, including television advertising of some types of drugs. At local and provincial levels, pragmatic expertise is offered limited scope for contributing to national debates. In a rapidly emerging free market, these mechanisms have been brushed aside or rendered practically useless.

The Local Politics of Drugs

Deregulation has left the local politics of drugs fractured into local, hospital, and provincial office-of-health fiefdoms, which are resistant to rationalization. Public sector procurement has fragmented, so that all levels, even down to the commune health station and its health workers, procure drugs direct from market suppliers. In each of these domains, there are financial and other rewards for maintaining personal and local control over procurement. At the national level, this situation has led to squabbles about essential drug lists between groups accusing each other of being in the drug companies' pockets. Not surprisingly, the quality of local drugs is a constant cause of concern for both consumers and clinicians. Borders are literally no barrier to cheap imports from the region, and there are endless rumors of fakes. Consumers are justifiably nervous.

Overlapping jurisdictions in Vietnam mean that individual departments and different levels of government regularly issue legislation that touch on and contradict other directives. In the case of drugs, in the Ministry of Health's own words, "Too many legal documents have been promulgated . . . some are outdated and no-one can tell whether they are still enforced or not, others are fragmented. . . . They are not approved by the highest legislative body, i.e. the National People's Assembly [sic]. Many regulations cannot be enforced due to weak enforcement structure and some strong cultural barrier" (Ministry of Health 1996b:12).

Despite the expressed hope that the NDP would remedy this situation, the finalized legislation remains very much a general charter for action and does little to reduce the regulatory burden borne by existing legislation, contained in some forty regulatory documents generated since 1975. Beyond this, the Vietnamese state faces many of the same difficulties as other developing countries seeking to implement an NDP: "internal and external pressures, the lack of resources, of a proper [sic] infrastructure and of the manpower required, weakness in the ministry of health, absence of management and planning ability" (World Health Organization 1988b, 106). The simple expense of an effective drug regulatory authority remains a major issue, in one of the world's poorer countries (Davis 1997:144).

Perhaps more significant, however, is the broader context in which the NDP has been enacted. Globally, drug regulation has come to depend increasingly on civil society: consumer activism, the threat of damages claims through the civil courts, often activated by an international consumer organization, with considerable media coverage and wide access to product information. Although there are nascent developments in all of these areas in Vietnam, civil law, the press, consumer organization and protection, and information have all long been bounded and constrained by state concerns over internal security, civil order, and sovereignty (Lu Phuong 1994; Marr 1994). The mechanisms that make regulation dependent on "consumer autonomy" work in other countries are simply not yet there in Vietnam.

On the other hand, the government has long lacked the resources to extend the sorts of health care, education, and public services that it would have wished to. Here, the state's dependency on the family to look after its own has been a constant strain in policy and rhetoric. User charges for health, and the promotion of traditional remedies at the household level, are examples drawn from two different periods of crippling state poverty (Nhan Dan 1977). Now, as in China, the state appears to be more and more overtly supporting traditional family values, as a reliable, conservative basis for political stability. Families in Vietnam have long been just the sort of autonomous, self-regulating subjects that emerging market-oriented governmental modes depend on.

The NDP Legislation and Implementation

Local input into framing the NDP came from nine large working groups, whose membership was primarily drawn from higher levels of health bureaucracy and clinical services. The meetings of these groups, some of which I was able to attend, proceeded with due deference to scientific and clinical "correctness," formal learning, and status, whereas members I spoke to expressed universally low assessments of the state and potential of popular knowledge.

The NDP's two aims are (a) to ensure a sufficient supply of good quality drugs to the people; and (b) to ensure rational, safe, and efficacious use of drugs (Ministry of Health 1996a). The nine objectives that follow reflect both mainstream essential drug policy concerns, and a socialist commitment to equity of access. The desire to maximize national self-sufficiency, build human resources, and bring the market into line; the "special importance" of traditional medicine; and current fears about drug safety are all written into the text in various ways.

Consumers and rational use of drugs receive uneven treatment in the document and in the accompanying "Masterplan for Implementation" (Ministry of Health 1996b), reflecting bureaucratic and funding agendas on the part of implementing institutions. Although the second aim is explicit about rational drug use, there is no mention of it in the objectives of the final document. Neither aim—nor any of the objectives—mentions consumer education, and despite one of the nine core sections of both the VNDP and its masterplan being given over to drug information, only one of the seventy-five proposed activities focuses directly on consumers. The international advisers have, however, been emphatic about the need to strengthen public information on rational use of drugs, suggesting establishment of "a separate working group to support a separate section of the Masterplan devoted to public education" as a way through the troubled internal politics.

Private sector pharmacies, where by far the bulk of Vietnam's drugs are sold, are promised better access to information. But policy objectives to "raise the effectiveness of state management over the pharmaceutical sector," to "restructure the pharmaceutical sector to make it fit the new mechanism," and to "improve the technical knowledge and professional ethics of pharmaceutical personnel" are supported by very few activities focused on existing private pharmacies, beyond information and education. Private and quasi-private public sector drug prescribers will continue to have considerable autonomy at the point of sale, and, because of the revenues they generate, will continue to influence and even capture regulatory authorities at the local and clinical level. Mechanisms whereby consumers' complaints about private and public sector pharmacy practice can be turned into effective regulatory enforcement are unchanged and remain dependent on local enforcement.

The Village Gate: Orders of Local Knowledge and Practice

Like all globalizing rationalities, the "King's Law" of pharmacy regulation has run into difficulties on entering the local domains inside the "village gate." The regulation has had to negotiate and sometimes compete with dense, complex political and cultural fields, which are in many ways designed—at both national and local levels—to resist externally imposed governmental modes, and to appropriate only what they can practically use for local control.

I have suggested, however, that local knowledge and practice in drug use is a form of self-regulation, attuned to local and personal situations. Here, I want to give the reader some sense of the nature of this knowledge and practice in northern Vietnam. I aim to show both the distinctive characteristics of household drug practices and how this mode of everyday regulation converges with and diverges from global modes. What follows, however, is necessarily only a brief summary, drawn from my own ethnographic fieldwork, over some eighteen months in 1995–1996 (Craig 1997).

It is crucial that the qualitative differences between popular and institutional regulation of drugs be mapped out. Popular regulation, for example, happens within local settings, and within the scope of primarily oral culture. The popular discourse on pharmaceuticals in Vietnam is a kind of open-ended discussion, a debate between self-cultivating, autodidactic men over a low coffee table, or between worried women standing on a footpath beside a market. It is a discussion whose primary aim is the giving and getting of good information, the sorting out of the best from an unstable, confusing situation, the establishment of whatever kinds of certainty are available. It is a discussion in which everyone's experience counts for something, where doctors' and pharmacists' opinions are traded off against each other, and where trust and information ebb and flow around relations of personal familiarity and intimacy, personal introduction and recommendation. Which medicine is best for what, which one suits this child or that child, which one is light and which is heavy, what the comparative advantages are of "inside" (*nôi*: domestic) and "outside" (*ngoai*: foreign) medicines, this doctor and that doctor, traditional healers and pharmacists, northern, southern, eastern, and western medicine.

A Mostly "Eastern Medicine" Metaphorical Framework

Popular Vietnamese knowledge and practice draw heavily on the core concepts and the root metaphors of Eastern Medicine (*Dông Y*), which until very recently in Vietnam was the most widely available and reliable form of medicine.

It is not going too far to describe traditional "Eastern" medicine as a system of bodily self-regulation, where maintaining the stability and strength of internal bodily systems is the main concern. This stability and strength are popularly conceived as the body's best defense against the vagaries and changes of the external environment (heat, cold, wind, dampness, dryness). This regulation operates in terms of a series of core, closely related binary constructions: environmental, medical, nutritional; other factors inside (*nôi*) or outside (*ngoai*) the body tend to be either harmful (*dôc*) or nutritious (*bô*), alien (*di*), or familiar (*quen*) and compatible (*hop*). These concepts tend to be broad and are applied polythetically to new situations or objects (e.g., in antibiotics being classified as hot). The breadth and flexibility of these conceptions enhance the scope of family caregivers' control and offer some kind of certainty and rubric for action in most situations.

This popular regulation is tightly bound with the regular rhythms and resources of everyday life. Preparing and watching the children's diet and their general thermal state, keeping them out of the way of harmful winds and medicines—these are the day-to-day activities of family life. In Vietnam as elsewhere, all of these core concepts and concerns, and the bodily practices associated with them, are closely related to wider social and cultural formations of bodily self-regulation, covering diet, exercise, sexuality, emotion, place in the family, and place in wider hierarchies of age, learning, and position. Whereas Western and other medical traditions (germ theory, antibiotics) have been accreted onto these basic understandings, it is still fair to say that for most Vietnamese, these kinds of concepts and practices are still at the heart of everyday life and health.

Together, these concepts tend to be applied in ways that balance regulatory notions of social correctness and order with those of personal compatibility and situational specificity. The balance between two moments of regulation is neatly captured in the two preeminent Vietnamese terms for medical regulation: *dieu chính* (to correct), and *dieu hoà* (to harmonize). Hence the concern often heard in Vietnamese families, both to apply the correct dose, and at the same time to give medicine that is individually compatible with a particular person. Hence also the almost universal concern to balance the harmful and hot properties of antibiotics with the perceived cooling ones of vitamin C, and the digestive strengthening ones of vitamin B.

Uneven Structures of Medical Authority and Household Practice

Crucially, however, Eastern medicine has provided no systemic clinical authority, and no monopoly over the prescription and sale of medicines. Traditional medicine, like today's "Western" medicine, offered scattered, variously reliable points of resort: Someone you know, for example, might know of and recommend a particular recipe, or might recommend a healer in a particular part of town or the country, whose family-guarded remedies would be said to heal a range of related (and sometimes unrelated) conditions. "If you know a medicine (or a doctor), then please recommend it," the popular saying goes. People take pride in having "passed on," "recommended," or "introduced" remedies or healers to neighbors and families. This geographical and personal unevenness of medical authority has persisted through into today's Westernized medical and pharmaceutical system, and as we have seen, people cope with its unregulated vagaries and establish their own certainties in the same ways.

The result is a high degree of local variation, within broad themes. Thus, for example, while "beating wind" (*danh gió*) to expel harmful influences and restore internal order is practiced throughout Vietnam, techniques vary widely, even between next-door neighbors. One will use a bottle top and a "wind oil," another ginger, urine, and a crumpled hair, another an egg white and a silver ring to achieve the same ends. In the case of many herbal remedies, the variations are related to local and seasonal availability of various herbal ingredients. Many mothers know a number of variations on a single herbal recipe and are thus able to act to cool, warm, or expel wind or excess water wherever and whenever the need arises.

Unevenness and Hybridity, Attuned to Locality

Unevenness and difference, then, are written into household knowledge and practice. This has a practical, controlling basis and effect. The differences accrue along lines of practical experience, or according to practical logics of association. Vitamin C, for example, is popularly seen as cooling because of its association with lemons and oranges. Vitamin C is used not just to balance the heat effects of antibiotics, but is, for example, also injected in solution intravenously by many Vietnamese women in summer, to prevent heat rash and boils. Drug taxonomy and rationalities often follow aesthetic logics of color, drawn from traditional medicine. These logics thus connect core concepts and practice in innovative ways—including metaphorical ones—to give popular medicine its polythesis, its epistemic slipperiness, and its empirical ability to improvise and create a kind of order and control in new and local situations where one or other remedy might not be available.

Viewed from the normalizing perspective of the high medical traditions, these practices might be called "hybridities," characterized by a "confusion of spheres" (Bourdieu 1985:110; Trinh Thi Minh Ha 1992; Bhabha 1994). Hybridity seems to be a basic dimension of popular household knowledge and practice, and one with crucial implications for the promotion of "rational drug use." Other popular Vietnamese hybridities include the popular reconciliation of germ theory with ideas of strength and weather. Heavy, humid weather, for example, is seen by many as ideal for the development and spread of germs, which are thought to be carried by steam. Vitamins are understood to be similar to traditional understandings of tonics and as such ascribed humoral qualities and relation to particular bodily systems, such as nerves (B6) and digestion (B1). Chloramphenicol tablets, prescribed by many for sore stomach and diarrhea, were used by some fishermen I talked with as a prophylactic against seasickness.

Again, however, these hybridizations all have a practical, regulatory dimension: they allow the accretion of new dimensions of effective medicine onto proven existing ones. For practical purposes, systematicity is nowhere near as important as overall and/or perceived effectiveness, and the return of the body to strength and control.

Mnemonic Rules of Thumb and Embodied Practice

Regulation at popular level is often realized by the rule of thumb. As oral traditions, popular knowledge tends toward the mnemonic, and therefore toward the formulaic, the rhythmic, the pithy structure of story (old wives' tales) and maxim (epithets and rules of thumb) (Ong 1982). In Vietnam, in the absence of an accessible, literate, authoritative medical practice at the local level, the oral tradition has survived strongly to the present day. These pieces of medical memory circulate in rhythmic herbal recipes and antibiotic dosages: "Take herb, pound it, strain it, take the juice, drink it, cures cough." Or "Ampicillin, take two pills, twice a day." The recipes are recited rhythmically, the elements often counted off against the joints of the little finger. Oral memories are prodigious: in my fieldwork, it was common to meet mothers who knew, with remarkable accuracy, the names, broad indications, and dosages for a dozen different antibiotics. These bits of knowledge are at least as much a part of the body's memory as the mind's, and accompany their user wherever she travels, always ready to hand.

Their form makes them highly transmittable, while their content gives them currency and reliability wherever health is a concern. In fieldwork, caregivers' recall of antibiotic doses was found to be remarkably accurate: for example, forty-five out of fifty-six mothers knew correct daily doses for ampicillin (Craig 1997). Again, it might be argued that by their very hybridic, mnemonic form, practical knowledge empowers household caregivers to regulate their own and their household's health. Popular medical concepts, both traditional and "Western," are graspable and operationalizable by caregivers, and applicable wherever the caregivers find themselves. They construct the caregiver as responsible, partly by locating the caregiver in relation to socially shared and normative practice, reinforced by family and neighborhood scrutiny, and a local medical hierarchy. They relate to locally available resources and seek to standardize these by repeated resort to the personally proved.

Familiarity, Personalization, and Authority

Oral, practical knowledge is not just technical knowledge, nor is it evaluated only by technical criteria. Rather, the abstract universally "correct" is held up against the authority of personal experience and is regulated by familiarity and emotion. Locally mediated through fairly intimate social relations, practical medical knowledge is affectively valued and located within the dense texture of sensibility provided by moral and aesthetic values of family, village, body, and mind. Traditional medicine, for example, has a positive affective value for many and is linked with concepts of identity, familiarity (*quen*), and compatibility (*hop*). For some, it is "our medicine" (*thuoc ta*), Eastern as opposed to Western medicine, appropriate, compatible; whereas Western medicine is harmful and hot, needing to be restricted. These affective valuations are weighed against other, technical considerations, but are still important for practice, "cultural safety," and placebo reasons.

Oral, practical knowledge travels within rather than outside the close confines of significant social relationships. Thus, it travels "up" into professional knowledges, very slowly, and travels best within the circle of the familiar, the known (*quen*): known people, recognized local authority, known source of medicine. Hence in Vietnam its association with the gerontocracy (*các cu*) (Ong 1982:41), and with traditions passed down from the old days (*co truyen*), including traditions of nationalism, and of defining insiders against outsiders. Hence again its role in social regulation, as it locates its knowers within a hierarchy that defines normality of a range of bodily practices and emotional states. A particular healer or even a Western medicine might be regarded as better than others on the basis of a personalized evaluation of its efficacy and familiarity (cf. Lepowsky 1990).

Are Local Knowledge and Practice Rational and Governmental?

Like global rational use of drugs, local knowledge and practice can be seen as an attempt to reconcile and regulate mind, body, and drug. Here, however, the location of the body is different: The body is not interpolated in a clinical setting, or within an epidemiological population, or a clean, rational space of public health and hygiene. Rather, it is in a local contingent place, environment—a family. In relation to drugs, it is a particular body, related to particular drugs, to familiar antibiotics. Popular knowledge and practice is specifically, locally, personally governmental, and therefore, in some important ways, not universally governmental. These personal and localized dimensions of popular knowledge and practice are crucial, in that they mean that there are basic ways in which popular knowledge and practice cannot be "scaled up" into a wider population, family, community, or national drug rationality. They limit the ways in which popular knowledge and practice can be retrieved for wider governmental and regulatory projects. They are the governmentality of a particular subject in a particular place at a particular time.

Symbiotic Rationality?

"The empirical foundation for analysis of what is good regulatory policy is acceptance of the inevitability of some sort of *symbiosis* between state regulation and self-regulation" (Ayres and Braithwaite 1992:3).

I have argued that local knowledge and practice, clinical biomedicine, and National Drug Policies are differently concerned with "regulation": all are, in different ways and forms, a regulation of the subject. These regulatory modes already exist in an unequal, de facto symbiosis, with each dominant in different situations. But could local and global orders of rationality and regulation be brought together, to make drug regulation a universal, level playing field for globally manageable subjects? If there are aspects in which local and personal health knowledge and practice cannot be scaled up, can other aspects of local subjectivity be retrieved for wider governmental projects?

The differences between the regulatory forms are starkly evident. Biomedical rationalities and the drug regulation they support are by definition global, locating control and stability in clinical dominance and exacting compliance to universal norms. Global drug rationality cannot surrender any part of its systemic order to local contingency and culture, without becoming internally contradictory. Unable to accrete, hybridize, or appropriate and build on local formations, it ends up dependent on centralized initiative to push its rationalities further out into local practice.

Popular Vietnamese bodily regulation, too, involves notions of correctness and order. But, as we have seen, it also works from an individualized, aestheticized, gendered, emotional regulation of the body, based on the preservation of inner integrity and harmony in a changing world that includes the spiritual. It is difficult to imagine how most of these vital aspects might be effectively subjected to national or international regulation.

The articulation of these different modalities of pharmaceutical rationality and regulation could perhaps be managed on the basis of recognition of the basic integrity and durability of each. However, as global pharmacy rationalities rush to establish "hard" rational forms, including global indicators, benchmarks, and algorithms, they become increasingly nonnegotiable by local and popular knowledge. Intervening regulatory mechanisms (National Drug Policies, local institutional biomedicine) appear less than agile in their ability to bring the two together. However, emerging modes of subjectivity and governmentality, supporting consumer autonomy with a populist approach to information, may constitute a ground on which some of these differences can be worked through. But in Vietnam, there are still many reasons these don't yet exist.

Where and How Local and Global Knowledge Might Be Able to Work Together

If local and global rationalities are to be symbiotic in Vietnam, they will have to be reconciled primarily at the household level, if only because household rationalities rarely travel much farther abroad. Local household rationalities and practice are in no position to grasp the totality of global rationalities. From their peripheral position, only partial, uneven, and hybridic appropriations (dosages, broad indications) are possible, and these are made according to the very different priorities (relational, aesthetic, humoral) of local culture.

If global rationalities are to travel into and articulate successfully with the modalities of local regulation and practice, they will need to take on a form that will travel locally as well, and as far as the drugs they regulate. Here they might learn something from the drugs themselves, whose form, packaging, and recognized value enable them to go into and be understood within domains of household practice. Perhaps global drug regulations need to become take-home, ready-to-hand rationalities, user friendly, family size, deliberately constructed to be appropriated by households and turned by them into practical regulatory action. They may need to mimic the modalities of existing household drug regulation, by taking on, for example, the simple formulaism of popular drug mnemonics, so that they can travel within local, oral-discursive formations. They will need to be scaled down, reordered, and repackaged into rules of thumb, maxims, polythetic concepts, simple binaries. They will need to become practical logics (Bourdieu 1990), operationizable by individuals at the household level, designed to be embodied, localized, to travel with traveling subjects.

If this can be done, drug rationalities will travel, in a simple, durable form, along with other medical knowledge, in conversations between mothers, and between mothers and daughters, in family conferences, in advice given by local and family medical authorities in oral situations. Evidence elsewhere (see, e.g., Craig 1995) suggests they may also travel well in the Vietnamese media, in thirty-second sound bites, and in the images and slogans consumers repeat when they go to the drugstore to buy medicine.

Can international drug rationalities be scaled down in this sort of way? It seems likely that lay diagnosis will continue to depend on overly broad indications, such as cough, sore throat, and combinations with fever. On the other hand, correct dosages travel fairly well in Vietnamese household medical culture. Local practical logic may not be able to be transformed into global, systemic logic, but it can transmit global rationalities, if in small, memorable pieces, and if robust enough to emerge intact from hybridizing, mix-and-match nosologies.

Will Vietnamese families emerge as the semiautonomous subjects of emerging pharmaceutical governmental modes? In a sense, global and national government machinations aside, they already have. In 1977, during a period of acute shortage of medical resources, a *Nhan Dan* columnist wrote that "on the basis of the existing pharmaceutical sources in the localities, and with the meticulous guidance of the public health cadres who continually care for their health, the people may easily become their own doctors and know how to prevent disease and promptly take medicine" (Nhan Dan 1977). Today a strong tradition of autodidacticism, transmission, and appropriation of knowledge in family health, clear notions of maternal responsibility to "know," and a widespread hunger for accurate drug knowledge continue to reinforce the contention that the family is the place to send drug information.

The reinvention, then, of the Vietnamese consumer as the globalized subject of universal drug rationalities is under way, ironically spurred by a lack of effectiveness in national regulatory mechanisms. Despite Vietnam's nominal adoption of a globally accepted National Drug Policy, household practices are likely to remain the dominant mode of drug regulation, forming a resistant local topography in the face of the globalizing will for a level playing field of rational drug use and drug regulation.

Notes

1. Ampicillin. Vietnamese mothers have shortened, two-syllable terms for most antibiotics, and these form a part of mnemonic formulae that help them remember correct dosages.

2. "Phép vua thua lê làng," a popular Vietnamese political saying, is literally translated "The king's law loses out to village custom," or, as reflected in the title of this chapter, "The king's law stops at the village gate."

3. These countries have worked together on the International Conference on Harmonization of Technical Requirements for Registration of Pharmaceuticals for Human Use, an ongoing, highly influential manufacturing standards setting body.

4. For example, the International Network for the Rational Use of Drugs (INRUD), Health Action Information Network (HAIN), and their regional and national associates.

5. The state sector accounts for only some 14 percent of all pharmaceutical expenditure, with some 83 percent coming from private pockets (Lalvani et al. 1997). Correspondingly, an estimated 80 percent of drug purchases are made through the private sector (Ministry of Health 1996b).

References

Akin, J. S. 1987. *Financing Health Services in Developing Countries: An Agenda for Reform.* Washington, DC: International Bank for Reconstruction and Development.

Atkinson, M. M., and W. D. Coleman. 1992. "Policy Networks, Policy Communities and the Problems of Governance," *Governance: An International Journal of Policy and Administration* 5(2): 154–180.

Ayres, I., and J. Braithwaite. 1992. *Responsive Regulation: Transcending the Deregulation Debate.* Oxford: Oxford University Press.

Bates, D., ed. 1995. *Knowledge and the Scholarly Medical Traditions.* Cambridge, England: Cambridge University Press.

Bhabha, H. 1994. *The Location of Culture.* London: Routledge.

Boston, J., J. Martin, June Pallot, and P. Walsh, eds. 1991. *Reshaping the State: New Zealand's Bureaucratic Revolution.* Auckland: Oxford University Press.

Bourdieu, P. 1985. *Outline of a Theory of Practice.* Cambridge, England: Cambridge University Press.
———. 1990. *The Logic of Practice.* Oxford: Polity Press.
Boyd, G. R. 1997. "Sustainable Pharmaceutical Expenditure," *Australian Prescriber* 20(supp. 1): 95–96.
Brudon, P. 1997. "Monitoring and Evaluating National Drug Policies: Where Are We Today?" *Australian Prescriber* 20(supp. 1): 67–69.
Chetley, A. 1990. *A Healthy Business? World Health and the Pharmaceutical Industry.* London: Zed Books.
Chowdhury, Z. 1995. *The Politics of Essential Drugs. The Makings of a Successful Health Strategy: Lessons from Bangladesh.* London: Zed Books.
Conrad, P. 1985. "The Meaning of Medications: Another Look at C Compliance," *Social Science and Medicine* 20(1): 29–37.
Craig, D. 1995. *Haiphong Health Financing for Primary Health Care Project: IEC Evaluation Report.* Hanoi: Save the Children Fund.
———. 1997. "Familiar Medicine: Local and Global Health and Development in Vietnam." In *Research School of Pacific and Asian Studies.* Unpublished Ph.D. diss. Canberra: Research School of Pacific and Asian Studies, Australian National University.
Davis, P. 1997. *Managing Medicines: Public Policy and Therapeutic Drugs.* Buckingham, UK: Open University Press.
Escobar, A. 1988. "Power and Visibility: Development and the Invention and Management of the Third World," *Cultural Anthropology* 3(4): 428–443.
Fforde, A., and D. Porter. 1994. "Public Goods, the State, Civil Society and Development." In *Assistance in Vietnam: Opportunities and Prospects. Doi Moi, The State and Civil Society: Vietnam Update 1994.* Canberra: Research School of Pacific and Asian Studies, Australian National University.
Gordon, C. 1987. "The Soul of the Citizen: Max Weber and Michel Foucault on Rationality and Government." In *Max Weber, Rationality and Modernity,* S. Lash and S. Whimster, eds. London: Allen and Unwin.
———. 1991. "Governmental Rationality: An Introduction." In *The Foucault Effect: Studies in Governmentality,* G. Burchell, C. Gordon, and P. Miller, eds. London: Harvester Wheatsheaf.
Hardon, A. P. 1992. "That Drug Is Hiyang for Me: Lay Perceptions of the Efficacy of Drugs in Manila, Philippines," *Central Issues in Anthropology* 10: 86.
Hoggett, P. 1991. "A New Management in the Public Sector?" *Policy and Politics* 19(4): 243–256.
Lalvani, P., M. Murray, et al. 1997. *Report of a Ministry of Health/WHO/SIDA Joint Mission for Development of a Masterplan for the National Drug Policy.* Hanoi: World Health Organization.
Lepowsky, M. 1990. "Sorcery and Penicillin: Treating Illness on a Papua New Guinea Island," *Social Science and Medicine* 30: 1049–1063.
Lu Phuong. 1994. *Civil Society: From Annulment to Restoration. Doi Moi, The State and Civil Society: Vietnam Update 1994.* Canberra: Research School of Pacific and Asian Studies, Australian National University.
Lupton, D. 1995. *The Imperative of Health: Public Health and the Regulated Body.* London: Sage.
Maloney, T., and B. Paul. 1993. "Rebuilding Public Trust and Confidence." In *Through the Patient's Eyes: Understanding and Promoting Patient-Centered Care,* M. Gerteis, S. Edman-Levitan, J. Daley, and T. Delbanco, eds. San Francisco: Jossey-Bass.

Marr, D. 1994. *The Vietnamese Communist Party and Civil Society. Doi Moi, The State and Civil Society; Vietnam Update 1994,* Canberra.

Mills, A., and A. B. Zwi. 1995. "Health Policy in Less Developed Countries: Past Trends and Future Directions," *Journal of International Development Special Issue: Health Policies in Developing Countries* 7(3): 299–328.

Ministry of Health. 1995. *National Drug Policy of Vietnam.* Hanoi: Ministry of Health.

———. 1996a. *Vietnam's National Drug Policy.* Hanoi: Ministry of Health.

———. 1996b. *Masterplan for Implementing Vietnam's National Drug Policy.* Hanoi: Ministry of Health.

Morris, L. S., and R. M. Shulz. 1991. "Patient Compliance: An Overview," *Journal of Clinical Pharmacy and Therapeutics* 17: 283–295.

Murray, M. 1995. "Australian National Drug Policies: Facilitating or Fragmenting Health?" *Development Dialogue* 1995(1): 148–192.

Nguyen Xuan Hung. 1997. "Improvement in Drug Procurement in the 'Renovation' (Doimoi) Period in Vietnam," *Australian Prescriber* 20(supp. 1): 86–87.

Nhan Dan. 1977. "Better Home Medical Care Urged." *Nhan Dan* (Hanoi), April 23, p. 1.

Ong, W. J. 1982. *Orality and Literacy: The Technologizing of the Word.* New York: Methuen New Accents.

Popkin, S. L. 1979. *The Rational Peasant: The Political Economy of Rural Society in Vietnam.* Berkeley: University of California Press.

Porter, G. 1991. *Vietnam: The Politics of Bureaucratic Socialism.* Ithaca: Cornell University Press.

Rose, N., and P. Miller. 1992. "Political Power Beyond the State: Problematics of Government," *British Journal of Sociology* 43(2): 173–205.

Roter, D. 1995. "Advancing the Physician's Contribution to Enhancing Compliance." In *Advancing Prescription Medicine Compliance: New Paradigms, New Practices,* J. E. Fincham, ed. New York: Haworth Press.

Sackett, D. L., and J. C. Snow. 1979. "The Magnitude of Compliance and Noncompliance." In *Compliance in Health Care,* R. B. Haynes, D. W. Taylor, and D. L. Sackett, eds. Baltimore: Johns Hopkins University Press.

Silverman, M., P. R. Lee, and M. Lydecker. 1992. *Bad Medicine: The Prescription Drug Industry and the Third World.* Stanford: Stanford University Press.

Smith, D. L., and L. R. Basara. 1995. "Advancing the Contribution of the Patient and the Caregiver to Prescription Medication Compliance." In *Advancing Prescription Medicine Compliance: New Paradigms, New Practices,* J. E. Fincham, ed. New York: Haworth.

Tan, J. G. 1997. "The Philippines National Drug Policy Programme: Reviewing a Nine Year Experience," *Australian Prescriber* 20(supp. 1): 41–45.

Trinh Thi Minh Ha. 1992. "From a Hybrid Place." In *Framer Framed.* New York: Routledge.

Trostle, J. A. 1988. "Medical Compliance as Ideology," *Social Science and Medicine* 27(12): 1299–1308.

Turner, B. S. 1997. "From Governmentality to Risk: Some Reflections on Foucault's Contribution to Medical Sociology." In *Foucault, Health and Medicine,* A. Petersen and R. Bunton, eds. London: Routledge.

UNDP (UN Development Programme. 1995. *Process Consultation: Systemic Improvement of Public Sector Management.* New York: UNDP Management Development Programme).

Van der Geest, S., and S. R. Whyte. 1988. "The Charm of Medicines: Metaphors and Metonyms," *Medical Anthropology Quarterly* 3(4): 345–367.

WHO (World Health Organization). 1988a. *Guidelines for Developing National Drug Policies.* Geneva: WHO.
———. 1988b. *The World Drug Situation.* Geneva: WHO.
World Bank. 1993. *Investing in Health: World Development Report, 1993.* Oxford: Oxford University Press.
World Health Organization Action Programme on Essential Drugs. 1995. *Report of the WHO Expert Committee on National Drug Policies.* Geneva: WHO.
Wunsch, J. S. 1991. "Institutional Analysis and Decentralization: Developing an Analytical Framework for Effective Third World Administrative Reform," *Public Administration and Development* 11(5): 431–451.
Zwi, A. B., and A. Mills. 1995. "Health Policy in Less Developed Countries: Past Trends and Future Directions," *Journal of International Development* 7(3): 299–328.

6

The Business of Medicines and the Politics of Knowledge in Uganda

Susan Reynolds Whyte and Harriet Birungi

The increasing and worldwide availability of medicines as commodities is one of the most striking health phenomena of our time. The lively sales and ready use of *materia medica* to solve health problems have led researchers to speak of the "commerciogenic" nature of health care (Ferguson 1988); the "commodification" and "pharmaceuticalization" of health (Nichter 1989); the commercialization of health care (Reeler 1996); and the "medicalization" of social, political, and personal problems (Zola 1972; Illich 1975; Scheper-Hughes 1992). The "drugging of the Third World" (Silverman et al. 1982) is recognized as an inundation.

Against this rising flood of medicinal commodities, international organizations, donors, and progressive forces in the corridors of health ministries are trying to construct meager dikes under the banner "Rational Use of Drugs." To this end the World Health Organization established the Drug Action Programme, which encourages member states to adopt essential drug policies. Efforts usually focus on national regulation of the types of drugs available, and on improving the knowledge and practice of health workers in the formal sector. But in most countries of Asia, Latin America, and Africa, pharmaceuticals are widely sold outside of government-recognized health units (Helling-Borda and Quick n.d.). Vendors peddle medicines in buses (Alubo 1985), pharmacists function like doctors K. Logan 1988), injectionists serve people at home (Birungi 1994a), and local provision shops stock medicines along with household supplies (Hardon 1991). To be effective, rational drug use initiatives would need to address the gap between formal, professionally formulated policies and the daily practices of businesses (small and large) and ordinary people striving for health.

The business of medicines poses questions about the distribution and politics of knowledge. How do people know about the array of medicinal products they use? Who has the right to know what about medicines? And based on whose rationality? These can be uneasy questions for anthropologists balancing between sympathy for local perceptions and respect for the potential of biomedicine to improve health. In this chapter we examine the situation in Uganda where medicinal commodities are freely available, but professional knowledge about their use is restricted in policy and practice.

We write from the ongoing experience of a project looking for ways to change people's knowledge and practice concerning drugs. But we are convinced that neither the global discourse on rational use of drugs nor the Ugandan National Drug Policy provides adequate ways of understanding and dealing with these issues. It is by engaging the local context of action—and the conflicting interests of various participants—that we are learning about the complexity and unevenness of the Ugandan playing field. What follows is a description "from the ground," which we hope will serve to project a local world into national and international discourses on rational drug use (Kleinman and Kleinman 1996:18). It is also an attempt to offer a more differentiated and pragmatic approach to anthropological assessments of the commodification of health. We argue that seeing Ugandans merely as unfortunate victims of capitalist forces is as problematic as adopting the view that local knowledge is always right.

The spread of manufactured pharmaceuticals throughout the world, whether through the efforts of international development aid or of multinational drug companies, is almost a prototype of globalization. But so is the effort to promote rational drug use through new policies, regulation, and training—as David Craig (Chapter 5) also argues. Both processes can be seen as global phenomena impinging on national realities that must be grasped in order to understand the local adequately (Chapter 3). Yet analyzing drug business and knowledge in terms of globalization tells us little about what practical steps might be taken to improve health care. Kleinman and Kleinman (1996) raise issues about the pragmatics of representation: they suggest that the way in which the media—and the anthropologist—represent problems of suffering and health carries implications for action. In this chapter, we want to push that pragmatic approach even further, basing our analysis on our own experiences on the "playing field," with an eye toward the kinds of futures that we and our partners envision.

Drug Use in Uganda

Medicinal substances are central in Ugandan health care, and presumably they have been for a very long time. Medicines made from plants, minerals, animal parts, and other items were probably never limited to those available in the immediate vicinity. The attraction of foreign medicines was evident in the interest in transformative substances from the East African coast, like the reputedly powerful ones from the island of Pemba and the exotic Islamic texts dissolved in water and used as medicine, brought inland by Swahili and Arab traders (Whyte 1988). Thus, although scholars like Vaughan (1991) emphasize the imposition of Western medicine and discourses on health as part of the colonial enterprise, it is well to remember that local people were not simply passive objects in this process. With a few exceptions, Western drugs, like other exotic medicines, were received with enthusiasm when they were first introduced by missionaries (Foster 1970:12).

By their nature as things, medicines easily become commodities for exchange and commercial trade (Van der Geest et al. 1996). But in the first hundred years of Western medicine in Uganda, most European medicines were what Appadurai (1986) called "enclaved commodities"—they were heavily controlled by Europeans, and later by Ugandans employed in health care facilities. True, there were proprietary brands of painkillers, antimalarials, and tonics available in local provision shops. And wherever there is enclaving, there are attempts at diversion; local entrepreneurs managed to get around restrictions and supply injections on convenient terms to desiring customers (Birungi 1994b:60–61). But the scale of this medicinal business was limited, even in the first decade or two after independence in 1962.

The Ugandan health care system of the 1960s has been praised as one of the best in sub-Saharan Africa (Dodge and Wiebe 1985). It consisted of an excellent national referral and teaching hospital, and a hierarchy of government health units and district hospitals, as well as many mission-run facilities. Until the time of Idi Amin's coup in 1971, health care was free at government units. This included medicines; the variety was limited, but there was almost always medicine. In 1969–1971, when Susan Whyte was doing her first fieldwork in eastern Uganda, government health centers were heavily used. Patients were sometimes referred to hospitals in town for more specialized care, but no one was referred to shops to buy drugs not provided by the public services. Indeed, there were no drug shops in rural areas. Chemist shops were an urban phenomenon, as was private biomedical care.

All this changed during the "time of regimes"—between 1971 and 1986. In 1972 Amin expelled the Asians, and many Ugandan professionals fled the country. This meant the loss of most trained pharmacists and many doctors (Scheyer and Dunlop 1985:34). Rural health centers and dispensaries (which never had pharmacists or doctors anyhow) continued to function for a time, but insecurity and lack of resources led to a marked fall in attendance. From 1976 to 1988 numbers of patients in government health units fell by half; some units were scarcely used at all because of lack of drugs. By the 1980s Ugandans were working out new channels for obtaining health care, especially medicines. Small private clinics and drug shops sprang up in trading centers and in the vicinity of government health units. When UNICEF started supplying drug kits to some public health facilities in 1981, an early evaluation pointed out that the antibiotic capsules and injectables supplied in the kits disappeared quickly from the health centers, but were readily available at nearby drug shops (Mburu 1985:90).

The privatization of health care was described (and decried) by the Health Policy Review Commission of 1987, which wrote of the "mushrooming" of private clinics and medicine shops all over the country. The metaphor of efflorescence was apt; rapid growth in the business of medicines is the dominant feature of health care as a whole in recent times. In the small town of Busolwe (population under two thousand) in eastern Uganda, for example, there were no shops or clinics specializing in the sale of drugs in 1971; by mid-1997 there were twelve. The business of medicine is truly flowering. The drug shops are supposed to be licensed and are legally permitted to sell only "Class C" drugs—that is, nonprescription medicine. In reality, there are practically no legal "Class C" drug shops in the country; even licensed shops sell antibiotics, injectables, needles and syringes, and chloroquine. The formal system actually depends on these commodities being available in nearby shops, because they often run short in government facilities.

After the accession to power of the National Resistance Movement in 1986, donor support to Uganda's health care sector poured into the country. Aside from contributions to preventive and health promotion initiatives such as the AIDS Control Programme and the Expanded Programme of Immunization, there was assistance to curative care. Renovation of health units, strengthening of district health services, vertical programs for sleeping sickness, tuberculosis, and diarrhea, a blood bank system, and other treatment programs were funded by the European Community, the World Bank, and U.S., German, Italian, and Swedish aid agencies (see Macrae et al. 1996). Perhaps most important, DANIDA (the Danish International Development Agency) financed the Uganda Essential Drugs Management Programme, which ensured the supply of basic drugs to every government and nongovernmental organization (NGO) outpatient unit in the country. The drug kits gave government units the means to attract patients again, but attendance figures have never regained the levels of 1971. Despite DANIDA's conditionalities and its strong role in shaping a comprehensive drug policy, private sales of all kinds of drugs continue to flourish (Okuonzi and Macrae 1995:128–129).

In reviewing these developments, it is important to bear in mind that the felt need for health care in Uganda is extremely high. Nationwide, 20 percent of children die before their fifth birthday—mostly from malaria and acute respiratory infections (Barton and Wamai 1994). The fevers and coughs that families are medicating are potentially deadly. Worm infections, anemia, diarrhea, eye diseases, tuberculosis, and AIDS and other sexually transmitted infections are common. Many health problems could be avoided in the long run with better economic conditions and public health measures, but in the short run people are sick and want curative care in the form of medicines. In this environment of high mortality and morbidity from infectious diseases, drugs assume a high value for health professionals as well as for ordinary people.

The Community Drug Use Study

In the 1980s and 1990s, researchers began to focus on issues of drug use. Studies initiated by the Uganda Essential Drugs Management Programme highlighted problems of polypharmacy, incorrect prescribing, and mismanagement within the nonprofit units receiving drug kits (Christensen 1990; Kafuko et al. 1996). Although most attention was given to the formal, nonprofit sector, a few researchers addressed the growing private, often unauthorized sale of medicine and the self-medication that it facilitated (Whyte 1990; Birungi 1994a, 1994b; Okello et al. 1997; Asiimwe et al. 1997). There is increasing recognition that from the user's point of view, the "informal" sector is an important alternative to the formal one (Ndyomugyenyi et al. 1998).

In 1992 this broader approach was applied in the Uganda Community Drug Use (CDU) project, a collaborative study with parallels in Mali, Pakistan, and the Philippines.[1] The project took a consumer, rather than an institutional, perspective on drug use, asking how people used drugs and where they got them. Fieldwork was carried out in three different parts of Uganda (Arua, Mbarara/Ntungamo, and Tororo districts) over fifteen months by fieldworkers who lived in local communities and spoke local languages. This included a survey of 450 households with six weekly recalls of symptoms and treatment. In addition to documenting consumer patterns, the project aimed to relate them to the overall health care system and to evaluate rational drug use interventions in the country. Although this first two-year phase was primarily a research project, we wanted to stimulate awareness and encourage discussion of drug use issues on the part of users, providers, and policymakers. The ultimate goal was to work out suggestions as to how drugs might be more effectively used to improve health care. To these ends, workshops and meetings were held at national, district, and community levels at the outset of the project, and at the conclusion, when we had results and ideas to present. The report was made available as a small book entitled *Popular Pills* (Adome et al. 1996).

The quantitative material showed that in Uganda today the first line of treatment for the most common health problems is pharmaceuticals, not "traditional medicine." Health care is thoroughly commodified in the sense that people depend on medicinal products they cannot produce locally.[2] We found that almost 90 percent of treatments for fever, cough, worms, and diarrhea relied on manufactured medicines.

Health care is also commercialized. Seventy-five percent of the drugs used came from small private clinics, drug shops, and ordinary provision shops—the ubiquitous *dukas* that sell sugar, tea, matches, and cooking oil in every neighborhood. The most common drugs sold are antimalarials (chloroquine was the most popular of all drugs), analgesics (paracetamol and aspirin), and antibiotics (cotrimoxazole, penicillin, tetracycline). About 75 percent of antibiotics and antimalarials were obtained through commercial sources.

This is not a matter of filling prescriptions. Most drugs (about 73 percent) were used in self-medication. This includes drugs that are restricted (prescription only) in Uganda; 67 percent of antibiotics and 64 percent of chloroquine were self-medicated. High levels of self-medication were facilitated by the commercialization of drug provision.

These survey results, together with what we learned through long-term participant observation and studies of various rational drug use interventions, presented a paradoxical picture. The Essential Drug Management Program and most systematic attempts to ensure effective curative care focused on the formal sector's nonprofit health facilities. But most treatment was in fact provided through the brisk business in medicines, much of which was informal in that it was unlicensed and illegal. Although donor agencies have contributed heavily to rehabilitating the government health system, utilization of the formal sector remains relatively low. The country's National Drug Policy (adopted by parliament in 1993) is progressive; relevant institutions, such as a national drug authority, national medical stores, and assistant drug inspectors in every district, have been put in place. But the gap between policy and practice is enormous. Although health planners, professionals, and administrators emphasize the need for rational drug use, people buy all kinds of drugs and use them in ways that are reasonable according to their own lights.

Anthropological Perspectives

Broadly speaking, anthropologists might take three views of such situations. We say "might take" advisedly, because most of us do not take a clear stand. We straddle several of these perspectives, as do the authors from whose texts we have plucked the following examples. But for the sake of exposition, we suggest that we can take a populist, an "enlightened," or a pragmatic approach to the business of medicines and the politics of knowledge.

The populist approach, fundamental to anthropological research, attempts to understand the viewpoints of the lay users of medicines. It portrays sympathetically their perceptions of symptoms and medicines. Rational drug use? Users have their own form of rationality. For example, ethnographers show how cultural reinterpretations of pharmaceuticals are made on the basis of indigenous semantics (Tan 1994) and the significance of qualities like taste, color, and tepidity (Bledsoe and Goubaud 1988; M. Logan 1973). Local notions of efficacy (Etkin 1988), and of the way medicines fit individual constitutions, may influence use of medicines (Hardon 1994; Nichter and Nordstrom 1989).

The populist position emphasizes the agency of consumers of medicines. They act to resist the monopoly of professionals, to refashion creatively therapeutic relations, and to obtain medicines and knowledge on their own terms. One of the clearest examples of this position is Anne Reeler's work on medicine use in northeastern Thailand (1996). She shows how people, especially urban slum dwellers, appreciate the convenience and support of medicinal commodities, in the absence of adequate therapy managing networks. She goes so far as to say that they find the ability to purchase those commodities "empowering."

Populist approaches portray people's attempts to gain control of medicines and the authoritative knowledge of doctors, as in the report of this informant's words from Sri Lanka:

> Medicine cures, doctors control the knowledge of medicines and we are made dependent. We do not receive health education about medicines, only about using soap, drinking boiled cool water, and taking immunizations—things from which there is no profit. There are many things we want to learn, but they teach us only what they want us to know. Yet we are not helpless. Just as we have learned to use . . . (herbal medicines) so we will learn about *ingirisi* (allopathic) medicines through experience. (Nichter and Nordstrom 1989:367)

Our Ugandan research had a populist element. We documented people's dissatisfaction with nonprofit health care: the user fees, the poor service, the inconvenience, and the frequent shortage of drugs. Over the difficult years of war and economic crisis, people engaged in self-help. Commercialization was experienced as positive because it diminished people's dependence on poorly functioning institutions (see also Whyte 1990).

The populist view valorizes consumers' capabilities and agency. In contrast, the "enlightened" one doubts them. It reveals people's knowledge of medicines as inadequate; their medication practices are irrational, and they are likely to be victims of commercial interests. These criticisms are based on an informed position against which popular knowledge is measured and found wanting. Two different variants of this "enlightened" position may be distinguished: the professional and the critical.

Much applied anthropology takes an "enlightened professional" stance, almost of necessity. When we cooperate with biomedical planners, policymakers, and practitioners in projects whose aim is to improve health and health services, we often adopt biomedical standards for evaluating such practices as medication. Although "critical" medical anthropology deplores the tendency of anthropologists becoming the "handmaidens-translators to biomedicine" (Morsey 1996:32), such criticism needs to be specific and contextualized. There are situations and health problems where it is important to compare people's knowledge and use of drugs to biomedical orthodoxy. Social scientists working on programs to control specific diseases, such as malaria, diarrhea, and acute respiratory infections (Kendall 1990:185; Pelto and Pelto 1997), examine perceptions and practices with an eye to what is effective and what is risky in biomedical terms.

In such an "enlightened professional" vein, our Ugandan research identified problems in the ways people were using drugs. A professional assessment of treatments suggested that most were not medically appropriate. Although chloroquine was commonly self-medicated, practically no layperson knew the recommended dose. Because of the danger of development of chloroquine resistance, the common practice of underdosing is a grave concern. Oral rehydration therapy, promoted as the treatment of first resort, was used in only 11 percent of diarrhea cases. We were critical of the overuse of pharmaceuticals; the "pill for every ill" approach encouraged polypharmacy. So did people's unwillingness to wait and see whether a treatment worked.

The "critical enlightened" position problematizes the knowledge and practice of *both* specialists and laypeople. The proliferation of medicines is related to a transformation in consciousness whereby professionals and laypeople alike come to believe (or know) that medicines are the answers to their problems. From this position one speaks of "false consciousness" generated by health commodification—the belief that health can be secured through medicinal commodities (Nichter 1989:235–236). Notions of ideology, hegemony, and complicity are invoked in discussing the medicalization and pharmaceuticalization of suffering. Health professionals play the role of intellectuals, "sustaining commonsense definitions of reality through their highly specialized and validating forms of discourse" (Scheper-Hughes 1992:171). Laypeople are "complicit" in that their everyday knowledge and practice—indeed, their bodily experience—are oriented toward medicinal commodities as solutions to their problems. The knowledge and practices of both users and providers of medicines are found wanting.

Against what standards are they measured? Neither Nichter nor Scheper-Hughes is explicit about this. But it seems safe to say that their criticisms are based on classic public health principles: recognition of the social/political/economic bases of health, social justice, disease prevention and health promotion, and rational drug use (therapeutic efficacy plus economic efficiency).

There are not many traces of the "critical enlightened" approach in the community drug use research. We agree that people often have unrealistic expectations—or hopes—about medicines. There are also many grounds to criticize the practices of the providers of medicines, both within and outside health institutions. In some cases, there is overuse of medicines—the "pill for every ill" orientation is strong among health workers, who tend to medicate symptoms rather than evaluate the whole patient and situation in order to address the cause. Lack of diagnostic examinations enforces the tendency to presumptive (shotgun) treatment (Whyte 1997:212–13) to cover all possibilities. But just as often, there is underuse or misuse of medicine; the problem is not simply that providers and users delude themselves that they can medicate their way to health.

Much of the "critical enlightened" view of medicines is directed against situations where people are using tonics, vitamins, or other drugs deemed unnecessary, rather than taking steps to change the political economy of health. The critique is just as relevant to the use of "indigenous" medicines. As Charles Leslie once wrote:

> The bottom line in the discussions . . . is how much choice people in poor countries should have in spending their pennies. Of course health care planners believe that they should not buy tonics to prevent premature ejaculation, or to make their sons more intelligent. They should deal realistically with the terrible problems in their countries, with malnutrition and infectious disease. (Leslie 1988:xii)

In Uganda people also spend money on love medicines, cough mixtures, and appetite stimulants. But most of the pharmaceuticals consumed cannot be dismissed as biomedically useless. The CDU survey found that 77 percent of drugs used in households were on the essential drugs list. In the formal units the figure was 97 percent (Kafuko et al. 1996:33). One of the reasons for this is probably that the "pharmaceuticalization" of health care in Uganda was strongly promoted through donor-supported programs and the formal health system. Patterns of treatment established there were popularized.

Here, as always, global processes must be analyzed in local situations. The general critique of commodification and medicalization seems less relevant in this environment of heavy morbidity from infectious diseases.

Given the high rates of malaria and acute respiratory infection, it seems perverse to criticize wholesale the commodification of health. Selected commodities, properly used, would help. Medicalization of some kinds of problems is justified.

The Community Drug Use project obtained funding for a second phase of research with the purpose of developing and pilot-testing interventions to improve the use of drugs. It is this mandate to engage in the politics of knowledge ourselves that has pushed us toward a more differentiated, pragmatic, and processual approach. Having to work out a plan of action has required us to distinguish categories of actors, specific kinds of knowledge, and particular ways of obtaining it. Discussing and negotiating in order to work with different people and agencies has brought us face-to-face with the politics of information. Notions of hegemony and false consciousness are less useful here than an appreciation of differentiated interests, power, and authority. In order to illustrate the elements of such a pragmatic approach, we shall briefly describe the logistics of obtaining knowledge about drugs in local settings. We can then turn to the existing policies about dissemination of knowledge about drugs.

The Logistics of Knowledge

In rural areas, where 90 percent of Ugandans live, there is little advertising of drugs; some families have working radios, but this is far from universal. Television and newspapers are not common in the countryside. Sources of knowledge about pharmaceuticals include nonprofit health units, private clinics and shops, and family and friends.

Sick people attending health units in Uganda answer the health worker's questions about their symptoms. They are not informed about their diagnosis or the name of the drug prescribed. Nor do most people expect that they will be told much in these situations (Munene et al. 1997:36). The health worker (usually a medical assistant or a nurse) writes the complaint or presumed diagnosis and the prescription on a form (the Medical Form Five), which is taken to the dispensing counter. Patients seldom ask questions. In a study on quality of care in Tororo district, it was found that only 13 out of 160 exiting patients had asked any questions during their consultation (Nshakira et al. 1996:49). One woman, responding to a query about why she had not posed questions, asked, "Why should I? He had already written on the paper." Another said, "The health worker told me to go and get tablets and that the injection was not there. What else should I ask him? What should I want to know?" (Nshakira et al. 1996:35).

From experience, people have learned to expect tablets, capsules, and injections for fever. Drugs are not provided in original packaging, but are counted out from large containers into small envelopes or paper cones. Instructions are given orally and usually also are written on the envelope in abbreviated form such as "2 x 3," meaning take two tablets three times a day. Given a high rate of illiteracy, especially among women, written instructions may have to be deciphered by someone else. Other studies have found that fewer than half of exiting patients are able to repeat the dosage instructions correctly (Nshakira et al. 1996; Kafuko et al. 1996).

These problems of communication in the formal nonprofit health care system are not unique to Uganda. In a review article on compliance in developing countries, Homedes and Ugalde (1993:294) observe: "Low income patients, who constitute the vast majority, seldom ask for clarification and additional information, much less question practitioners. . . . In the third world, to transform the poor from passive to active patients when they receive modern Western care is an interesting, and probably urgent, but little discussed issue."

Customers at private shops and clinics are in a different situation from patients at public health units. They are more in control, can decide whether or what to buy, and how much they want to spend. They can leave their patients at home, which is often highly convenient, given transport difficulties, and buy medicine to take back. Moreover, in rural areas, customers often know the proprietors as neighbors, friends, or relatives. There is a tendency to personalize relations with private providers; people refer to shops and clinics by the name of the owner or attendant, and they have distinct individual preferences (Birungi 1994b:116). The attendant must try to please them in order to keep their patronage, but also because they are more than just customers.

Here too most drugs are sold loose, wrapped in paper cones made from pages torn from school exercise books on which is written the dosage (e.g., 1 x 4). There are no package inserts to study at home; information must be sought and given orally. But the social relations of private care are such that customers are in a stronger position to ask questions. Roughly half of them ask what the attendant recommends for the symptoms; some use the opportunity to learn the names of drugs and to compare their relative merits. They can look at the drugs or check about the ones they used last time. If someone has been to the government unit and been told that some of the drugs they need are out of stock (a common situation), they show the Medical Form Five to the proprietor and ask what it says.

The attendants at commercial drug outlets themselves have various sources of knowledge. Proprietors of clinics and "Class C" drug shops often have medical training or experience. Licensed facilities are usually owned by doctors, medical assistants, nurses, or midwives. They have formal training behind them, although it is only recently that nurses and midwives have been taught diagnosis and prescribing as part of their formal course. Equally important, they have experience from formal facilities, where many of them are still employed and where certain patterns of drug indication and prescription are established. When they are not behind the counter, however, less qualified attendants may see patients and customers; the trained license holders are supposed to instruct and supervise these attendants. Unlicensed drug shops and clinics are sometimes owned by medically trained people; having a license may depend on ability to pay the steep fee more than qualifications. But others, particularly in remote areas, are owned by nursing aides or dressers, or people with less medical experience. Lacking systematic training, they pick up knowledge as they can. Some informally ask for information from trained health workers whom they happen to know. Proprietors of ordinary provision shops, a major source of drugs, seldom have any special experience, much less training, in the use of pharmaceuticals. The medicinal products they sell are commodities like the others in the shop, and they feel no responsibility for instructing people in how to use them. As one shopkeeper commented, "I don't tell people how to use the sugar they buy either."

One source of knowledge that drug shops in Ugandan rural areas do *not* have is the sales representative from pharmaceutical companies. In India, Sri Lanka, and the Philippines, researchers have reported that these "reps" provide information (or misinformation) on products, and may be important discussion partners for small-scale drug retailers (Carpenter et al. 1996; Wolffers 1988; Nichter 1989:235-36; Kamat and Nichter 1997). Ugandan rural drug shops are often stocked from larger shops in towns, where some information on drug indications and dosages may be obtained. But some of the drugs they sell are smuggled, stolen, or resold by someone who has a surplus—and the retailer has little opportunity of getting information from these more dubious sources.

The last important source of information for users of drugs is other laypeople—family and neighbors. Participant observation has shown that people seek advice from those they consider more knowledgeable. Someone who has lived in town or traveled might be consulted by neighbors. Anyone who has ever worked at a health facility, even as support staff, may serve as a channel of information to relatives and friends. Many of those who know how to give injections at home learned from a family member who was a health worker. The health workers themselves probably disseminate more information on drugs in this informal way than they do within the formal setting of the health unit. People who are younger and better educated often know more names of drugs than their less schooled elders, although they are not actually taught about them in school. They seem more interested in seeking out this kind of knowledge and ask more informed questions in commercial settings, thus increasing their expertise (Katahoire 1998).

The Politics of Information

When we started the Community Drug Use project in 1992, policymakers and ministry of health officials expressed consternation at the extent to which medicines have become a business. Since colonial times, national policy has required the licensing of drug retailers and prohibited them from selling restricted drugs like antibiotics. Officially, even chloroquine is to be dispensed on prescription only. Gatekeepers are notable for enforcing this policy or restricting the free flow of all kinds of pharmaceutical commodities. But they can restrict the dissemination of knowledge to drug retailers and the public, thus declining to legitimize private provision of drugs and self-medication. (In the United States and Scandinavia, the situation is the opposite: access to drugs is controlled, but information about them is readily available.)

In the early 1990s, a government health center in one of our study locations had no medicine for six months. The shops in the nearby trading center responded by stocking up on basic medicines; there was no other source in that rural area. The shopkeepers as a group requested that the health unit give them some training about the medicines they were so briskly selling. The health workers asked the district medical officer for permission to do so, but he turned them down.

Public education about drug use was nonexistent until the establishment of the Uganda Essential Drugs Management Programme. As part of its support to this program, DANIDA financed a public education initiative through the Uganda Red Cross to encourage rational use of drugs. The agency followed official policy, which was to encourage people to seek treatment at formal health units and to obey instructions given there. This meant that public education was all about how *not* to use drugs. Messages disseminated in connection with the Essential Drugs Management Programme were mostly warnings: Do not ask for injections. Do not share drugs. Do not self-medicate. Do not consult "quacks." There were no posters or radio broadcasts or community meetings about how to use pharmaceuticals properly.

Likewise, the community health worker projects that the CDU researchers examined in Tororo and Arua districts did not instruct village health workers or traditional midwives about the use of medicines. Nor were they supplied with drug kits as is the case in many other countries; this had been tried in some Ugandan programs earlier and abandoned. Their work was seen as preventive and promotive, not curative. The only "medicine" about which they were taught was oral rehydration solution. They were to refer cases needing treatment to health units. Many were dissatisfied with the situation. They received nothing from their neighbors for their advice about nutrition and sanitation; like the woman from Sri Lanka interviewed by Nichter and Nordstrom, they had only been taught "things from which there is no profit." A few of the more entrepreneurial health workers had set up small drug shops in order to gain an income from their health work.

In 1993 the Uganda Red Cross made a modest and careful step in a new direction. They decided to integrate teaching about drugs in their primary health care activities and included in their training of community health workers information on indications and dosages for selected medicines. These included chloroquine (for malaria), mebendazole (for worms), paracetamol and aspirin (for pain), magnesium trisilicate (for ulcers), oral rehydration therapy (for diarrhea), and ferrous sulphate (for anemia). Plans were to try this approach in six pilot areas. In these areas, drug retailers were also to be offered training in these same indications and medicines.

Although the work with community health workers went ahead in most of the pilot areas, the training of drug sellers lagged behind. When it did take place, the facilitators of the training sessions put great emphasis on clarifying the regulations concerning drug shops, which frightened some of the participants. Many were not registered—they claimed they could not afford it. All were reminded that it was illegal to sell antibiotics, though this was an important part of their business. Still, the Red Cross initiative was an important turning point in the politics of information about drug use. When the Community Drug Use project ended its two-year research phase, we concluded that this combination of public education and retailer training was the way forward.

Workshops were held at national, district, and local levels to present the findings of the Community Drug Use study, and to discuss plans for an action research phase to try an intervention—which we thought should focus on the private sector and self-medication. We found strikingly different attitudes toward the politics of information at the various levels. Local consumers and community leaders were eager that teaching on the use of all kinds of drugs be given to shopkeepers and the public. They saw no problem in being given more systematic information about the drugs they were buying in any case. However, representatives of the National Drug Authority, the Ministry of Health, and the Essential Drug Management Programme at the national level had firm reservations on two points.

First, they did not want instruction about indications and dosages for antibiotics to be given to retailers or the public, despite our figures about the commercial sources of and levels of self-medication with these drugs. Their argument was that this would legitimate self-medication and that wrong use of antibiotics would contribute to the growing problem of drug resistance. Interestingly, the same argument could be made about chloroquine, but the authorities were more willing to accept that people should be taught about antimalarials. Second, they did not want teaching offered to unlicensed shop owners—thus effectively excluding most of those selling drugs, and many in greatest need of training.[3] They claimed that this would amount to recognition and would work against their efforts to control and regularize the sale of drugs.

The district authorities were caught in the middle. They were well aware of the gap between policy and practice. Some took the populist view that knowledge should be provided to everyone who wanted it; they saw no reason that it should be the monopoly of professional groups when laypeople were so busy buying and selling medicine. Other district health officials were concerned about their power struggle with the shopkeepers and did not want to give them any form of acknowledgment. They reckoned that an invitation to a training session would constitute a sign of approval.

Playing on the Field

Our objectives in the first phase were to delineate the contours of the problem, as seen from different positions, and to bring the issue of drug use to wider attention and debate. Through the research itself, which involved many people, through the workshops, through our little book, and not least through the efforts of Richard Odoi Adome in making video films and regular television programs about use of medicines, the Community Drug Use project did contribute to awareness of patterns of drug availability and use. Other forces were at work in the same period. Most important was a growing recognition on the part of policymakers and authorities that commercial sources of drugs and self-medication would continue to play an important part in health care. Despite the enormous influx of donor money to the health sector, the government health system remains weak—whether because of lack of state resources, World Bank policy, corruption, or the patterns of self-help established during the "time of regimes." The question now is, How and how much should the politics of information change to accommodate the realities of drug use?

When we obtained funding from DANIDA for an intervention phase of the Community Drug Use project, it was our intention to form alliances with established institutions. As academic researchers we can document problems and design interventions. But it is unlikely that our effort will be sustainable if it is not part of some bigger program. In fact, we might not be able to do it at all. We intended to work with the Uganda Red Cross to build upon their attempts to integrate teaching about drugs in their community health activities. However, they were in the process of restructuring their whole organization—at the behest of their donors—and it seemed doubtful that public education on drug use would have much of a profile in their future.

Meanwhile a heavier player had emerged on the field in the form of the National Drug Authority. Established under the new National Drug Policy passed by parliament in 1993, the NDA has a broad commission. It has authority to regulate the import, manufacture, export, quality, storage, and sale of pharmaceuticals. As part of its control over sales, it develops sensitization workshops for drug retailers. Representatives of the NDA had attended our national dissemination workshop and expressed their reservations about training. They made it clear that they were concerned about enforcing the registration of drug shops and would like to close unregistered ones—a policy that had not worked previously and indeed seemed open to misuse in some areas where payoffs were made.

At the same time, the new NDA was trying to develop more realistic approaches. It was planning to remove chloroquine from the list of restricted drugs, and to include information about chloroquine in the workshops offered in the future to registered drug retailers. Other projects and programs were also pushing the NDA to review its policies, especially as international programs moved toward emphasizing easy availability of drugs to promote early treatment. For example, after protracted negotiations with the NDA, a Social Marketing for Change project gained permission to distribute kits for treatment of male urethritis through drug shops—even though the kits contained antibiotics (which drug shops were not supposed to handle). These shifts in the politics of knowledge were modest in proportion to the dimensions of the business of medicines. But they were important in that they provided openings for dialogue. The Community Drug Use project was committed to an alliance with the NDA, although it was not always easy. NDA staff were very busy and were unable to be involved in the development of the CDU action plans to the extent we had once envisioned. Still, they hope that they will be able to incorporate our materials and experiences in their future training and educational activities.

Other alliances were also important. In 1998 the Malaria Control Unit under the ministry of health started to publicize information on the correct dose of chloroquine. For the first time, the radio and newspaper carried announcements about the recommended course of chloroquine. With this new policy, they expressed an interest in cooperation with our project to develop ways of conveying this information effectively.

Given the policy of decentralization in Uganda, district health teams were key players in determining and implementing local health activities. We originally planned to try out programs of public education and drug retailer training in the three districts in which we had worked in the first phase. We had to make compromises: One district medical officer did not want any training of retailers in his district. We decided to concentrate our efforts in the district where the authorities seemed most committed to the project. That district was quite liberal—we would say realistic—in its views of what was needed. But the district health team took pains not to offend the NDA, which was more restrictive.

In working together with local drug shop owners and users of drugs to assess their needs and wishes for information, we clearly saw that they wanted guidance on more kinds of drugs than the NDA thought they should be using. Local people wanted to know how to give safe injections of penicillin; drug shops do a big business in septrin (cotrimoxazole) for respiratory infections. The NDA did not want to accept this reality, but, rather, to work for a future where antibiotics will be controlled by professionals. This is a political issue we had to learn about through the experience of playing on the field.

The Community Drug Use project did a needs assessment and a baseline survey of drug shops and communities in all three of the original districts. Training modules for providers and community members were developed and tested, as were public education strategies to reach schoolchildren, church congregations, and other local groups. The researchers were closely involved in all the interventions in order to evaluate the process and will carry out follow-up surveys to measure changes in knowledge and practice.

But just as important as this evaluation of an intervention was the more general principle of participant observation. Being active participants put us in a position to try out ways of improving drug use. Moreover, being part of the process also allowed us to experience the workings of authority, interest, and contrasting perspectives firsthand. One of our objectives in this phase of our work was to document the negotiations we undertook and the problems we encountered in trying to carry out our intervention. By playing on the playing field, we explored its unevenness. By defining a specific problem for action, discussing plans, forming alliances, choosing strategies, and learning from our successes and failures, we were able to refine and differentiate our understanding of the field.

Conclusion

Although the worldwide spread of manufactured pharmaceuticals may be taken as a prime example of globalization, solutions to problems of drug misuse must be worked out locally. What is possible and relevant in one country is not necessarily replicable elsewhere. Nepal was a pioneer in developing a program for training drug retailers; licensing requires participation in the course and passing an examination (Kafle et al. 1992). Those who have done so are authorized to fill prescriptions. Together with Richard Odoi Adome we visited this project in 1996. Though it gave us many useful ideas, we realized that the structure of professional interests in Uganda would make it impossible to duplicate the program there. In Kenya, the Ministry of Health/Kenya Medical Research Institute/Wellcome Trust project to train keepers of ordinary provision shops about malaria treatment has been another source of direct inspiration. Members of the CDU team visited Kilifi, and Ane Haaland and John Muturi brought their experience from that project to our work in Uganda. But in Uganda it was not politically possible to train the owners of *dukas* as an explicit target group—even though our research showed they were the single most important source of drugs.

What is the role of anthropology in addressing the "pharmaceuticalization" of health care? Both of us have done long-term ethnographic studies on health in Uganda (Birungi 1994b; Whyte 1997) in which we adopted a "populist" perspective, emphasizing the perceptions and practices of laypeople. Through work with the World Health Organization, the International Network for the Rational Use of Drugs, and medical colleagues, we are also aware of the "professional enlightened" perspective on the dangers of drug misuse and emerging resistance of microbes to antibiotics and antimalarials. But neither of these perspectives provided the platform we needed to apply anthropology to the problems of morbidity and mortality in the particular historical circumstances of Uganda. For that we have taken the anthropological commitment to participant observation into an attempt to improve knowledge about pharmaceuticals—involving ourselves in an initiative and trying to reflect on the experience we gained. We had to deal with particular interests, configurations of authority, and the gap between policy and practice.

Applying anthropology in this case has meant a long-term engagement with a set of problems in one country. Time is important; we have been able to follow changes as they unfolded, and to feel that our project was a part of them. Applied anthropology should be processual but is too often squeezed into the narrow time frame of a funding cycle.

This kind of research, funded from Denmark and integrated in networks of researchers working on similar problems elsewhere, is itself a product of globalization. Like so much of current research in Uganda, it is externally funded. But it is firmly anchored in a Ugandan academic setting and has given high priority to building up alliances with relevant players in the Ugandan field. When the funding for the Community Drug Use project is finished, it will leave behind experienced and knowledgeable researchers who will continue to work on health issues in Uganda. It will have developed training materials, and relationships with agencies that can use them. We hope also that by getting involved in the politics of knowledge, it will provide some needed information to people who were not receiving it.

Notes

1. The overall collaborative study was funded by the European Commission and coordinated by Dr. Anita Hardon of the Medical Anthropology Unit at the University of Amsterdam. The Ugandan study was supported by DANIDA and based at Makerere Institute of Social Research, with Dr. Richard Odoi Adome, head of the Department of Pharmacy, as principal investigator. Fieldwork in Uganda was carried out by Enoch Ezati, Xavier Nsabagasani, Joseph Owor, and Lisbet Årtenblad. Ane Haaland and Spencer Birungi, who are experienced with information, education, and communication interventions, joined members of the original team. We gratefully acknowledge the support and contributions of them all.

2. "Traditional" treatment forms are more embedded in local contexts and less subject to massive commodification than manufactured pharmaceuticals. Herbal and Islamic medicines—even dealings with spirits—are commercialized to some extent. But in Uganda, "African medicines" are not mass produced and marketed on a large scale; local communities are self-sufficient in "traditional medicines."

3. The extent of the licensing problem was revealed in a baseline survey of drug shops undertaken as part of the current intervention phase of our project. A total count was made of all the drug shops in eight parishes in three different districts. Of the thirty-five existing drug shops, only five were licensed.

References

Adome, Richard Odoi, Susan Reynolds Whyte, and Anita Hardon. 1996. *Popular Pills: Community Drug Use in Uganda.* Amsterdam: Het Spinhuis.

Alubo, S. Ogoh. 1985. "Drugging the Nigerian People: The Public Hazards of Private Profits." In *The Impact of Development and Modern Technologies in Third World Health,* Barbara E. Jackson and Antonio Ugalde, eds. Williamsburg, VA: Studies in Third World Societies, no. 34.

Appadurai, Arjun, ed. 1986. *The Social Life of Things: Commodities in Cultural Perspective.* Cambridge: Cambridge University Press.

Asiimwe, Delius, Barbara McPake, Frances Mwesigye, Matthias Ofumbi, Lisbeth Ørtenblad, Pieter Streefland, and Asaph Turinde. 1997. "The Private-Sector Activities of Public-Sector Health Workers in Uganda." In *Private Health Providers in Developing Countries: Serving the Public Interest?* Sara Bennett, Barbara McPake, and Anne Mills, eds. London: Zed Books.

Barton, Tom, and Gimono Wamai. 1994. *Equity and Vulnerability: A Situation Analysis of Women, Adolescents and Children in Uganda.* Kampala: National Council for Children.

Birungi, Harriet. 1994a. "Injections as Household Utilities: Injection Practices in Busoga, Eastern Uganda." In *Medicines: Meanings and Contexts,* Nina L. Etkina and Michael L. Tan, eds. Quezon City, Philippines: Health Action International Network.

———. 1994b. "The Domestication of Injections: A Study of Social Relationships of Health Care in Busoga, Eastern Uganda." Ph.D. diss., Institute of Anthropology, University of Copenhagen.

Bledsoe, Caroline, and M. F. Goubaud. 1988. "The Reinterpretation and Distribution of Western Pharmaceuticals: An Example from the Mende of Sierra Leone." In *The Context of Medicines in Developing Countries: Studies in*

Pharmaceutical Anthropology, Sjaak van der Geest and Susan Reynolds Whyte, eds. Dordrecht: Kluwer.
Carpenter, H., L. Manderson, M. Janabi, G. Kalmayem, A. Simon, and G. Waidubu. 1996. "The Politics of Drug Distribution in Bohol, the Philippines," *Asian Studies Review* 17(1): 35–52.
Christensen, F. R. 1990. "A Strategy for Improvement of Prescribing and Drug Use in Rural Health Facilities in Uganda: A Report of an Assignment Carried Out Under the Auspices of UEDMP." Entebbe: Ministry of Health.
Dodge, Cole P., and Paul D. Wiebe, eds. 1985. *Crisis in Uganda: The Breakdown of Health Services.* Oxford: Pergamon Press.
Etkin, Nina. 1988. "The Cultural Construction of Efficacy." In *The Context of Medicines in Developing Countries: Studies in Pharmaceutical Anthropology,* Sjaak van der Geest and Susan Reynolds Whyte, eds. Dordrecht: Kluwer.
Ferguson, Anne. 1988. "Commercial Pharmaceutical Medicine and Medicalization: A Case Study from El Salvador." In *The Context of Medicines in Developing Countries: Studies in Pharmaceutical Anthropology,* Sjaak van der Geest and Susan Reynolds Whyte, eds. Dordrecht: Kluwer.
Foster, W. D. 1970. *The Early History of Scientific Medicine in Uganda.* Nairobi: East African Literature Bureau.
Hardon, Anita. 1991. *Confronting Ill Health: Medicines, Self-Care and the Poor in Manila.* Quezon City, Philippines: Health Action International Network.
———. 1994. "People's Understanding of Efficacy for Cough and Cold Medicines in Manila, the Philippines." In *Medicines: Meanings and Contexts,* Nina L. Etkina and Michael L. Tan, eds. Quezon City, Philippines: Health Action International Network.
Helling-Borda, Margretha, and Jonathan D. Quick. N.d. "The Other 'Prescribers': International Perspectives on Self-Medication, Pharmacy Practice, and Rational Drug Use." In *International Experience in Rational Use of Drugs,* vol. II, Ranjit Roy Chaudhry, ed. Bangkok: College of Public Health, Chulalongkorn University.
Homedes, Nuria, and Antonio Ugalde. 1993. "Patients' Compliance with Medical Treatments in the Third World. What Do We Know?" *Health Policy and Planning* 8(4): 291–314.
Illich, Ivan. 1975. *Medical Nemesis: The Expropriation of Health.* London: Calder and Boyars.
Kafle, Kamud, Shrestha Madden, Das Karkee, and Quick Pradhan. 1992. "Drug Retailer Training: Experiences from Nepal," *Social Science and Medicine* 35(8): 1015–1025.
Kafuko, Jessica M., Christine Zirabamuzaale, and Danstan Bagenda. 1996. *Rational Drug Use in Rural Health Units of Uganda: Effect of National Standard Treatment Guidelines on Rational Drug Use.* Entebbe: Uganda Essential Drugs Management Programme.
Kamat, Vinay R., and Mark Nichter. 1997. "Monitoring Product Movement: An Ethnographic Study of Pharmaceutical Sales Representatives in Bombay, India." In *Private Health Providers in Developing Countries: Serving the Public Interest?* Sara Bennett, Barbara McPake, and Anne Mills, eds. London: Zed Books.
Katahoire, Anne. 1998. "Education for Life: Mothers' Education and Children's Survival in Eastern Uganda." Ph.D. diss., Institute of Anthropology, University of Copenhagen.
Kendall, Carl. 1990. "Public Health and the Domestic Domain: Lessons from Anthropological Research on Diarrheal Diseases." In *Anthropology and Primary Health Care,* Jeannine Coreil and J. Dennis Mull, eds. Boulder, CO: Westview Press.

Kleinman, Arthur, and Joan Kleinman. 1996. "The Appeal of Experience," *Daedalus* 125(1): 1–24.

Leslie, Charles. 1988. "Preface." In *The Context of Medicines in Developing Countries: Studies in Pharmaceutical Anthropology,* Sjaak Van der Geest and Susan Reynolds Whyte, eds. Dordrecht: Kluwer.

Logan, Kathleen. 1988. "'Casi como doctor': Pharmacists and Their Clients in a Mexican Urban Context." In *The Context of Medicines in Developing Countries: Studies in Pharmaceutical Anthropology,* Sjaak van der Geest and Susan Reynolds Whyte, eds. Dordrecht: Kluwer.

Logan, Michael. 1973. "Humoral Medicine in Guatemala and Peasant Acceptance of Modern Medicine," *Human Organization* 32(4): 385–395.

Macrae, Joanna, Anthony B. Zwi, and Lucy Gilson. 1996. "A Triple Burden for Health Sector Reform: 'Post'-Conflict Rehabilitation in Uganda," *Social Science and Medicine* 42(7): 1095–1108.

Mburu, F. M. 1985. "Evaluation of Government Rural Health Centres and UNICEF Essential Drug Inputs." In *Crisis in Uganda: The Breakdown of Health Services,* Cole P. Dodge and Paul D. Wiebe, eds. Oxford: Pergamon Press.

Morsey, Soheir A. 1996. "Political Economy in Medical Anthropology." In *Handbook of Medical Anthropology: Contemporary Theory and Method,* Rev. Ed., Carolyn F. Sargent and Thomas M. Johnson, eds. Westport, CT: Greenwood Press.

Munene, John, Tobias Onweng Angura, Harriet Birungi, Betty Kwagala, Patrick Orone, and Pieter Streefland. 1997. *Revitalization of Primary Health Care in Uganda: A Study of the Interface of Basic Health Services and the Community.* Kampala: Makerere Institute of Social Research.

Ndyomugyenyi, Richard, Stella Neema, and Pascal Magnussen. 1998. "The Use of Formal and Informal Services for Antenatal Care and Malaria Treatment in Rural Uganda," *Health Policy and Planning* 13(1): 94–102.

Nichter, Mark. 1989. *Anthropology and International Health: South Asian Case Studies.* Dordrecht: Kluwer.

Nichter, Mark, and Carolyn Nordstrom. 1989. "A Question of Medicine Answering: Health Commodification and the Social Relations of Healing in Sri Lanka," *Culture, Medicine and Psychiatry* 13(4): 367–390.

Nshakira, Nathan, Susan Whyte, Jessica Jitta, and Gonzaga Busuulwa. 1996. *An Assessment of Quality of Out-Patient Clinical Care in District Health Facilities, Tororo District.* Kampala: CHDC Document.

Okello, David, Joseph Konde-Lule, Rosalind Luganga, John Arube-Wani, and John Baptist Lwanga. 1997. *Aspects of the Private For-Profit Health Sector in Uganda: An Appraisal of Scope and Impact.* Kampala: Uganda National Council for Science and Technology.

Okuonzi, Sam Agatry, and Joanna Macrae. 1995. "Whose Policy Is It Anyway? International and National Influences on Health Policy Development in Uganda," *Health Policy and Planning* 10(2): 122–132.

Pelto, Pertti J., and Gretel H. Pelto. 1997. "Studying Knowledge, Culture, and Behavior in Applied Medical Anthroplgy," *Medical Anthropology Quarterly* 11(2): 147–163.

Reeler, Anne. 1996. *Money and Friendship: Modes of Empowerment in Thai Health Care.* Amsterdam: Het Spinhuis.

Scheper-Hughes, Nancy. 1992. *Death Without Weeping: The Violence of Everyday Life in Brazil.* Berkeley: University of California Press.

Scheyer, Stanley, and David Dunlop. 1985. "Health Services and Development in Uganda." In *Crisis in Uganda: The Breakdown of Health Services*, Cole P. Dodge and Paul D. Wiebe, eds. Oxford: Pergamon Press.

Silverman, M., P. R. Lee, and M. Lydecker. 1982. *Prescriptions for Death: The Drugging of the Third World.* Stanford: Stanford University Press.

Tan, Michael. 1994. "The Meaning of Medicines: Examples from the Philippines." In *Medicines: Meanings and Contexts,* Nina L. Etkina and Michael L. Tan, eds. Quezon City, Philippines: Health Action International Network.

Van der Geest, Sjaak, Susan Reynolds Whyte, and Anita Hardon. 1996. "The Anthropology of Pharmaceuticals: A Biological Approach," *Annual Reviews in Anthropology* 25: 153–178.

Vaughan, Megan. 1991. *Curing Their Ills: Colonial Power and African Illness.* Oxford: Polity Press.

Welbourne, F. B. 1961. *East African Rebels.* London: SCM Press.

Whyte, Susan Reynolds. 1988. "The Power of Medicines in East Africa." In *The Context of Medicines in Developing Countries: Studies in Pharmaceutical Anthropology,* Sjaak van der Geest and Susan Reynolds Whyte, eds. Dordrecht: Kluwer.

———. 1990. "Medicines and Self-Help: The Privatization of Health Care in Eastern Uganda." In *Changing Uganda,* Holger Bernt Hansen and Michael Twaddle, eds. London: James Currey.

———. 1997. *Questioning Misfortune: The Pragmatics of Uncertainty in Eastern Uganda.* Cambridge: Cambridge University Press.

Wolffers, Ivan. 1988. "Traditional Practitioners and Western Pharmaceuticals in Sri Lanka." In *The Context of Medicines in Developing Countries: Studies in Pharmaceutical Anthropology,* Sjaak van der Geest and Susan Reynolds Whyte, eds. Dordrecht: Kluwer.

Zola, Irving B. 1972. "Medicine as an Institution of Social Control," *Sociological Review* 20: 487–504.

PART 3

Relocating Bodies and Body Parts

7

Bodies Transported: Health and Identity Among Involuntary Immigrant Women

Lenore Manderson, Milica Markovic, and Margaret Kelaher

> Bodies that are in the way . . .
> Bodies marked to be transported, relocated, dispersed.
> —Alfonso Lingis, 1994

Discussion regarding globalization has focused conventionally on its economic rather than its political face, describing the processes concerned particularly with the movement of commodities—material and informational—across national and cultural boundaries to enable market expansion with this free flow of goods. But globalization also influences the political environment of both importing and exporting countries (e.g., the United Kingdom and Ireland and Israel). Commerce is protected by shows of muscle: political, economic, or military action legitimized by claims to the moral role of highly industrialized, democratic states to protect, in other states, individual rights, civil society, and an open market. This includes direct involvement in, and control of, economically dependent states by the richest industrialized countries via the international machinery of the United Nations, its Security Council, and its forces. Iraq and Yugoslavia are contemporary examples of countries under the UN's scrutiny. This international governmental environment is the starting point of this chapter.

Conceptually and governmentally, health extends well beyond the administrative fields as represented internationally by the World Health Organization (WHO) or nationally by ministries of health, and it is often at the periphery of medicine that the links between health and globalization are most evident. Environmental issues are one example where economic interests continue to exploit resources and intergovernment agencies lack the mechanisms to prevent or control this exploitation. Consider the political economy of the bushfires and consequent air pollution in Southeast Asia; the United States' or Australia's refusal to comply with the international measures to reduce greenhouse gas emissions; or the role of the United Nations Environment Programme (UNEP) indirectly in protecting people's health through its explicit mandate of the global management of natural and cultural environments. Or consider the use of child labor and outwork in poor countries by large multinational corporations, the efforts to regulate this within the industry and by agencies such as the UN Children's Fund (UNICEF) and International Labour Organization (ILO), and the uncertain impact on the health and well-being of children so involved when their only means of income is stripped from them (Bissell and Sobhan 1996). Or, of direct relevance to this chapter, the role of the UN High Commissioner for Refugees (UNHCR) and the UN Security Council in local economic and political conflicts that erupt into little wars of extraordinary terror and violence.

The international agencies in this action operate (and have to operate) on the basis of global culture, and at the level of the state on the assumption of a policy of multiculturalism, although, practically, there is often no such policy. That is, international policies are developed and implemented on the supposition of "one globe," within which people as well as commodities can flow with minimum disruption. In addition, it is supposed that mobile cultures carry with them certain local traditions (and language), and this difference is accommodated and even valued. Hence it is implicitly assumed that positive aspects of culture travel, but, contradictorily, that negative local features are diluted by globalization and rendered irrelevant with migration.

Australia's Humanitarian Program

The composition of the Australian population over the past two hundred years of immigration—with regard to gender, race, ethnicity, religion, and so on—has changed, bringing new health-related issues into focus. Colonization of Australia and its immigrant intake have always been closely related to international political and economic events, particularly in Europe, but more recently also in Africa, Asia, and Latin America. Local problems in other countries (e.g., economic depressions, unemployment, civil wars, dictatorial regimes) and world wars made people cross national boundaries, and Australia used these factors to its own economic and strategic advantage.

In the context of international agencies taking care of refugees, the UNHCR appeals to countries that offer resettlement to humanitarian settlers and assigns the applicants to the program of a particular country.

Industrialized countries, including Australia, respond to their humanitarian obligations by setting annual quotas for refugees. The federal government makes decisions regarding the immigrant intake, but these are political decisions, influenced by various interests such as government departments, the media, public polls, lobby groups, political parties, members of parliament, industry, unions, and the international community (Kabala 1993). In light of UNHCR guidelines, not all people who fear for their safety would fall under the refugee category, and Australia has introduced the special humanitarian (1981) and the special assistance (1991) categories in its humanitarian programs. In January 1993, the Australian government separated the humanitarian program from the migration program. Apart from refugees, other humanitarian settlers need to have community/family links in Australia who will undertake support (Australia Department of Immigration 1994).

Australia admitted refugees long before the international agencies were involved. From the early twentieth century Australia received refugees from war-torn countries[1] and, unlike most Western European countries, offered permanent resettlement in order to attract immigrants. World War I and the Russian revolution displaced persons, and Jews from Europe after 1938, were the first humanitarian settlers (Australia Department of Immigration 1994). Until 1972, as a result of restrictions on immigration under the White Australia Policy, the people who arrived both as refugees and as economic immigrants were primarily European; thereafter, a substantial proportion of refugee and humanitarian immigrants were from Indochina. In the 1990s, in response to the current political events around the globe, many humanitarian program entrants were from the former Yugoslavia, the Horn of Africa, and the Middle East. As a result of war in the former Yugoslavia, 3.5 million people were displaced. This is the largest number since World War II (Australia Department of Immigration 1994), and Australia responded to this conflict by admitting humanitarian settlers and refugees, in addition to enabling the continued selective settlement of other immigrants from this origin.

Since the 1980s, women predominate among the settlers in Australia, but not significantly (Hugo 1994). However, the proportion of females admitted under the humanitarian program has been lower than the proportion of men in the same category (Bureau of Immigration statistical data). The introduction of "Woman at Risk" into Australia's humanitarian program in 1989 partly addressed this gender bias.[2] This category was the response of the Australian federal government to the appeal of the international body (UNHCR) to protect "refugee women in particularly vulnerable situations" (Australia Department of Immigration 1996c). The Woman at Risk category has been applied to women, with or without children, whose partners have been killed or are missing. Not all women with this experience are brought to Australia under this category, however, and Australian missions undertaking offshore assessment for humanitarian settlement are encouraged to use visa categories pragmatically. In the absence of a husband or other "responsible" male, the state assumes the role of patriarch, but subsequently takes on no special role for the well-being of these women. Yet the circumstances of immigration and resettlement indicated to us that women were still at risk physically, emotionally, socially, and economically, with implications for their own and their children's health.[3] Social networks reduce the risks of immigration (Tilly 1990). These women by definition lack them, and this affects their early stages of resettlement. Vulnerability and isolation are real and possible outcomes, and for some women the risks that justified their immigration—the threats to their person—continue, even if the source of "risk" is changed and the environment different (Manderson et al. 1998). However, although the Woman at Risk program targets women without men, those with husbands are not necessarily without risk either before or after immigration. They may be exposed to maltreatment because of their husband's ethnicity, political affiliation, religious denomination, and so on (Reid and Strong 1987). Furthermore, upon immigration women with husbands may be at risk because of the violence of their husbands who were tortured in their country of origin, the trauma of their children (Pittaway 1991; Allotey 1992), or male unemployment, which affects the family dynamics, as our research has indicated.

Difficulties and adjustments are associated with resettlement for all people who come to Australia to escape war or the threat of persecution. Migration itself is a significant and life-altering event involving uprooting from a familiar social setting, severing networks, a possibly dangerous travel to a refugee camp and/or the country of destination, and ultimately adjusting to a host society (Siem 1997). Forced or involuntary movement or resettlement encompasses factors that differ somewhat from voluntary and planned migration, including because the former migrants usually have less opportunity to collect relevant information and consider all available options, advantages, and disadvantages.

Stresses of migration and resettlement affect men and women in different ways (Tyhurst 1951; Westermeyer et al. 1984; McSpadden and Moussa 1993). For some people there may be an increased risk of mental illness (Minas 1990; Klimidis et al. 1993; Minas et al. 1996); there may also be short- and longer-term physical health problems. Under war conditions, refugees and displaced persons frequently face food shortages, have limited access to medical supplies and services, live in crowded camp/temporary accommodation conditions, and are subject to assault and/or abuse both in flight and while temporarily sheltered (e.g., McSpadden and Moussa 1993:212–13; Macklin 1995:220, 226). Those who spent the war in Sarajevo lived in a divided city with restrictions on mobility and access to information, in an environment under constant shelling. Women in all environments may have experienced nutritional, gynecological, and/or mental health problems. Furthermore, although refugees like all other migrants to Australia must pass routine health assessments, including both clinical and radiological examination, and be considered well and able to work, these criteria do not include an emotional health cost associated with forced migration. In addition, health status indicators may be waived for humanitarian settlers for compassionate reasons (Australia Department of Immigration 1994).

Rationales and Methods

In this chapter, we consider the politics of identity following migration and resettlement, and how women from the former Yugoslav republics manage alternative identities in order to maximize their well-being. The selection of the study population enabled us to explore how the context of the country of emigration and the opportunities in the country of destination interplay in immigrant experiences (Grasmuck and Grosfoguel 1997). Immigrants' experience in the host country (that is, the country to which they immigrated) is affected by their prior experience of sociopolitical and economic systems, the reasons that influence their immigration decisions, their personal/social and economic position and skills, and the local conditions in their new country (e.g., labor market opportunities, availability and access to government and nongovernment organizations, the existence of established ethnic communities). Thus, immigrant health policy and service delivery in Australia may not be applicable in other countries whose immigration policy stands on different premises. Further, world health policy that targets refugees from developing countries needs to address issues other than those addressed by policies and programs oriented toward refugees fleeing from reasonably developed countries.

The data presented here were collected during 1996–1997, from fifty-two in-depth interviews and a survey among 118 women from the former Yugoslavia who arrived in Australia after the commencement of the war in 1991. In terms of their socioeconomic background, these immigrants are considered to be a different wave of immigrants compared with those who settled during the rapid expansion of Australian industry, with the 1991–1995 war providing a very different context of emigration. Participants in this study were recruited from among women resident in southeast Queensland, via snowball sampling, with introductions to women by other community members, community health and welfare workers, service providers, and personal contacts. The interviews were conducted in the mother tongue of women by the second author of this chapter, who herself is an immigrant from Yugoslavia. They addressed six major areas of interest, including:

- Immigration experience.
- Qualifications and access to employment and professional development.
- Social support and social networks.
- Relationship issues.
- Perceptions and use of health services.
- Cultural perspectives on health and maintenance of health.

The survey questionnaire derived from the Longitudinal Study of Immigrants to Australia (LSIA), Mothers in a New Country (MINC) study, the main questionnaire of the Australian national study on women's health,[4] and consultations with community workers. It contained sections on mental health, physical health and health service utilization, life events, settlement experience, and language and demographics. The questionnaire was pretested and then reviewed by multicultural workers. Questions about income were replaced by a question about health care cards (provided by the federal government to welfare recipients), and questions on eye and dental care were added. Questions on occupation, employment, social networks, and social support were also added.

Study Population

Issues of adaptation and settlement are made complex by differences in social structure and institutions in Australia, and by different cultural experiences and expectations, and are moderated by individual differences in terms of personal adaptation, resilience, responsibility for others, and resourcefulness. Such differences can include the educational and social status of women in their home country. For example, a highly educated woman from an urban center in the Middle East will, on resettlement, have rather different needs from rural women without formal education from the same region. Cultural and language similarities need to be understood against differences in worldviews, perceptions, and experiences, and these may include English-language competence, experience of travel, contact with peoples of different cultures, and interaction with the outside world, including government services and agencies.

Other humanitarian settlers in Australia (e.g., women from the Horn of Africa) arguably face greater problems than those from the former Yugoslavia in terms of adaptation to a new social and cultural environment and different language, institutions, and services; they are also less likely to have a preexisting community from which to gain information and support.

Several factors facilitate the adjustment of the study population. First, there are some similarities in the cultures of immigrants from the former Yugoslav republics and the majority Anglo-Australians. Both are part of Western (European) civilization, and share certain parts of history, values, social heritage, and way of life (Gordon 1978).[5] Second, immigrants from the former Yugoslavia have settled in Australia since the nineteenth century, and they make up the second largest non-English-speaking background group (Australia Department of Immigration 1998). They are characterized by strength of family and kin chains (Tisay 1985), and a number of authors argue that the provision of ethnic social support positively affects the settlement process (Roth and Ekblad 1993; Hugo 1994; Menjivar 1997). However, all immigrants face settlement problems. The political circumstances that resulted in flight and resettlement for women from the former Yugoslavia raise issues of the impact on health and welfare of all such immigrants, but their experiences, too, provide evidence of how globalization now functions to smooth over some of the upheavals associated with forced migration.

Immigrants from the former Yugoslavia are heterogeneous. Divisions relate to age; gender; educational and occupational backgrounds; personal, economic, and political circumstances influencing decisions to migrate; time of migration; religion; and ethnic/national identity. Basic demographics of the sample are shown in Table 7.1.

Differences in visa category overlap with these social and demographic categories. A woman's immigrant status is influenced, too, according to whether she has migrated as part of a family unit that includes a husband/partner, as a couple without other family members, or as an individual to be reunited with her family, partner, or parents from whom she was separated during the war. Women migrating alone with or without children but without partners may be either independent immigrants or immigrants covered by the gender-specific Woman at Risk visa subcategory (Manderson et al. 1998). Our data suggest that women without partners are disadvantaged in terms of health, help from the government, social support, and socioeconomic status (see Table 7.2).

Informal Social Support

The economics of migration and understandings of ethnicity are substantially different for those who came to Australia in the 1970s and 1980s and those who came more recently. Immigrants sponsored by informal networks are expected to be welcomed by their family or friends and usually access relevant government services via these networks. A sponsor should be prepared to undertake the following tasks for newly arrived settlers during the

Table 7.1 Sample Demographics

Variable	Level	Percentage
Age	Under 20 years	1.7
	20–29 years	14.4
	30–39 years	45.8
	40–49 years	22.8
	50 and above	15.3
Education	Primary	16.1
	High school	61.9
	Tertiary	22.0
Current partner	Yes	78.8
	No	20.2
Children	Yes	82.1
	No	17.9
English proficiency	Excellent/very good/good	44.1
	Fair	28.0
	Poor	19.5
	Not at all	8.5
Social Security source of income	Yes	57.6
	No	42.4
Employed women with access to commensurate employment	Yes	22.5
	No	77.5

Table 7.2 Differences Between Women with Partners and Women Without Partners

Variable	Response	Current Partner (%)	No Current Partner (%)	X^2	$pr > X^2$
Impairment of functioning due to physical health in the last 4 weeks	Yes	31.18	64.00	7.30	0.007
	No	68.82	36.00		
Finished less due to mental health in the last 4 weeks	Yes	24.18	56.00	8.46	0.004
	No	75.82	44.00		
Have nightmares	Yes	33.70	46.52	4.44	0.035
	No	66.30	43.48		
Received help from government employees	Yes	63.74	36.00	3.74	0.05
	No	36.26	64.00		
Social support-made new friends since immigrating	Yes	94.62	80.00	5.79	0.02
	No	5.38	20.00		
Social support-give help to people I socialize with	Yes	93.55	72.00	5.29	0.02
	No	6.45	28.00		
Social support-satisfied with the frequency of socialization	Yes	75.27	52.00	5.63	0.02
	No	24.73	48.00		
Earned money in Australia	Yes	57.00	24.00	5.95	0.015
	No	43.01	76.00		
Transport via own car	Yes	61.30	92.00	6.09	0.014
	No	38.71	8.00		

first two years: (a) provide support as required to enable them to attend appropriate English-language courses; (b) ensure they have adequate accommodations; (c) provide any necessary financial assistance; and (d) provide information and advice to help them settle in Australia (Australia Department of Immigration 1996b). In addition to informal support, government information is provided via a "Settlement Information" booklet (produced by the department of immigration in all states) and settlement information officers. For privately sponsored immigrants, access to information depends initially, at least, on family or friends who are very often recent arrivals themselves. However, even long-established settlers prove sometimes to be of little assistance to newcomers because different waves of immigrants have different access to resources in the receiving country, and, as Menjivar (1997) notes, the context of the social world and the immigrants' backgrounds generate different immigrant experiences. The responsibility taken on by immigrants' family/friends is enormous, and sometimes it results in friction, questioning the official supposition that immigrants with families in Australia have no need of institutional support:

> *It was very difficult living with my husband's uncle and aunt. They would not let us do anything. Since everything is new to you and they somehow helped you in coming here, you don't want to make any problems. . . . My psychological health is being ruined by the relationship with my relatives in Australia.* (Ljerka; September 12, 1996; born in Bosnia and Herzegovina; thirty-three years old; married; migrated in 1993; sponsored by her husband's uncle)

> *Our relatives rarely call us. The first night we moved here we did not have any food and we slept on the floor. . . . You can't rely on relatives. They can talk and give pieces of advice, but nothing hurts them, only us.* (Tijana; September 16, 1996; born in Bosnia and Herzegovina; thirty-eight years old; widow with two children; migrated in 1994; sponsored by her uncle)

In addition to failing to provide expected emotional support, informal ethnic networks also pass to recent immigrants inaccurate information, which unnecessarily leads to disadvantage: "In the beginning I was not registered with the CES [Commonwealth Employment Service]. My sister's husband said there was no need" (Dana; September 13, 1996; forty-one years old; Bosnia and Herzegovina; married; sponsored by her sister). This is an apparent example of a woman being discouraged from accepting assistance from a government department during resettlement, and in this case informal networks actually narrowed the alternatives of migrants (Pohjola 1991). Immediate registration with the CES is important, because depending on the number of months registered with this department, an unemployed person is eligible for different types of assistance, which increase his or her prospects for finding a job.

Government Support

Because earlier settlers are not always capable of fulfilling the role of assisting recently arrived immigrants, complementary support is needed if immigrants are to make the most of available services in Australia. These case histories have clear policy recommendations in terms of recognizing a need for complementary government support. Women appear to be dependent and expect to be fed information about entitlements from the government, rather than rely on their personal skills and sponsors. Their request for institutionally organized access to services also means that immigrants themselves want to hold the power of knowledge to access government and nongovernment support. Initially, because of low language skills and unfamiliarity with the system, women have little control over access to services, which puts them in a subordinate position in mainstream society:

> *I think that people who came through the Department of Immigration were in a better position. Sometimes people with whom you settle are not sufficiently able to assist a migrant with settlement. It's not that they don't want to, but that they don't know how. Even though my relatives came here a year before us, I think that we have solved problems and know more things than they do. If you settle with a relative, it's not a guarantee that you will get what you need. Employees from the Department of Immigration provide all information to settlers sponsored by the Australian Government. It would have been better if we had had a person from that Department. How can someone who works take you to the CES or DSS [Department of Social Security]? Those things must be done during the day, during working hours.* (Petra; November 18, 1996; born in Bosnia and Herzegovina; thirty-seven years old; married; migrated in 1995)

The Migrant Resource Center, responsible for information provision to refugees sponsored by the federal government at the time of conducting this study, lacked the resources to organize sessions for those privately sponsored. Accordingly, it was the responsibility of sponsors and immigrants to seek information.

Poor linguistic skills of women are not necessarily a barrier to seeking information independently. In theory, for the cost of a local call, women can access any agency they need with the help of the Telephone Interpreting and Translating Service. Some do not initially know of this service, however, or are not always aware that it is also a referral agency. Thus, the mechanisms of achieving an integration of immigrants into a host society need to be developed at the local level, taking into account the circumstances of emigration, available funds, and long-term consequences of barriers immigrants face in their resettlement. Unless the playing field is even for all immigrants, regardless of their particular entry category, which is ultimately only an administrative issue and does not necessarily correspond to the real context of emigration, tensions may occur between immigrants who are eligible for different types of government and nongovernment support.[6] Budgetary cuts may result in lack of government interest in advertising its programs widely, but this is a short-sighted approach because the lack of formal support in the early stages of resettlement may result in problems that are harder to deal with when they become chronic (e.g., long-term unemployment, psychological distress).

Barriers to Psychosocial Adjustment

Preimmigration Stressors

Of particular relevance to refugees and humanitarian settlers is post-traumatic stress disorder (PTSD). People who have been exposed to torture, trauma, and fear for their lives, typically associated with war, or people who have experienced violent events such as rape, abuse, domestic violence, and natural disasters, may suffer from PTSD (Kinzie et al. 1984; Reid and Strong 1987; Kalucy 1988; Tran 1993; Cheung 1994). Not all people who have had such experiences will develop PTSD, however, and age, personality, previous health, and available post-traumatic support are related to this (Thompson and McGorry 1995). PTSD is manifested through such varied problems as emotional numbness, depression, sense of helplessness, feelings of guilt, insomnia, problems in concentration, panic attacks, recollection of traumas, and nightmares. These are considered normal reactions to abnormal and severe life events. The symptoms may disappear in time without treatment, but for some victims, support from informal networks is inadequate, and the traumatic experience may have long-term effects, causing psychosomatic and mental dysfunction over many years (Reid and Strong 1987).[7]

During the interviews few women chose to recount their experiences during the war in great depth, and these issues were not pursued in the question line. Because of the sensitivity of the issue, women who participated in the survey were not asked whether they had a direct experience of war, torture, and/or trauma. However, women did report that they felt like crying all the time (59 percent) and had nightmares (38.3 percent), panic attacks (35.6 percent), and sleeping problems (34.7 percent). Although these health problems are usually identified as PTSD symptoms, some women interviewed reported suffering from them even though they had left Croatia or Bosnia and Herzegovina before the war started. Thus, even when people do not have direct experiences with war or trauma, they may still suffer from symptoms associated with PTSD (Kalucy 1988). In addition, symptoms usually associated with PTSD may derive from other causes, and in this present study they were related to women's perceived difficulties in maximizing their well-being in the host country, that is, postimmigration stressors. Women believed that service providers sometimes assumed preimmigration traumatic experience, which they considered a useful tool to discredit their postimmigration problems:

> When the tribunal called me to a commission [workers' compensation], they asked me if I was affected by the war in Bosnia. I did not understand how that related to my injury at work; anyway, I left the country before the war started. (Aida; October 30, 1996; government-sponsored refugee; a nurse in Bosnia)

This case sheds light on the interplay of gender, ethnicity, and immigrant status in women's experiences in the host country. Hence, although host countries need to introduce services for immigrants likely to have PTSD symptoms, generalizations in terms of attributing mental and physical health problems predominantly to preimmigration traumatic experiences rather than postimmigration stressors will negatively affect their well-being (see also Jayasuriya et al. 1992).

Postimmigration Stressors

Women from the former Yugoslavia share with other humanitarian settlers certain common problems: separation from normal social networks and supports; often the first time being alone, or alone with children; needing alternative forms of support for their children and themselves. Beyond the practical problems of settlement and everyday life, too, are fear for those left behind, the uncertainty of any reunion, the pain of experiences from the past, and the loss of former status and identity. In general, humanitarian immigrants have usually lost family and social networks, as well as social and occupational status, and they face social isolation due to language difficulties, cultural differences between home and host societies, lack of personal contacts, and fear (Sommers 1993). It is difficult for these immigrants to build new social networks (Allotey 1992); they experience nostalgia and suffer geographic isolation both within the new country and from family overseas and are further isolated when they are sole parents, a particular issue for woman-at-risk immigrants. However, even women with partners in Australia find it hard to rebuild their lives because members of their extended family networks could not accompany them:

> It was very hard for me when we came, because of my parents who did not have any other choice but to return to Sarajevo, and their apartment

is in a Moslem part of the city. I think about the time I spent in Sarajevo, about my parents who are there. The distance affects me . . . distance from my family. (Jana; September 4, 1996; forty-eight years old; married; migrated in 1996)

Forming alternative support networks is a central factor in resettlement. For women who migrate alone, establishing a trusted and reliable network assists in the process of resettlement and provides a source of emotional support. As Wellman and Wortley (1990) note, in traditional communities neighbors are considered to be a potentially good source of support, and people easily access them. However, due to frequent spatial mobility, people in industrialized societies may have less opportunity to develop relationships with their neighbors. Greider and Krannich (1985:68) argue that people may be "maintaining a level of polite but non-committed involvement with neighbors while withdrawing into more disaggregated and personalized social networks of social support." In addition, life orientation in contemporary societies concentrates on individualism rather than solidarity, so neighbors are not necessarily a part of informal networks.

In this study, women from larger cities in the former Yugoslav republics, especially capital cities where close acquaintance with neighbors has already begun to disappear, did not find it strange that they had little contact with neighbors in Australia. On the other hand, immigrant women who had lived in smaller towns and villages, where communal life has stayed partly intact (Suvar 1970; First 1981), experienced difficulties in adjusting to being isolated from their Australian neighbors:

We don't socialize with neighbors. We say hi to each other, which is strange to us, because we come from a country where relationships with neighbors were very well developed. Neighbors would come for a cup of coffee, a piece of cake. (Tina; August 30, 1996; lived in a small city in Bosnia and Herzegovina; thirty-two years old; married)

It is strange that you don't know your neighbors, you don't communicate with them. It's not that back at home I knew all neighbors or that I would like to visit my neighbors here every day, but it's strange that I haven't the faintest idea who lives in my neighborhood. (Tanja; September 18, 1996; single; thirty-seven years old; lived in a small city in Bosnia and Herzegovina)

Adjustment was particularly difficult for women accustomed to relying on social support from neighbors, who at the same time did not have ethnic social support. The absence of daily socialization with people from their country of origin/ethnicity was predominantly related to spatial dispersion of community members, which for many women made Australian-born neighbors the only potential source of social support. Accordingly, they were particularly disappointed that their neighbors showed no interest in their well-being:

> *Australians do not mix with their neighbors. I don't know whether they don't like to have contact, or that's their mentality, or they don't like foreigners. I remember when I first moved in my city to another flat. Neighbors I had never seen before came on the very first day to greet me and ask me if I needed any help. When I now think about that I see that probably they came when it might have not been suitable for me, but it still shows our [ex-Yugoslavians'] warmth as a people. Here, none of my neighbors even say hello to me. Once, I asked a neighbor to come to my place to help me with a problem I had. The other neighbor did not even bother to come to the gate when I called. The other one came, she helped me, sat here for a while, but after that, she never ever said a single word to me. There were days when I was trying to greet her first, even though I am older, but she was just keeping her head down, as if purposely avoiding me.* (Javorka; September 26, 1996; fifty-eight years old; divorced; lives in an outer suburb with poor public transport; does not drive)

> *In the middle of the night a car hit our house. None of our neighbors came out to see what happened or if maybe we were hurt.* (Jelena; January 25, 1997; migrated without a husband; with two children; no community members in the suburb)

Migration is both an international and a personal experience. Unique strengths and weaknesses are exacerbated by a major life experience such as migration or the refugee journey. The ability of the migrant woman to interact with the new host community and form or create new social networks and support systems also is individual. Some women risk social isolation because of the commitment of their time with their children (particularly if sole parents). Others are isolated because they cannot quickly acquire new language skills, either due to lack of access to such programs or because of their inappropriateness to particular women (e.g., illiterate women). The following remarks demonstrates how, in addition to sadness because of the effects of the civil war, isolation from the society and perceived lack of social support led Javorka, the immigrant woman from Bosnia and Herzegovina quoted above, into despair and depression.

Javorka retired a few months before the war started. Instead of being surrounded with friends with whom she developed close relationships over the years, and enjoying a secure financial position, she had to migrate to Australia. This resulted in socioeconomic, environmental, and cultural changes that negatively affected her well-being:

> *I simply cannot stand this way of life in Australia. It's completely disappointed me. I don't have contact with cultural activities, civilization,*

there is no urbanization, no public transport, contacts with people. . . . Before I immigrated to Australia I always enjoyed it when we were going for a holiday and passed through mountains, hills, greenery. But now, I am sick of seeing only nature, I want the sights of the city in front of me, concrete. . . . A psychologist helped me. I was talking to her both about my sorrow for what I lost in Bosnia and problems I faced here. It's hard to plant roots in another part of the world, in a different country, among different people, on a different continent, different culture, especially at my age. . . . Too many changes have happened to me, starting from the dwelling, then the city, country, continent, environment, and I am not that young to easily overcome the sorrow. . . . I feel totally isolated. I am without neighbors, friends. . . . Weekends are the worst time in the week. They really drive me crazy. During the week you go to school and time passes quickly. On weekends I become depressed. It's not that I don't have things to do. I work in the garden, house, play with my grand-daughter, but everything is so empty, without content. . . . At home I was at a hairdresser's every Monday, before my work started. I was tidy, with makeup, dressed in fine clothes. That's Europe, that was normal for us. When I came here, I virtually became a savage. I cannot live like I was used to. . . . At the beginning I had a desire to make myself beautiful, you get used to doing so, and then I saw it was not important. . . . Who can see me here?—only the birds and the lizards. (Javorka; September 26, 1996)

Javorka believed that her mental health in Australia would have been much better if she had had friends around her to whom she could lament. However, although she managed to establish new friendships in Australia (as was the case with 91.5 percent of survey participants), she was reluctant to share her disappointment with them: "I can't share my feelings with my friends. I see around me people who are in the same situation as I am. Nobody wants to put their load on to another person. You try to spare others from your problems, because they can't help you, they have their own problems." (Javorka; September 26, 1996)

Socioeconomic Adjustment

Differences among immigrants in various ways all complicate the process of resettlement and adaptation, with impact on women's mental and sometimes physical health. Financial hardship and economic vulnerability, for which the social welfare provides a "safety net," introduces a further element of dependence on the state. In general, sociodemographic differences pre- and postimmigration appear to affect women's health after arrival in Australia. A logistic regression was conducted comparing women who had reported that their health had worsened since arrival to women whose health had stayed the same (see Table 7.3). Socioeconomic status in Australia appeared to be an important determinant of women's self-perceived

Table 7.3 Logistic Regression Comparing Women Whose Health Has Deteriorated Since Being in Australia and Women Whose Health Has Stayed the Same or Improved

Variable pr	Response	Deteriorated (%)	Same/Improved	X^2	OR 95%	CI
Long term condition	Yes	88.64	82.43	0.81	0.09–2.42	0.37
	No	11.36	17.57			
Source of income—social security	Yes	75.00	47.30	5.31	1.19–9.00	0.02
	No	25.00	52.70			
Transport via own car	Yes	18.18	46.52	4.44	0.09–0.94	0.04
	No	81.82	43.48			
Problems communicating with doctors	Yes	50.00	17.14	7.67	1.51–11.5	0.01
	No	50.00	82.86			

health. Women who believed that their health had deteriorated were more likely to have a social security benefit as a source of income and were less likely to have a car.

As a widespread phenomenon in highly industrialized developed countries, unemployment has attracted attention in relation to its implications on health. Studies in Australia and elsewhere have documented that the unemployed have a higher prevalence of physical and psychological morbidity, and that they are at greater risk of death (Kerr and Taylor 1992; Bartley 1994;[8] Hammarström 1994; Ferrie et al. 1998). The consequences of unemployment include stress, a sense of worthlessness, poverty, and social isolation. An unemployed person loses social status, his or her personal contacts shrink, consumption patterns differ from those of the employed, and there is no sense of belonging to society (Kerr and Taylor 1992). Accordingly, anxiety, depression, disturbed sleep, nervousness, and so on occur.

Women in our study also identified unemployment as one of the main negative events that followed immigration to Australia. Survey results indicate that 73 percent of women were unemployed, and it was the case with 24 percent of women immediately before immigration. Other studies (Inglis et al. 1992; Macintyre and Dennerstein 1995) have also confirmed that immigrant women consider unemployment a reason for being dissatisfied with life in Australia. It is hard for women to accept a sudden change in their socioeconomic position. Immigrants came to Australia planning to work, and unemployment results in a sense of great disappointment, because opportunities for enriching one's life are limited:

> People here are very nervous. You feel you are worthless. You can't find a job. . . . You know you do not need to be on welfare, you know you are capable of working. You want to work but the circumstances are against you. (Tina; August 30, 1996; high school; twelve months unemployed)

It's hard for me because I don't work. If I were working it seems to me that I would be better, feel healthier, it would be easier. I would be psychologically healthier. When you are at home you work from day to day doing the same thing. You think about problems, about the worst. If I were working . . . even at a routine task filling out forms . . . you keep thinking about the situation in Yugoslavia. (Mila; September 2, 1996; a professional cook; thirteen months unemployed)

I am in prime age for working and not sitting at home. When you work you have money, you can buy things you need or like, travel, see new things. A lot of things are beyond my income: I can't afford them. (Jadranka; December 16, 1996; an entrepreneur in Bosnia and Herzegovina; during two years in Australia, only a three-month job from which she was sacked)

On the other hand, women unable to find work similar to that which they did prior to immigration resorted to noncommensurate employment. Immigrants were motivated to undertake employment in order to achieve economic security. This is a coping strategy among humanitarian settlers and refugees who came without material means of subsistence (Hauff and Vaglum 1993). Thus, the circumstance of their immigration made them choose noncommensurate employment, rather than devote time to other activities, such as acquiring higher education or gaining new skills, which in the longer term may offer them a better alternative. In many cases, social displacement due to unemployment and underemployment has negatively affected women's mental health:

I am an economist, but I was working as a cleaner. That made me feel very unhappy, I was crying and going to work. I felt like a woman of a lower value. (Dana; September 13, 1996)

I owned a shop in Bosnia and Herzegovina. I was always a boss and now the time has come for me to become a servant. I had never been in a position to beg for something. I was the one to whom other people were coming. (Jadranka; December 18, 1996; was employed as a hotel cleaner)

Women hoped to find in Australia what they lost due to a civil war, that is, a life full of good events, friends with whom to socialize, support in everyday chores, and a way of putting behind bad memories. Instead, they experienced displacement in Australian society: spatial, as a result of affordability of housing in outer suburban areas with inadequate public transport, and social, as a result of unemployment and underemployment. Accordingly, their mental health worsened. Because unemployment, noncommensurate employment, geographic isolation, and so on have a negative impact on health, it is necessary when developing immigrant health policy in Australia and elsewhere to move from the narrowly defined medical connotations of health. Concrete circumstances in a particular country will delineate policy needs in this regard.

Limits of Formal and Informal Support

Survey results indicate that 12.7 percent of women believe that if they were in need, they would lack social support. However, social support is multidimensional and relates to the individual's perception of available people who can be called upon for a particular reason, such as information, instrumental help, or emotional support (McColl et al. 1995). In interviews, women indicated the reasons behind their perceptions of unavailability of social support. Most problems among immigrant families derive from economic stress, and respondents tried to avoid "burdening" network members, to minimize further stress on them, by not asking for support (Wellman and Wortley 1990:568). In addition, given that most families establish horizontal ties, that is, ties with people from similar economic background who are themselves subjected to financial difficulties and associated mental health problems, immigrants perceive that members of their informal networks are incapable of providing support (Ball 1983). Hence, social support from informal networks has limited effects on the well-being of recipients (Janes 1990; Oakley et al. 1990; Smith et al. 1993), as our data show. This has implications for settlement policy in general and in wider terms of immigrants' well-being. However, only qualitative research on immigrants' settlement experience in the particular host country provides an understanding of the factors people identify as threatening their well-being, which will determine policy at the level of the country, state, and urban-rural area.

Isolation from the community as a whole and/or from fellow immigrants from the same language/ethnic group is, for some women, self-imposed, the only means by which they believe they can move outside the politics of ethnicity and the personal tragedies so engendered. Other immigrants believe that crossing national boundaries does not necessarily or automatically narrow other gaps that exist among people who have fled a common country of origin. Ethnic identity, which became important with the rise of nationalism in the former Yugoslavia and eventually resulted in war, is a base for divisions among recent immigrants and ultimately leads to lack of social support. Women from mixed marriages and those who do not want to take sides in the ethnic conflict feel isolated from their fellow countrymen:

> *School was a way of meeting friends. However, the political situation [back home] affects people here. We (her husband and herself) were seeking company, we felt isolated.* (Dana; September 13, 1996; Croatian married to Serbian)

Even new immigrants from the former Yugoslavia separate from each other:[9]

In school groups are formed. I was always alone during breaks in school. (Tijana; September 16, 1996; survived in Sarajevo due to help from a friend of different ethnic origin)

In the beginning I was reserved toward Bosnians, because of the fear we all brought with us, because we were not familiar to each other. Eventually, you find countrymen who you think suit you best. (Diana; January 7, 1997; Muslim from Sarajevo)

At the same time, often working against the value of preexisting social networks and communities, immigrants hold a range of expectations of migration. Consider the expectations of a Serbian who immigrated in order to put ethnic conflict behind her, who must come to terms now with the condemnation of Serbs from the international and the Australian-Croatian and Bosnian (Muslim) communities, and who must make assessments about the representation of the conflict.[10] Or consider the couple of a mixed marriage who encounter prejudice in Australia similar to that which they would have faced had they not migrated. Given that governments in Australia fund ethnic community projects, this has implications on service utilization. Individual immigrants who do not want to "find themselves labeled as belonging" (Pettman 1995:77) to particular communities, because of discrimination they encountered or witnessed toward other ethnic groups in their country of origin, may lack access to government and nongovernment support. Accordingly, it may well be that ethno-specific services are counterproductive for the well-being of immigrants (Jayasuriya 1993).

Conclusion

Governments are confined by the instruments and mechanisms under which they operate. The humanitarian visa categories are the effective intellectual technology of government that manages the legal and political processes of assisting humanitarian applicants to Australia. These categories are signposts to the possible needs of people once they begin settlement in Australia but neither predict nor describe those needs. As already noted, women entering Australia as part of its humanitarian program are not a homogenous group in terms of their presettlement history or ease of resettlement, and this is the case regardless of commonality of social or cultural background prior to migration. Migration is a unique experience for each individual involved. Although themes of migration are similar for many women and their families, it is difficult to generalize their experiences, perceptions, and reactions.

Learning the language, arranging schooling for children, gaining employment and securing an adequate income to meet family needs, recognition of qualifications or possible retraining, and organizing housing, health care, and services are some of the basic needs with which women (and all immigrants) must deal. Although they are often mundane and routine tasks, they are complicated because of the inability to communicate, unfamiliarity with the system, transport barriers, and family obligations.

The emphasis on economic processes and technologies somewhat overdetermines the role of the large highly industrialized states and multinational corporations, while ignoring other political media that sustain globalization. We have noted already the roles (not always effective) of international agencies, and it is important to acknowledge there were important rehearsals of the notion of one-world government pre-World War II (via the League of Nations, especially, although also, of course, via European imperialism).[11] Raw material, capital, manufactured produce, and communication systems are the tools of globalization, but so too is the movement of people, directly as dictated by the varying labor force needs at different sites, or by the movement of people in the consumption of leisure and cultural tourism, or as a consequence of international agency.

In this chapter, we have focused on women caught up in the processes of global government, regionalization, and notions of universal moralities. These moralities are that human rights exist for and are similarly recognized regardless of gender, age, race, or class; that the protection of these rights is a global responsibility that overrides national and cultural boundaries; and that those not caught up in local conflicts or local cultural and political environments have the right to comment and act upon perceived human-rights breaches. Global movements against human rights, such as limits of agency, unjust internment, and violence against the person (e.g., Amnesty International), or against specific practices and controls (e.g., female genital mutilation), assume this moral imperative and responsibility. In the face of breaches, particularly those that threaten to destabilize the wider economic and political sphere, or that are flagrant and horrifying breaches of common ethics, other countries and/or international forces may intervene and, where this occurs, take responsibility for the welfare of individuals directly affected by such circumstances. Hence the moral basis of the machinery of humanitarian resettlement and the organized movement of peoples. However, as we have argued, this does not take account of the difficulties that follow when governments cede duty of care after the migration of individuals.

Notes

1. Although the policy was motivated by humanitarian concerns, there were also distinct economic advantages for Australia, which faced labor shortages during a period of rapid industrialization.

2. According to Macklin (1995:216), the Netherlands was the first state to acknowledge gender-specific aspects of persecution. The UNHCR introduced Guidelines on the Protection of Refugee Women in 1991, and the Canadian Immigration and Refugee Board (IRB) introduced its Guidelines on Women Refugee Claimants Fearing Gender-Related Persecution in 1993. Guidelines on Gender Issues for Decision Makers were introduced in Australia in 1996 (Australia Department of Immigration 1996a) and supplement the understandings of gender that were already reflected operationally in the visa subclass of Woman at Risk.

3. We are very grateful to Kerrie McManus, who first drew our attention to the problematic nature of the Woman at Risk category.

4. The study was jointly undertaken by the University of Newcastle and the University of Queensland and was funded by the Australian Commonwealth Government (Brown et al. 1996). The University of Queensland research was conducted with populations who would be underrepresented in the national cohort study because of their small size and demographic structure, and probable low response rates to the standard mail questionnaire. This included indigenous and non-English-speaking background communities.

5. In a study of ex-Yugoslavian refugees who lived in Dutch households, Van Leer (1997:7) noted that "cultural differences were mostly denied by hosts and guests alike."

6. People arrive under different visa categories depending on circumstances at time of application to migrate: where they were geographically at a particular time (determines status), and other considerations such as health and personal history. Entrants arriving under the categories of 200 (refugee), 203 (emergency rescue), or 204 (woman at risk) are fully funded and are referred directly to DIMA (Department of Immigration and Multicultural Affairs) to participate in settlement programs. People in the 202 category (global special humanitarian program) may be referred to CRSS, but must pay their own airfares. People who arrive under the 209 category (special assistance category—SAC) from former Yugoslavia (for persons considered to be in special need but not meeting the definition of refugee) go directly into the community without any formalized activities/programs provided.

7. In a study on Latin American refugee women in Western Australia, Allotey (1992) revealed that women whose husbands were tortured were more likely to be abused by them, which points to the fact that the health of family members of a person diagnosed with PTSD may deteriorate as well.

8. Although poor health may result in unemployment, longitudinal studies have demonstrated that unemployment causes poor health (e.g., lung cancer, ischemic heart disease) (Bartley 1994).

9. The point implied in this comment is that frictions between earlier settlers from the former Yugoslavia existed because some were political refugees rather than economic immigrants. The other example is the conflict between communities in the early 1970s, when Croatians (*ustashi*) in Australia developed military camps in order to send soldiers to fight for the independence of Croatia.

10. A Serbian journalist gives an example of the Australian magazine, *The New Weekly*, in which, under a picture of the destroyed bridge in Mostar, there is text implying that it was blasted by the Serbs, whereas in fact it was ruined by the Croats during the fight for this city with the Muslims. Later the magazine apologized for this mistake, stating that this information was forwarded "by a *leading European news source*" (Gladanac 1995:49; emphasis in the original).

11. With regard to international health government, see Weindling 1995.

References

Aboagye-Kwarteng, T., L. Manderson, and R. Msiska. 1997. "Reviews and Strategic Planning for HIV/AIDS Prevention and Care: Anthropology and the Expanded Response to AIDS," *AIDS and Anthropology Bulletin* 9(2): 1, 8–10.

Allotey, P. 1992. "Perceived Health Status, Health Needs and Utilisation of Health Services Among Latin American Refugee Women in Perth." M.Med.Sc. diss., University of Western Australia.

Altman, D. 1995. "The New World of Gay Asia." *In Meridian: Asian and Pacific Inscriptions,* Surendrini Perera, ed. Melbourne: Meridian Press.

Australia Department of Immigration and Multicultural Affairs. 1994. "Refugees and Humanitarian Issues: The Focus for Australia." Canberra: AGPS.

———. 1996a. "Guidelines on Gender Issues for Decision Makers for Refugee and Humanitarian Visa Applicants." Internal document. Canberra: DIMA.

———. 1996b. "Department of Immigration and Multicultural Affairs, Migrating to Australia: Sponsorship." Form 961i, McMillan Print.

———. 1996c. "Woman at Risk." Information Sheet 965i. Canberra: DIMA.

———. 1998. "Population Flows: Immigration Aspects." Canberra: DIMA.

Ball, R. E. 1983. "Family and Friends: A Supportive Network for Low-Income American Black Families," *Journal of Comparative Family Studies* 14(1): 51–65.

Bartley, M. 1994. "Unemployment and Ill Health: Understanding the Relationship," *Journal of Epidemiology and Community Health* 48(4): 333–337.

Bissell, S., and B. Sobhan. 1996. "Child Labour and Education Programming in the Garment Industry of Bangladesh: Experiences and Issues." Education Section, Occasional Papers. Bangladesh: UN Children's Fund.

Brown, W., L. Bryson, J. Byles, A. Dobson, L. Manderson, M. Schofield, and G. Williams. 1996. "Women's Health Australia: Establishment of the Australian Longitudinal Study of Women's Health," *Journal of Women's Health* 5(5): 467–472.

Cheung, P. 1994. "Posttraumatic Stress Disorder Among Cambodian Refugees," *International Journal of Social Psychiatry* 40(1): 17–26.

Eisenbruch, M. 1991. "From Post-Traumatic Stress Disorder to Cultural Bereavement: Diagnosis of Southeast Asia Refugees," *Social Science and Medicine* 33(6): 673–680.

Ferrie, J. E., J. Shipley, M. G. Marmot, S. Stansfeld, and G. Davey Smith. 1998. "The Health Effects of Major Organizational Change and Job Insecurity," *Social Science and Medicine* 46(2): 243–254.

First, R. 1981. *Seoska porodica danas: kotinuitet ili promjene* [The rural family today: continuity or change], Institut za drustvena istrazivanja Sveucilista u Zagrebu, Zagreb.

Gladanac, Z. 1995. "Media Misrepresentation of the War in the Former Yugoslavia and Tudjman's Book and Jasenovac." In *Responding to the Serbs: A Challenge to the Multicultural Ethos,* Serbian Conference Papers, July. St. Albans: Australian-Serbian Community Services Inc., 49–54.

Gordon, M. M. 1978. *Human Nature, Class, and Ethnicity.* New York: Oxford University Press.

Gove, S., and G. H. Pelto. 1994. "Focused Ethnographic Studies in the Programme for the Control of Acute Respiratory Infections of the World Health Organization," *Medical Anthropology* 15(4): 409–424.

Grasmuck, S., and R. Grosfoguel. 1997. "Geopolitics, Economic Niches, and Gendered Social Capital Among Recent Carribean Immigrants in New York City," *Sociological Perspectives* 40(3): 339–363.

Greider, T., and R. S. Krannich. 1985. "Neighboring Patterns, Social Support, and Rapid Growth: A Comparative Analysis from Three Western Communities," *Sociological Perspectives* 28(1): 51–70.

Hammarström, A. 1994. "Health Consequences of Youth Unemployment: Review from a Gender Perspective," *Social Science and Medicine* 38(5): 699–709.

Hauff, E., and P. Vaglum. 1993. "Integration of Vietnamese Refugees Into the Norwegian Labor Market: The Impact of War and Trauma," *International Migration Review* 27(2): 388–406.

Hugo, G. 1994. "Demographic and Spatial Aspects of Immigration." In *Australia Immigration: A Survey of the Issues,* 2nd edition, Mark Wooden et al., eds. Canberra: Bureau of Immigration and Population Research, AGPS.

Inglis, C., J. Elley, and L. Manderson. 1992. *Making Something of Myself: Educational Attainment and Social Economic Mobility of Turkish-Australian Young People.* Canberra: Department of the Prime Minister and Cabinet, Office of Multicultural Affairs, AGPS.

Iredale, R., C. Mitchell, R. Re-Pua, and E. Pittaway. 1996. *Ambivalent Welcome: The Settlement Experience of Humanitarian Entrant Families in Australia.* Canberra: Department of Immigration and Multicultural Affairs.

Janes, C. R. 1990. *Migration, Social Change, and Health: A Samoan Community in Urban California.* Stanford: Stanford University Press.

Jayasuriya, L. 1993. "The Facts, Policies and Rhetoric of Multiculturalism." In *Four Dimensional Social Space: A Reader in Australian Social Sciences,* 2nd ed., T. Jagtenberg and P. D'Alton, eds. Pymble: Harper.

Jayasuriya, L., D. Sang, and A. Fielding. 1992. *Ethnicity, Immigration and Mental Illness: A Critical Review of Australian Research.* Canberra: Bureau of Immigration Research, AGPS.

Kabala, M. 1993. "Immigration as Public Policy." In *The Politics of Australian Immigration,* J. Jupp and M. Kabala, eds. Canberra: Bureau of Immigration Research, AGPS.

Kalucy, R. S. 1988. "The Health Needs of Victims of Torture," *Medical Journal of Australia* 148(7): 321–322.

Kerr, C., and R. Taylor. 1992. "Grim Prospects for the Unemployed," *Australian Journal of Public Health* 16(4): 338–339.

Kinzie, J. D., R. H. Fredrickson, R. Ben, J. Fleck, and W. Karls. 1984. "Posttraumatic Stress Disorder Among Survivors of Cambodian Concentration Camps," *American Journal of Psychiatry* 141(5): 645–650.

Klimidis, S., G. Stuar, I. H. Minas, and A. W. Ata. 1993. "Immigrant Status and Gender Effects of Psychopathology and Self-Concept in Adolescents: A Test of the Migration Mobility Hypothesis," *Comparative Psychiatry* 35(5): 393–404.

Lingis, A. 1994. *Abuses.* Berkeley, Los Angeles: University of California.

Macintyre, Martha, and Lorraine Dennerstein. 1995. *Shifting Latitudes, Changing Attitudes: Immigrant Women's Health Experiences, Attitudes, Knowledge and Beliefs.* Carlton, Australia: Key Centre for Women's Health, University of Melbourne.

Macklin, A. 1995. "Refugee Women and the Imperative of Categories," *Human Rights Quarterly* 17(2): 213–277.

McColl, M.A., H. Lei, and H. Skinner. 1995. "Structural Relationships Between Social Support and Coping," *Social Science and Medicine* 41(3): 395–407.
McSpadden, L. A., and H. Moussa. 1993. "I Have a Name: The Gender Dynamics in Asylum and in Resettlement of Ethiopian and Eritrean Refugees in North America," *Journal of Refugee Studies* 6(3): 203–225.
Manderson, L. 1981. "Cultural Aspects of Loss and Grief," *New Doctor* 21: 33–36.
Manderson, L., M. Kelaher, M. Markovic, and K. McManus. 1998. "A Woman Without a Man Is a Woman at Risk: Woman at Risk in Australian Humanitarian Programs," *Journal of Refugee Studies* 11(3): 267–283.
Menjivar, C. 1997. "Immigrant Kinship Networks and the Impact of the Receiving Context: Salvadorans in San Francisco in the Early 1990s," *Social Problems* 44(1): 104–123.
Minas, I. H. 1990. "Mental Health in a Culturally Diverse Society." In *The Health of Immigrant Australia: A Social Perspective,* J. Reid and P. Trompf, eds. Sydney: Harcourt Brace Jovanovich.
Minas, I. H., T. J. R. Lambert, S. Kostov, and G. Boranga. 1996. *Mental Health Services for NESB Immigrants: Transforming Policy into Practice.* Canberra: AGPS.
Oakley, A., L. Rajan, and A. Grant. 1990. "Social Support and Pregnancy Outcome," *British Journal of Obstetrics and Gynaecology* 97(2): 155–162.
Pettman J. J. 1995. "Race, Ethnicity and Gender in Australia." In *Unsettling Settler Societies: Articulations of Gender, Race, and Ethnicity,* vol. 11, Daiva Stasiulis and Nira Yuval-Davis, eds. London: Sage Publications.
Pittaway, E. 1991. *Refugee Women Still at Risk in Australia: A Study of the First Two Years of Resettlement in the Sydney Metropolitan Area.* Canberra: Bureau of Immigration Research, AGPS.
Pohjola, A. 1991. "Social Networks—Help or Hindrance to the Migrant," *International Migration* 29(3): 435–443.
Reid, J. C., and T. Strong. 1987. *Torture and Trauma: The Health Care Needs of Refugee Victims in New South Wales.* Sydney: New South Wales Department of Health and Cumberland College of Health Sciences.
Roth, G., and S. Ekblad. 1993. "Migration and Mental Health: Current Research Issues," *Nordic Journal of Psychiatry* 47(3): 185–189.
Siem, H. 1997. "Migration and Health: The International Perspective," *Praxis* 86: 788–793.
Smith, C. A., C. J. Smith, R. A. Kearns, and M. W. Abbott. 1993. "Housing Stressors, Social Support and Psychological Distress," *Social Science and Medicine* 37(5): 603–612.
Sommers, M. 1993. "Coping with Fear: Burundi Refugees and the Urban Experience in Dar es Salaam, Tanzania." Selected Papers on Refugee Issues, vol. 2, M. Hopkins and N. D. Donnelly, eds. Arlington, VA: American Anthropological Association.
Suvar, S. 1970. "Kulturne promjene u selima Jugoslavije" [Cultural changes in Yugoslav rural communities], *Sociologija sela* 8(29–30): 117–129.
Thompson, M., and P. McGorry. 1995. "Psychological Sequelae of Torture and Trauma in Chilean and Salvadorean Migrants: A Pilot Study," *Australian and New Zealand Journal of Psychiatry* 29(1): 84–95.
Tilly, C. 1990. "Transplanted Networks." In *Immigration Reconsidered: History, Sociology, and Politics,* Virginia Yans-McLaughlin, ed. New York: Oxford University Press.
Tisay, L. 1985. "Yugoslav Families." In *Ethnic Family Values in Australia,* D. Storer, ed. Sydney: Institute of Family Studies, Prentice-Hall.

Tran, T. V. 1993. "Psychological Traumas and Depression in a Sample of Vietnamese People in the United States," *Health and Social Work* 18(3): 184–194.

Tyhurst, L. 1951. "Displacement and Migration: A Study in Social Psychiatry," *American Journal of Psychiatry* 107: 561–568.

Van Leer, M. 1997. "Hospitality, Inclusion and Exclusion: Dutch Households Sheltering Ex-Yugoslavian Refugees." Paper presented at the European Sociological Association Conference, University of Essex, United Kingdom, August 27–30.

Weindling, P., ed. 1995. *International Health Organisations and Movements, 1918–1939*. Cambridge, England: Cambridge University Press.

Wellman, B., and Wortley, S. 1990. "Different Strokes from Different Folks: Community Ties and Social Support," *American Journal of Sociology* 96(3): 558–588.

Westermeyer, J., M. Bouafuely, and T. F. Vang. 1984. "Hmong Refugees in Minnesota: Sex Roles and Mental Health," *Medical Anthropology* 8(4): 229–245.

8

Poverty, Pity, and the Erasure of Power: Somali Refugee Dependency

Christina Zarowsky

Globalization occurs through the interactions of institutions and discourses in particular contexts. One important set of institutions and discourses has to do with refugees and, more broadly, humanitarian aid. Interactions related to refugees and aid affect millions of people around the world every year. Local histories and circumstances are addressed through, and affected by, models and algorithms developed by transnational agencies based primarily in the West, to the extent that "refugees" are seen as a generic, global category with a common "refugee identity" and amenable to generic "durable solutions"—voluntary repatriation, settlement in the host country, or third-country resettlement, in order of decreasing desirability from the perspective of key agencies such as the Office of the United Nations High Commissioner for Refugees (UNHCR) and the donor governments that fund the agencies. Humanitarian aid is a large industry and can be examined in terms of the economic and political interests typically explored under the rubric of globalization. However, globalization is not purely economic. Comaroff and Comaroff (1997) argue that British colonialism cannot be understood solely in terms of political economy. Similarly, attention to the symbolic or cultural framework and history of humanitarian aid is essential for understanding the mechanisms through which this facet of globalization exercises its cultural, political, economic, and health effects. An important dimension of this symbolic framework is a long-standing European moral discourse of charity, based on pity.

This moral dimension of globalization is not limited to institutions that explicitly espouse moral agendas, such as the protection of human rights and provision of humanitarian aid. The justification offered for military intervention in recent wars—Kuwait, Somalia, Kosovo—was moral:

the imperative to prevent genocide, protect human rights, prevent starvation. Although each of these interventions also had important, and often overriding, economic or geopolitical implications for key actors, a moral rhetoric was essential to the mobilization of economic and political resources. In the case of refugee relief, the moral imperative is central to the existence of large institutions and global programs affecting millions of people around the world. The potential and real conflicts between institutional interests and moral objectives are recognized within the humanitarian field (Minear and Weiss 1995). This chapter argues further that moral models based on pity contribute to inequality, both in particular instances of humanitarian aid and globally. Humanitarian aid is based in historically contingent models and practices of charity, and it continues to manifest the conflicts and ambiguities present in the practice of charity over the last two to three centuries. The increasing use by humanitarian agencies of mental health language about trauma or dependency syndrome, in place of a moral language of pity and charity, does not overcome the ambivalences and inequalities integral to older models of charity. Rather, it masks them. This ambivalence toward charity and especially its recipients, and its implications for refugee well-being and the possibilities of "leveling the playing field," are often eclipsed by the urgency of humanitarian crises and by the real transfer of resources and relief of suffering that occur through humanitarian aid. The ambivalence toward beneficiaries and the role of pity in maintaining, rather than erasing, inequality are more clearly visible in the widespread concern and rhetoric over "refugee dependency."

This chapter situates current concerns about "refugee dependency" in the context of the history of charity in Europe and the United States, and in contrast to some ways in which the term "refugee" (in Somali *qoxoti* or *qaxooti*) is understood by selected populations of Somalis in Ethiopia. The rhetoric of refugee dependency and, more broadly, refugee suffering and refugee mental health tends to situate political and social processes in individual psychopathology, and it plays a role in a global process of economic and social polarization. The ways in which Somali refugees and returnees discuss refugee issues do not privilege individuals, either individual psychobiology or individual suffering. Rather, Somali refugee rhetoric emphasizes social relations, politics, and duty. Attention to this Somali discourse, and to the historical antecedents of both the rhetoric and the practices of modern humanitarian aid, may help practitioners and scholars in the Western tradition to revisit some of the assumptions at play in the global discourse of refugees, and of refugee suffering and mental health.

I argue, with Boltanski (1993), that pity—and not, say, a sense of justice—is a central dimension of the perception among Western audiences and donors of an obligation to help refugees, and of the structures and practices involved in "helping," from fund-raising to the rhetoric of "refugee dependency." As Kleinman and Kleinman (1997) argue with respect to the representation of misery in general, this centrality of pity has troubling implications. I suggest that a globalizing discourse that conflates refugee distress and experience with a view of mental health that privileges the individual, the private, and the psychological as the "really real," erases, in the process, both individual and collective identity, and history, and power. This chapter therefore addresses the specific European histories that laid the groundwork for both humanitarianism and the welfare state, and that also set out key conflicts still enacted today. This chapter also attends to the particular circumstances in which some Ethiopian Somali refugees find themselves, and through which their lifeworlds intersect with the homogenizing language of refugee relief and refugee dependency. These lifeworlds and the concerns of particular populations can serve as a foil for the scrutiny of Western assumptions, but they are primarily important in their own right.

"Refugee" and *Qoxoti*

The dominant discourse about refugees is that of Western states and the United Nations and nongovernmental agencies, through which donor interests are pursued and, at times, challenged. This discourse is based formally on international conventions[1] and treaties defining rights and obligations, and it serves as an important political arena for various actors.[2] However, the specific meanings and stakes of "refugee" and other words in the lexicon of refugee relief are constructed and contested in concrete interactions or language games, where participants bring in assumptions, memories, and expectations around words, ideas, and issues, and negotiate or hammer out new social realities and new networks of meaning (Ulin 1984:26–41). These interactions occur in many settings, including refugee camps, United Nations and agency meetings, research projects, therapists' offices, media reports, scholarly publications, and so forth. It is through these concrete language games that both "refugees" and the refugee relief system or refugee regime are made real and significant. It is also through these language games that dominant assumptions are naturalized, resisted, transformed, or rejected, by one or more parties to the interaction.

The semantic network around the word "refugee" has two dimensions or axes: (1) geopolitical, evoking words such as "nation," "borders," "migration," "sovereignty," "denationalization"; and (2) moral-experiential, having to do with rights and obligations, notions of the self, experience, and evoking words such as "persecution," "suffering," "duty," "charity," "dependency," "humanitarianism." The two axes are rhetorically and pragmatically interconnected. Both axes are important to the globalization of this word, to its institutionalization transnationally, and to its translation and practical manifestations in very different contexts around the world.

The Somali word *qoxoti* (*qaxooti*; *Xoog*—power, strength, force; *xoog ku qabsi*—conquer) is relatively new. Although I have not traced its genealogy in detail, older informants have stated that it was not used or did not apply before the wars of the 1970s and possibly the 1960s, whereas younger people simply use the word as part of their vocabulary. Historical research might reveal whether *qoxoti* was used in discussing the nineteenth-century wars of the Somali leader Mohammed Abdille Hassan against the British and Abyssinians,[3] or indeed the sixteenth-century war of Muslim expansion of Ahmed Gureh, known by Ethiopians as Ahmed Gran (see Trimingham 1965:85–91). The general sense among my informants, at least, was that this was a relatively new word referring to the relatively new phenomenon, in Somali experience, of wars between states or cities. Its meanings are shaped both by Somali notions and experiences of flight, war, justice, and need, and by outside notions and social organization—specifically, by the UN Convention definition of "refugee," and by the experience of refugee camps and refugee relief agencies. The word *qoxoti* in its strictest Somali sense may be glossed as "people who flee before the mouth of a gun" (Sidney Waldron, personal communication). It implies dislocation, forced migration, and fear, but also dispossession and poverty that are outside the normal framework of mutual assistance, or the possibility of recovery through mechanisms such as livestock raiding. Central images are of destitution on the one hand, and on the other hand of the appropriateness of looking to outsiders for assistance. The latter aspect reflects the fact that the civil and other wars in which the category *qoxoti* evolved also featured highly visible involvement by international relief agencies.

Both implicit and explicit meanings of *qoxoti* indicate the close relationship to "Western" notions of refugee. The core components of *qoxoti* are forced flight from one's homeland because of war; destitution; and a right to protection and assistance from international bodies. Emotion, politics, and duty are engaged in attempting to convey what *qoxoti* means. *Qoxoti* is a political arena as well as a definition. Affective, political, and moral aspects are variously emphasized, depending on context: who is participating, to what ends, with reference to what history.

Refugee Dependency

Refugee dependency is one of the central preoccupations of many actors on the donor side of the global refugee relief system (von Buchwald 1994). Dependency is seen as a negative psychological state, somewhere between demanding laziness and learned helplessness, which arises from being unable to pursue gainful employment or subsistence activities because decisions and survival needs are controlled by the governments or agencies controlling refugee camps (von Buchwald 1994; Murphy [1955] 1995).

The dimension of laziness reflects the continuing influence of the discourse of the "deserving poor," which characterized the debates over charity in England since the seventeenth century (Cowen and Shenton 1996; McBriar 1987; Cunningham and Innes 1998) and justified the existence of the hospitals and workhouses of Britain and the United States in the eighteenth and nineteenth centuries (Risse 1986; Rosenberg and Charles 1987; Harrell-Bond et al. 1992). Christian charity obliged the wealthy to help the poor, but the poor in turn were expected to work. Although the practice of charity in Europe in the late eighteenth and early nineteenth centuries was marked by "a widespread emphasis on the need to individualize and moralize the donor-recipient relationship through domiciliary visiting" (Cunningham 1998:6), a distinction between the destitute and the poor, and among the impotent poor, the able-bodied poor, and those refusing to work, was evident as early as 1601, with the formal codification of the English Poor Laws (McBriar 1987). A bulletin of the Charity Organisation Society (COS), an umbrella group of private charities formed in London in 1869, outlines the moral concerns central to charity debates in the nineteenth century and still visible in debates about welfare and refugee dependency today:

> The working man does not require to be told that temporary sickness is likely now and then to visit his household; that times of slackness will occasionally come; that if he marries early and has a large family, his resources will be taxed to the uttermost; that if he lives long enough, old age will render him more or less incapable of toil—all these are the ordinary contingencies of a labourer's life, and if he is taught that as they arise they will be met by State relief or private charity, he will assuredly make no effort to meet them himself. A spirit of dependence, fatal to all progress, will be engendered in him, he will not concern himself with the causes of his distress, or consider at all how the condition of his class may be improved; the road to idleness and drunkenness will be made easy to him, and it involves no prophesying to say that the last state of a population influenced after such a fashion will certainly be worse than the first. (Quoted in McBriar 1987:83)

Proponents of harsh deterrent measures assumed that the allure of evil and sloth posed grave threats to will and character (McBriar 1987:57). These concerns also characterized philanthropic endeavors in the United States. Individuals who were thought to have come upon hard times through moral error or sin—such as becoming pregnant out of wedlock—

were expected to do additional and overtly penitential work in exchange for receiving charity. For example, in the mid–nineteenth century both Massachusetts General Hospital and the Pennsylvania Hospital reduced the weekly charges—which were often paid through labor—of individuals initially admitted as venereal patients in cases where physicians discovered that they had been mistaken in the admission diagnoses (Rosenberg and Charles 1987:29).

The late-nineteenth and early-twentieth-century debates over Poor Law reform, which led to the formation of the twentieth-century welfare state in Britain, included many of the divergent positions evident today in the humanitarian field. Then, as now, some parties were strongly opposed to the characterization of the poor as lazy and ungrateful and of the charity provisions as excessive. Liberals and Socialists argued that a decent wage and livelihood were a right, but the majority view was articulated in the COS statement previously quoted (McBriar 1987; Cowen and Shenton 1996). Other characteristics of modern humanitarianism were also visible over the past two centuries: the increased moralization and individualization of charity already mentioned; an increased emphasis on the family and on either maintaining or intervening in the family unit; a view that at least some categories of the poor could be rehabilitated; and "evidence that rivalry between denominations was increasingly fought out, among other places, in the charitable arena" (Cunningham 1998:8). From the 1880s on, the terms "deserving" and "undeserving" were increasingly replaced by references to the "helpable" and "unhelpable" poor, the latter being the proper object of Poor Law relief. Although these references reflect an Enlightenment discourse of the potential perfectibility of all humans, they are more directly and explicitly rooted in Victorian Christian emphasis on self-help, and their use was explicitly moral. Key actors in the welfare debates wished to de-emphasize what were generally accepted to be the moral faults that had brought the destitute to destitution, in order to stress the presence or lack of sufficient character and will to draw oneself out of destitution.

In the refugee context, this moral discourse is usually covert. However, the emphasis on work and its salubrious or protective effects against the development of "DP (Displaced Person) apathy" (Murphy [1955] 1995) and "dependency syndrome" (von Buchwald 1994) remains, now couched in terms of offering refugees the possibility to "regain control" (von Buchwald 1994) or to be "consulted" in the planning of their care and activities (see Allen and Turton 1996 for a critical view). Though the moral discourse is less obvious today, it is so pervasive in the culture of refugee relief that critics of this notion from within the refugee regime do not cite specific examples in the literature but rather seek to disprove the general assumption (Wilson 1992). The overt model today is psychological, referring to Seligman and Maier's experiments on "learned helplessness," in which dogs in a metal cage receive electric shocks from which they cannot escape. Eventually the animals no longer try to escape, even though an exit is opened in the second part of the experiment (see, e.g., Sternberg 1995:258 for one introductory psychology textbook's treatment of this topic). "Refugee dependency" is thought to occur as the almost inevitable result of receiving rations and other forms of support from the UNHCR and other agencies in refugee camps or settlements. One author, writing on behalf of the Association of Red Cross and Red Crescent Societies, cites Seligman's own views of the relevance of learned helplessness:

> [U]ncontrollable and unforeseeable trauma seems to lead to a style of attribution of learned helplessness. This implies a cognitive, emotional and motivational disposition which favours the appearance of a passive reaction rather than initiative or a search for a solution to stress and danger. Learned helplessness, once established, can become a constant personality characteristic. (Seligman 1975:13, quoted in von Buchwald 1994:233)

However, von Buchwald is not referring to the repeated traumas that refugees may have experienced in the course of their flight, but rather stresses that

> refugees who are beneficiaries of assistance programs are often "over-institutionalized" and deprived of personal control over their circumstances. . . . Because of the lack of activities to fill their daytime hours, they may begin to lose self-confidence, and this eventually gives way to numbness and apathy. The refugees may begin to feel that there is nothing they can do to make a difference in their lives. (von Buchwald 1994:232–233)

Thus, animal experiments involving physical trauma are translated into a psychological helplessness (lack of effort to be materially "self-sufficient"), caused by the "trauma" of being given too many goods and too little work. A psychobiological mechanism is implied, in place of the more expressly moral concerns of philanthropists of the past century. This translation of animal experiments into human traumas, and then into apathy caused by a lack of daytime activities, reflects the influence of a generalized view of psychic trauma as at least analogous to, if not identical with, physical trauma (Young 1995, 1997). It reflects the implicit acceptance of individual psychobiology as the fundamental locus of causation, and hence as the appropriate level of analysis. Finally, one aspect is perhaps the most obvious from a critical perspective but almost invisible from either a medical/psychological or a "development" perspective: this model reflects the naturalization of a model of human nature based on theories corresponding to a capitalist mode of production. The "economic man" who is driven by internally generated needs and wants and who, more importantly, is independent of any social context or influence (Douglas and Ney 1998) is plainly visible. I do not wish to imply a simple functionalism or, even less, conspiracy, but it is clear that economics, politics, ethics, and medical thinking are interconnected in the most up-to-date scientific models of human behavior, as they are, in different ways and to varying degrees, in other models for explaining motivation, causation, and health.

Harrell-Bond et al. (1992) and Wilson (1992) address the notion of charity, which is central to the humanitarian dimension of the global language game of refugee relief. Harrell-Bond and colleagues argue that closer attention to traditional anthropological notions of "gift," namely, the creation of a particular relationship of debt and reciprocity between the giver and the recipient, would lead to a better understanding of the dynamics of the refugee system. Attention to social rules of gift giving might facilitate recognition of the social, cultural, and political nature of all human interaction. In particular, the relationships among refugees and various levels of donors could then be recognized as having attendant role expectations, including the expectation by donors of gratitude, compliance, and a certain degree of obsequiousness from recipients. Such a recognition might reframe both the "dependency" discourse, and condemnations of "demanding" or "dishonest" behavior by refugees. However, the absence in refugee relief discourse of the possibility of reciprocity on the part of the recipient, except for the expression of gratitude and indebtedness, suggests that gift exchange may not be a useful framework for understanding the dynamics of the system[4] beyond drawing attention to the fact that there are culturally determined behaviors expected from the recipients of gifts in any society. "Charity" may be a more useful explanatory construct than gift exchange. Charity is understood in this chapter as a form of redistribution analogous to clientage but set in motion by personal pity and altruism rather than by obligations perceived as structural.

Lemarchand (1968) and Foster (1967) stress that clientage is not primarily an interpersonal relationship, or in Lemarchand's terms a "lopsided friendship." Rather, it represents the enactments of recognized structural differences and culturally defined obligations by individuals from groups with differential access to resources. The models of charity in Late Antique and Medieval periods emphasized almsgiving as obedience to the law of God and did not imply criticism of the poor, and this view of charity as a right of the poor and duty of the rich remains the formal position of Muslim scholars today, even if the practice of charity in Islamic societies is experienced more ambivalently and more hierarchically (Kozlowski 1998). By the late nineteenth century in England, this charitable form of patronage was not seen as a structural obligation on the part of the wealthy, but rather as a gesture of generosity and kindness on the part of the donor. This vision of charity remains prevalent today.

An important component of the modern practice of charity is the emotion of pity and the mutual recognition of inequality that this emotion marks. The discourse of pity and charity invokes dyadic emotional ties, erasing the visibility of the structural inequality that makes these discourses possible. However, the practice of pity is not a private, interpersonal transaction. The long tradition of "Christian charity," of which humanitarianism is an important modern version, developed in a stratified society. Pity does not erase power differences, but reinforces them, by providing emotional and moral valuation of patron-client relationships. In Ethiopia, open appeals to pity were almost never made by even the poorest Somali refugees or returnees with whom I interacted, but were frequently made and almost always accompanied by physical gestures of subordination, such as bowing the head and making whimpering noises, by destitute Amharic returnees and beggars. Amharic society is much more stratified and hierarchical than Somali society (Levine 1974; Lewis 1961). The evocation of pity by Amharic beggars and refugees was an attempt to obtain assistance precisely through offering recognition, and reinforcement, of the stratification of Amharic society. The appeals to pity and expressions of pity by Western donors, individual and corporate, do the same thing on a global scale, but without the acknowledgment that this global society is structurally, and not simply accidentally and temporarily, stratified.

In addition to the perspective of the gift, the dependency theory sense of "dependency" could shed light on both the behaviors and relationships at issue, and the ways in which the rhetoric of refugee dependency is used.[5] Dependency theorists such as Gunder Frank (1988) argued that the requirements of capitalism led to the inevitable and unequal relationship between the center or core countries of Europe and later the United States, and the peripheral countries of the colonies. Although totalizing models of "dependency" have been rejected by many theorists, including dependency theorists (Roseberry 1988; Leys 1996), dependency theory nevertheless brings to the fore a historical and economic relationship that liberal theories systematically ignore. The invisibility of any structural economic relations between donor (center) and recipient (periphery) countries in refugee discourse in general and the rhetoric of refugee dependency in particular is striking, especially because development—which is firmly anchored in economics—is such an important context for the work of refugee agencies in poor countries. The absence of any economic analysis in refugee rhetoric stems in part from the origins of the modern refugee regime, which lie in state politics on the one hand, and theories of individual human rights on the other. This history and the position of the HCR in the UN system as *not* a development agency (Stein 1991) help to explain the reluctance of official spokespeople to accept openly the development work that, in fact, constitutes the majority of its efforts in countries such as Ethiopia. However, the absence of any structural economic analysis, despite the presence of community- and women-oriented documents (such as "A Framework for People Oriented Planning," United Nations High Commissioner 1991, and various reports and guidelines addressing the protection of women, e.g., United Nations High Commissioner 1990), also reflects the dominant development paradigm within which much refugee relief discourse remains situated, namely, modernization theory and its neoliberal avatars. In contrast to dependency theory, which emphasizes the logic and effects, at systemic levels, of a particular mode of production, modernization theories privilege individual behavior and mind-set as the preeminent locus of effect and change, even though the "conditions for takeoff" of an economy are largely systemic (such as rates of investment and transportation networks) in these same models (see Rostow 1971 for the classic exposition of what is at least clearly identified as a political, as well as economic, program: *The Stages of Economic Growth: A Non-Communist Manifesto*). Rostow's forthright agenda is much less clear in development—and refugee—discourse today. The focus on individual psychopathology in the discourse of war trauma and in the rhetoric of refugee dependency contributes to the invisibility both of structural economic and political relations, and of the interests of donors, experts, and other helpers (Bracken and Petty 1998).

Although it is acknowledged that refugees often have little choice but to accept both basic survival supplies and the extreme control of mobility and enterprise characteristic of many refugee settings in poor countries, "dependency" is nevertheless thought to occur, to be situated in the refugee, and to be a bad thing. Many social scientists have challenged this view. Kibreab (1993) states that refugee dependency has never conclusively been shown to occur in African refugee settings (see also Wilson 1992). Harrell-Bond (1986) documented how refugee relief was provided—in her words, imposed—in southern Sudan, leading to a structured relationship in which refugees were required to accept what was given, but nevertheless sought to avoid precisely this "dependency," primarily by avoiding camps or settlements whenever possible. In studies of self-settled versus scheme-settled Angolan refugees, Hansen (1990) acknowledges that "psychological dependency" did occur in scheme-settled populations. He believed that this reflected an accurate assessment of the real power situation faced by refugees. In her study of Burundian Hutu refugees in Tanzania, Malkki (1995) found two radically different modes of being a refugee. In the first, the label "refugee" and the fact of being together in a camp were critical to a population's efforts, through mythico-historical narratives, to define itself and to bring coherence as well as the possibility of collective restitution to the experience of attempted genocide. In the second, characterizing the "town dwellers," the label "refugee" was actively avoided in favor of more diffuse, cosmopolitan identities, in an effort to bring closure to the past and to facilitate the possibility of a better life in the future. The first, encamped community may be described as "dependent" in the sense that the camp and its structures and practices of control were critical to the mobilization and maintenance of a collective identity and collective project. This "dependency," however, was very different in its characteristics and its possible effects from the individual psychopathology of "refugee dependency syndrome." The outcomes of "refugee dependency" as previously discussed would seem to be more likely to fall into two groups: (1) despondent helplessness, isolation, and lack of initiative, often leading to depression (von Buchwald 1994), or (2) organized demands for continuing agency support. An organized political activism that has the experience of encampment—including its enforced "dependency"—as a core source of energy and ideology but that is directed at entirely different actors does not fit into the medicalizing model of "refugee dependency." Somali refugee experiences and rhetorics also shed new light on the discourses and practices of pity, charity, and refugee dependency. The Horn of Africa has been and continues to be the site of multiple intersecting waves of flight, migration, and return, as is also the case for other regions in Africa and elsewhere (see Lewis 1988; Markakis 1987).

There is no simple, uniform, universal "refugee experience." A catalog of some of the specific refugee movements affecting the individuals and communities with whom I interacted suggests the diversity of "refugee experience" even within apparently homogeneous categories such as "Ethiopian Somalis." My doctoral research in May-September 1995, and from December 1995 to October 1996, was directed at exploring local idioms of suffering, examining how "the refugee experience" was construed and represented by various groups of Somali refugees and returnees, in comparison with representations by development agencies and by scholars. The focus was primarily on returnees who had fled almost twenty years ago, in order to examine the historical dimension and significance of the experience of flight and return, and of the identity of "refugee." It turned out to be much less straightforward than I had thought to separate distinct episodes of flight. Fieldwork was conducted primarily with poor returnees and middle-class urban Somalis in and around the city of Dire Dawa. I also visited refugee camps populated primarily by urban refugees fleeing the conflict in the cities of the self-declared republic of Somaliland, the former British colony of Somaliland. Only a few individuals in this part of Ethiopia had been directly affected by the civil war around Moqdishu in the early 1990s. Most of those in and around the eastern Ethiopian city of Dire Dawa had experienced and fled the "Red Terror" of Mengistu Haile Mariam's Derg regime, as well as the 1978 Ogaden War between Ethiopia and Somalia. Many had also experienced and fled the relentless 1988 bombing of Hargeisa and other territories of the Isaaq clan by the forces of former Somali leader Siad Barre. In fact, a significant proportion of them had fled to Hargeisa and other areas to escape the fighting and terror in Ethiopia, only to flee back. Others, however, had instead fled to Djibouti in the 1970s, where they stayed for eight to twenty years, the last waves returning to Ethiopia in 1995 and 1996 under pressure from the Djibouti government. Other returnees had left Ethiopia in the chaos and violence accompanying the downfall of the Mengistu government in 1991, and still others left localized drought and famine before and after 1991. I spent several months working in and around one particular village, Hurso.

Hurso is home to about five thousand former fruit farmers and agropastoralists of the Gurgura clan, intermingled with and surrounded by Gurgura and Issa pastoralists and Oromo farmers. The center of the village lies along the railway, which leads from Djibouti to Addis Ababa. Here there are a few dozen mud-and-thatch shops and tea houses, and behind them are the typical Somali dome-shaped huts, some built solidly of mud, sticks, and cloth or plastic roofing, and others in varying states of decomposition as the wind and the rains tear the scraps of plastic bags, rags, and remnants of blue UNHCR tarps, which most people use for roofing. At one end of the "downtown" area (villagers refer to it as *magaala,* the city) are two large acacia trees, under which Oromo and Somali women sell tiny amounts of tomatoes, onions, fruit, and milk, and where the battered pickup trucks drop off and pick up passengers. A train leaves once a day in the direction of Addis, and in the opposite direction to Dire Dawa, some twenty-five kilometers away. The pickup trucks arrive sporadically, depending on demand from traders or other travelers who board at the town of Malka Jabdu, eighteen kilometers toward Dire Dawa. These pickups are "retired" from smuggling the mild drug *chat (Catha edulis)* to Djibouti, or have been banned from the larger city precincts because they are considered too decrepit even to travel the streets of a provincial African city. They are considered full when twenty-four passengers, with their goods, are in the bed, in the cab, and on the cab. These trucks would also be the way that sick people, or women in obstructed labor, would be transported to the hospital in Dire Dawa. The fare, one way, is 7 birr, or about 1 U.S. dollar, which represents an above-average daily wage. The trip, including transfer to another vehicle at Malka Jabdu, takes between two and four hours one way.

Around the central village, some few hundred meters away, are other homes, some in clusters, and others in groups of two or three huts surrounded by thorn fencing. A clinic with intermittent supplies of drugs, a school with intermittent supplies of teachers and materials, a new rural pharmacy, a mill, and the municipal offices—two mud-and-thatch rooms, recently expanded to three with a galvanized steel roof—are also a few hundred meters from the downtown. Behind the clinic, in the direction of the military base, is a separate string of some two dozen mud-and-thatch houses—these are the brothels that service the military base.

At the other end of downtown, immediately adjacent to the village and on either side of the railway, are the farms. These lands extend for several square kilometers, but villagers are not allowed to enter them, as the lands have been expropriated by the military. The lands are guarded by people from the surrounding area who are hired by the base. If livestock wanders onto the lands, the owners are required to pay a fine. About three hundred meters from downtown is the river, one of three all-season streams in this area. This river is the reason for this population having become increasingly sedentary over the past seventy years, gradually moving from having a few small fields of sorghum in addition to livestock, to planting orchards of citrus and mango with the assistance of Haile Selassie and of the Italian occupiers in the 1930s. The farms are held by families, and the individuals whose names are mentioned as the "owners" of the larger gardens are in fact trustees of land considered, in former times, to be available for the subsistence of extended families or entire lineages.

The village population fled almost in its entirety during the 1978 Ethio-Somali war and the subsequent confiscation of extensive orchards and farmlands by the Derg for a military base. The story of the flight and return was told by men and women, elders as well as youth who had been infants at the time. It goes as follows. In the aftermath of the war, the Ethiopian government decided to expand the military base near the village and began to expropriate farmlands. Some families were offered compensatory lands at Sodere, hundreds of kilometers away, but the majority refused. One day the military arrived. People were told to gather together. They were surrounded by soldiers who pointed their guns at the villagers, who were then asked if anyone objected to leaving. They were told to evacuate within twelve hours. Bulldozers arrived and destroyed the homes and shops, and people fled, some to Djibouti, others to Somalia, depending on contacts and the availability of transport at crossroads towns. A few stayed in the area, living in the acacia scrub forest or staying with pastoralist kin, returning to their lands and facing repeated beatings until, according to the villagers, the army realized these individuals were angry but harmless. A few families were allowed to stay, to service the military base and the train that stops in the village; these faced very strict controls on travel, visiting, and other activity during the period 1979–1991. The majority fled to Djibouti, where they stayed in UNHCR camps and, increasingly, in Djiboutiville itself, until 1988 or 1991–1995. The journey to Djibouti took between five and ten days on foot, traveling by night to avoid bombing raids by the Ethiopian air force. Refugees made their way with the assistance of Gurgura and Issa clan pastoralists in the area, who shared food and lodging and indicated the way to Djibouti for those travelers with no prior transhumance, trading, or smuggling history on which to draw for knowledge of the terrain. Villagers say that they were at risk from the Ethiopian military and from natural hazards, but not from the pastoralists residing in the area. At a time of war between Somalia and Ethiopia, interclan rivalries, which in other circumstances might lead Issa pastoralists, say, to prey on traders from another clan or lineage, were suspended in favor of the higher-level solidarity that the flexibility of the Somali segmentary lineage system allows, if necessary (see Lewis 1961). Although rape of refugee women is very common and has become of increasing international concern (Hyndman 1997; World Health Organization 1996), it was not spontaneously mentioned by my informants. When I asked directly, both men and women indicated that it did occur, and one woman in particular was named by several respondents as having been raped. However, rape was said to be a problem in Djibouti from non-Somali officials or soldiers. How much of a role is played by Somali ethnic solidarity in these assertions that it was safe for women to travel is uncertain, but blanket statements that all refugee women are raped, or that Muslim women cannot travel safely, are clearly not true in this area, where women do travel alone, frequently, over great distances.

With the fall of the Derg in 1991 came promises of the return of the farmlands, and most of the refugees returned. In 1998 the population was still waiting, negotiating, and trying to survive. Villagers identify the land as "Ahmed's garden," "Amina's garden," and so on, and express their impotent anger at watching the military "eat their lands," selling crops from expropriated orchards while allowing other orchards to become unproductive through neglect. The military base itself is critical to the survival of the village, as it is the main market for the shops, and the brothels serving the base are an important market for the firewood gathered by many villagers as their main source of livelihood. This, then, is a community that has been "repatriated" and "reintegrated," for whom, in the eyes of the refugee relief system, the identity of "refugee" has been extinguished. In the eyes of the community itself, however, the war is not yet over. In my early contacts with this community, individuals would often refer to themselves, collectively, as *qoxoti*. Responses to my asking respondents to explain what *qoxoti* means included:

> *the people who leave their home, and those who [lose] their property. Their homes are burned or [destroyed]. Those who have nothing else except Allah.*
>
> *Hurso was a big village, with many, many kinds of fruit—lemons, oranges, papayas, mangos. . . . We have a proverb: "Hurso, the Rome of the Gurgura [clan]." Today the people are returnees and refugees; women sell firewood, the life of the children is so hard. . . .* Qoxoti *means this kind of people.*

> Qoxoti *are a forced people. There was war, a bad situation was forced on them; they left their home and their property to save only their life.*

Not all wars produce refugees. Former conflicts between clans, such as those celebrated in Gurgura songs recounting wars between the Gurgura and Issa clans, are not considered to have produced *qoxoti*. In small civil wars, said the elders, you might lose your animals, then after a few months you might take another group's animals, or the elders may sit down and negotiate a peace and restitution. The wars between countries, or those in Moqdishu and Hargeisa, are different. They are city wars, or wars over land instead of animals. "War over land is hard," I was told; "if you have no land, where will you graze your animals?"

Poverty, powerlessness, and forced flight are central to the experience of *qoxoti,* and in this community, poverty is the dominant aspect most of the time. However, *qoxoti* was distinguished from two other categories characterized by poverty: *caid,*[6] or destitution, and *cabaar,* or drought, and from one radically different category, that of the person who may well "flee before the mouth of a gun," but becomes a liberation fighter. The liberation fighter has transformed his or her imposed powerlessness into power. *Cabaar,* drought, is a category also involving forced migration, poverty, and an expectation of government or agency assistance from outside the clan or local society, but it does not involve extensive fighting or war and is expected to resolve in one or two years, at which point agriculture or animal husbandry can resume. The expectation of short-term government assistance is relatively new, but has become naturalized and is now a taken-for-granted component of the semantic network around "drought."

Poverty, say these elders, can happen to anyone in any society. In the case of Gurgura Somali, "We have a culture. If someone loses his animals, he can go with his relatives to other relatives and get new animals, one by one." Relatives in the paternal line are expected to assist unexpectedly impoverished kinsmen to restock their herds. On the other hand, *qoxoti* is not only about poverty, for two closely related reasons: the dimension of sudden forced flight and the destruction of the social safety net, often in its entirety, make it impossible to resolve the crisis internally to the community. As one elder put it: "[*Qoxoti* are] not only poor, but [there was] war, or some people died, or [their] home [was] destroyed. *Qoxoti* is a sudden situation which makes both the poor man and the rich man flee."

Poverty, then, is understood to be a condition whose resolution is internal to the society. In these conversations, *qoxoti* was seen to be worse, because the conditions necessary to make resolution possible have been eliminated. However, *caid* in the strict sense—utter destitution, and not just poverty—was emphatically stated to be worse than *qoxoti* by some elders—perhaps *because* it is internal: it does not traditionally include an expectation of outside assistance as an implicit dimension of the concept. What is new and not yet naturalized in Hurso is a discourse of poverty that attempts to make moral claims on outsiders. These claims are based primarily on justice, secondarily on human solidarity and compassion, and only thirdly, angrily, on appeals to pity: "*Qoxoti* is not like a beggar; there is no shame to *qoxoti*."

Overall, however, the general gloss used in Hurso to explain *qoxoti* to me was not "those who flee before the mouth of a gun," but rather, "those who have nothing except Allah." The UN definition would fit the former gloss more closely, but this emphasis on emergency—reflected in Western legislation as well as in media reports and mental health programs that focus on the extreme, the sensational, and the horrific—masks the more widespread reality: poverty and chronic insecurity regarding basic needs such as food, without the drama that sells newspapers and relief programs. However, a bleak view of hopelessness also fails to capture the resilience and perspicacity of members of communities such as Hurso. Reactions expressed during accounts of this community's history were complex. They included a blackly humorous sense of its utter absurdity, where even those who once had thousands of fruit trees are now selling firewood—considered one step above begging in the local scheme of things. They included accounts and expressions of impotent rage—*marrora dillac*. The most frequently mentioned mood, however, was *niyed jab*—demoralization, hopelessness, brokenness. *Niyed jab* reflects the poverty in which the population lives. It reflects the openly acknowledged fact that this community has lost both the skills and the desire to live "in the countryside," as they put it, as nomads: health care, education, and farming—the core components of rural "development" goals—have been thoroughly incorporated into their notions of what constitutes a decent life, *nolol aadaminiimo,* the life of a human being. In the absence of teachers' salaries, clinic supplies, and, most important, the material and political conditions of livelihood—land, tools, seeds, livestock, and effective political representation or channels through which to press claims—they exist, for all intents and purposes, as *qoxoti*, those who once fled before the mouth of a gun and now have nothing except Allah. It is in this sense that families who had accepted compensatory lands near Sodere were stated *not* to have been *qoxoti* at the time—"They changed their homeland [and did not lose it]"—but now, having been evicted from those lands and returned "home" to their expropriated lands, are as close to being *qoxoti* as makes no difference. It is also because the cause of their poverty is identical to the cause of their flight that the villagers consider it justified to demand assistance from outsiders: they are politically and materially this poor because they were, and remain, *qoxoti.* Thus, the awareness of demoralization and the frequent discussion of this state with me did not primarily represent a statement about the emotional condition of individuals or the community. Instead, it was an accusation against those who had created or who might alleviate the conditions to which the only remaining response was *niyed jab*.

Dependency is part of this community's understanding of "the refugee experience." One woman, a tea seller, defined *qoxoti* as follows: "People who are gathered in one place and are dependent on government and the UN.... When you don't have a farm, or animals, or money, and when you are resettled and depend on the United Nations or government, that is *qoxoti*."

These definitions in terms of dependency, as well as the shifting among the terms *qoxoti, caid,* and simple poverty (*miskin*), are at once statements of fact, and not entirely explicit moral judgments. They are not judgments, however, of the psychological condition or degree of entrepreneurship of refugees or the poor. Rather, they are judgments of who should bear collective responsibility for the existence, and hence for the resolution, of a life they describe as "the last poverty."

Having said that, it must be added that the *rhetoric* of dependency was also used by my Gurgura interlocutors. When I asked what they thought of the comment that Somalis are lazy and just want to sit and eat rations, one elder said:

> There is a tribe which is very interested to get rations—Ogaden like to be *qoxoti* because they don't have farmlands, they have only camels. Nomads all want rations. If nomads hear there are rations, they will go and get rations. Ogaden were offered resettlement—they didn't take it. We have returned here and no one has given us rations or resettlement and we are surviving. We believe in work and Allah only.

This statement was delivered in a rhetorical style that was different from the general tone of our interview. It was a praise-song for the sedentarized Gurgura. More important, it was a political salvo in an ongoing struggle for power and representation among Somali clans in Ethiopia. On examination, however, this statement is different from a similar statement summarizing much of the rhetoric about dependency, which might go as follows: "If people hear there are rations, they will go and get the rations and stay in camps forever, refusing to be independent." The Gurgura elder's statement, even though intended to be disparaging of another clan and mode of subsistence, suggests a pragmatic resourcefulness more than an unenterprising dependency. It is also a sophisticated use of refugee relief system rhetoric, demonstrating the domestication of this global discourse into a new tool of local politics.

"Pull Factors" and Repatriation

One setting in which the meaning of "refugee" is contested is a holding camp for returnees—returning refugees—in the city of Dire Dawa in eastern

Ethiopia. The "returnee camp" (officially known as a "reception center") in question involves a three- to five-day stay in a soccer field belonging to the railway company managing the Djibouti–Addis Ababa railway, the construction of which in the early 1900s was the impetus for the development of Dire Dawa as a major Ethiopian city. Between September 1994 and November 1995, an official total of 11,682 families with 39,038 members were assisted to repatriate to Ethiopia through Dire Dawa (UNHCR Sub-Office Jigjiga Situation Report, December 19, 1995). On most Monday and Thursday nights in June through August 1995, a train would arrive in Dire Dawa between 9 P.M. and 2 A.M., carrying about a thousand refugees who had registered for repatriation in Djibouti. After a twelve- to fourteen-hour train ride across the semidesert, they would be met by representatives of UNHCR, the World Food Programme, and the Ethiopian Administration for Refugee and Returnee Affairs—the implementing partner of UNHCR. The returnees would make their own noisy, chaotic, and fearful way to the parking lot, where large trucks had been contracted to take them to the stadium. At the train station and over the following days at the stadium, complaints about thieves on the train and at the station were frequently heard. A number of scuffles occurred during the three nights that I went to observe the arrival of returnees.

On arrival at the stadium, families and groups of returnees would set up makeshift tents with the HCR tarps they had received in Djibouti along with 180 birr (U.S.$30.00) as part of the repatriation package. This making camp would often occur during a thunderstorm, as the summer months are the rainy season. A few hundred people could also fit in the large tent hall that had been set up for that purpose by the agencies and was left standing semipermanently. Local vendors sold tea, biscuits, and snacks, and families also cooked what they had brought with them or could buy in Dire Dawa, over kerosene stoves or fires fueled by wood purchased from other vendors. The next morning and for the following days the locus of structure and control was different. Vendors and family groups continued their business, but the focus of attention and the dominant organizing institution were no longer the returnee groups, but the distribution setup.

First, one or two aid workers began registering returnees, checking their names and photos on the Djibouti refugee cards against the list of returnees that had been faxed from Djibouti. Next, heads of households could go either to collect their ration—fifty kilograms of wheat and ten kilograms of lentils per person registered on that household's card—or to collect a further 30 birr (U.S.$5.00) cash payment. The food distribution was also checked against the lists of returnees and against the inventory in the storage sheds, and was distributed by local young men who had been hired for the job. This distribution was noisy and chaotic, with frequent complaints that the agencies were holding back goods, and occasional fights as individuals were accused of theft. Returnees had been promised nine months' rations. The agencies decided to give three months' worth in Dire Dawa, and the remainder later at the destination sites, in order to encourage people to leave the city. Many returnees were furious, as the rations were clearly insufficient for nine months, and there was no oil or sugar.

The cash distribution occurred on the terrace in front of the stadium cafeteria. Two officials sat at a table under the large acacia tree, while returnees lined up according to destination, under the supervision of guards armed with clubs or guns. At the table, the name would be checked again, and then one of the officials would take the hand of the returnee to make a fingerprint and stamp this signature next to the name, indicating receipt of the cash. Eye contact was almost never made. When I asked why the individuals did not do the stamping themselves, it was explained that they couldn't read, the lines on the paper were narrow, and time was short. Sometimes cash or food would run out because of problems elsewhere in the pipeline, and people would have to wait, with explanations circulating by rumor.

After receiving their package, returnees would arrange their own transport to their destination, with rumor or local middlemen supplying information about renting trucks or other vehicles. After each distribution, a small number of families would remain—they claimed to have lost their cards, or to have been omitted from one or another list. There was no formal complaint mechanism—individual appeals to whoever looked official (or white) were the norm, and individual reconsideration and resolution would occur. Some individuals stayed because they had spent the cash on food or other goods and could not afford transport to their destination. Individual appeals from these people also continued.

In addition to several dozen informal and about thirty-five semistructured interviews, I attempted to do a more formal survey, asking every third person in line for the cash payment to complete a brief verbal questionnaire. Of 119 respondents, only 28.5 percent explicitly offered war, famine, and the like as the reason for having left Ethiopia. The remaining respondents would thus usually be labeled "economic migrants." However, only about 15 percent could be thought to have "chosen" to go, that is, to have had the choice of staying and surviving. There seemed to be a clear distinction between those who wanted to improve their socioeconomic status, and those who believed that they could not survive in Ethiopia and had heard that life was possible in Djibouti. This is reflected in the answers to the question, "How did you make a living in Djibouti?" A third of the sample found regular jobs—17 percent as domestic servants, and 17 percent as mechanics, waiters, teachers, masons, and so on. In some of the longer interviews, I learned that young girls who worked as servants were often paid only part of the agreed salary, and sometimes nothing at all. Another third survived on the margins of the productive economy doing "odd jobs and selling," which included portering, sorting and selling garbage, selling plastic bags, begging and then selling bread, as well as irregular casual labor. Another 12.6 percent relied on relatives, and 16 percent said they survived by begging.

Five out of the 119 said that they had gone to Djibouti a few days or weeks previously with the express purpose of becoming registered as refugees—more precisely as voluntary returnees—in order to get ration cards and the repatriation package, and 11 percent of respondents identified the repatriation package as their chief motivation for returning to Ethiopia at this time. Aside from the 5 who had deliberately become official "refugees," only 2 out of the 119 identified having been UNHCR refugees, that is, having gone to refugee camps or sought UNHCR assistance. This low rate is supported by the answers to various probe questions in the longer questionnaire. This is not to say that hardly anyone was ever in refugee camps in Djibouti—tens of thousands were—but since at least the mid-1980s, Ethiopians had actively avoided the camps, which were seen as a major limitation on their economic and social possibilities. People registered as refugees and staying in camps were forbidden to work or travel elsewhere in Djibouti, in part because the refugee population represented a very large demographic and hence economic influx into a country whose entire population is estimated at less than one million.

One of the longer interviews was with Khadija, a twenty-eight-year-old woman who was accompanied by five children and was six months pregnant at the time of the interview, in July 1995. Khadija was married and mentioned her husband during the interview, but decisions related to her family's welfare and to the use of the repatriation package appeared to be made by her. Khadija did not want to return to Ethiopia, but the Djiboutian government said that if they didn't go back, there would be trouble. The family had gone to Djibouti four months prior to the interview. Here is an excerpt from the interview:

> Christina: *Why did you go to Djibouti?*
> Khadija: *The livestock died in a drought—we went to Djibouti to get some money.*
> Christina: *Why did you leave Ethiopia?*
> Khadija: *In Djibouti, even if you live like a beggar you get something to eat; here everyone is poor and you get nothing.*
> Christina: *Why Djibouti?*
> Khadija: *In Somalia, to get anything, I have to work; in Djibouti I don't have to do anything. I heard that children grow well. People come from Djibouti and they look rich.*
> Christina: *What did you do when you first got to Djibouti?*
> Khadija: *I made brooms out of sticks. Then I started to sell vegetables, then stopped because the government threw away everything we had, then got back to broom making.*

Neither individuals nor any relief agencies contacted her, but the police did.

> Christina: *How?*
> Khadija: *They came and bulldozed our shack as soon as we got to Djibouti. Then we slept by a wall for a few weeks, then we built a small house by the sea for three months, then the place was burned by the government because we were told that that land had been bought by Arab agencies. Then there was an announcement to go register yourself and go back. They made an announcement to leave. Since we didn't have Djibouti cards we went to the stadium to go home. We were there for six days. This was decided between the governments. . . . When the announcement was made we went to the stadium for six days, [then] to Shabelle camp for one night, waiting for the train to Dire Dawa. We couldn't stay any longer in Djibouti.*

The reasons Khadija offered for choosing Djibouti would seem to support the fears of moral decay articulated by philanthropists since the eighteenth century: she would have to work if she went to Somalia, whereas in Djibouti she wouldn't have to do anything; people look rich when they come from Djibouti. The reality she describes over the subsequent four months paints an entirely different picture.

What the questionnaire responses and longer interviews reveal is not the operation of a nefarious "pull factor" dragging people across borders to sit in refugee camps and demand rations (see Kibreab 1987:54, 269, for a nuanced discussion) but a pragmatic readiness to exploit any available source of livelihood. Indeed, these and other findings support Cassanelli's drought response model (1982), one of the characteristics of which is the low desirability of having no options—that is, of dependency—in particular when it involves social, economic, and political subordination. In the context of the returnee holding camp, the Somali returnees emphasize those dimensions of *qoxoti* that are likely to contribute to a better material outcome while safeguarding political and other options. The similarities with the publicly sanctioned meanings of "refugee" are offered back to the donors: "These are *your* values, so put your money where your mouth is."

"Dependency" and the Globalization of the (Anti)Welfare State

Charity and humanitarianism are not just rhetorical strategies cynically manipulated to achieve the "real" agendas of various actors. Humanitarian aid is seen as an obligation, on both moral and legal grounds. To this extent, it is redistributive of resources and delimits sovereignty, much as Hathaway (1991) argues that human rights law is primarily a way of delimiting state sovereignty. However, donors also seek to delimit the extent of obligation on them or, conversely, to delimit the rights of claimants, in this case refugees. The obligation of gratitude and the pervasive rhetoric of dependency, with its proposed remedy of cutting off aid out of concern for the recipients' dignity and mental health, are ways both of expressing the conflict and of attempting to resolve it in the donors' favor.

However, I wish to suggest a further point, namely, that the rhetoric of dependency contributes to what Mark Duffield (1992) refers to as the globalization of a socially polarized society, wherein one part exists in a state of permanent crisis. Duffield suggests a continuity between the permanent underclass in the West and the nexus of conflict, impoverishment, drought, and chronic large-scale food insecurity in, especially, sub-Saharan Africa. Duffield suggests that the perceived undesirability of "relief" as opposed to "development" tends to minimize awareness of the state of chronic emergency characterizing sub-Saharan Africa, even though the general orientation to Africa is one of welfare or relief. The conditions requiring continual "relief" are presented as temporary aberrations, "emergencies," rather than as the normal state of affairs for the past two to three decades.

Refugees, refugee discourse, and "dependency" play a particular role in this process. In addition to being an uncomfortable marker of nation- and statehood, refugees also represent the most visible part—literally, the homeless—of the global underclass. It is not surprising that with the internationalization of welfare, we should also see an internationalization of attempts to erase, through discursive, legal, or fiscal strategies, the structural links between the underclass—welfare bums, bag ladies, youth gangs, or refugees—and the rest of society. A pity-based discourse that zeros in on standardized individuals—both on the donor and on the recipient side of the relationship—who are stripped of social, political, or economic networks (let alone power) makes these structural links more difficult to see, while maintaining inequality between donors and beneficiaries.

"Dependency" could be understood as a simple description or assessment of the degree of choice (i.e., little or none) available to the recipient. However, in the context of debates over domestic safety nets and refugee relief, it is instead a discursive strategy that shifts the topic of debate from material and social inequality, to psychological and moral weakness. It reinforces the power of the donor to give or to withhold, by invoking scientific ("mental health") and moral authority to limit both the basis and the extent of claims that would-be recipients can legitimately make. "Dependency" in this sense may or may not reflect objective dependency, and may or may not be a "bad thing." It is located, however, not in the refugee, but in the rules that structure the language game where the meanings and significance of "refugee" and "humanitarianism" are contested.

The semantic and pragmatic networks around the Somali word *qoxoti* show the influence—indeed, incorporation—of important aspects of post–World War II Euro-American discourses of development and refugees.

However, they draw on indigenous notions of justice, need, and duty, and attempt to articulate a wider base of responsibility for formerly internal problems such as poverty, which are now inextricably linked to both the promises and the failures of development. Attention to these alternative networks suggests a different reading of "refugee dependency," and of its remedies.

Conclusion:
Pity, Mental Health, and the Erasure of Power

A recent WHO manual on the mental health of refugees (World Health Organization 1996), which mentions the primacy of securing basic needs and the importance of addressing cultural aspects of mental illness and of healing, nevertheless slips into the perhaps inevitable position of recommending and describing breathing exercises and relaxation techniques for managing the stress under which refugees often find themselves (World Health Organization 1996:16–31). Despite frequent reference to the material and political risk in which people live, healing in this manual is limited to activities that are thought to improve the emotional state of the individual. Thus, although religious rituals, meditation, and traditional healing practices are cited as possibly beneficial interventions, their benefit is tacitly assumed to lie in helping to calm or heal the individual. Social action, or even individual action, directed primarily at social, political, or economic conditions is not mentioned as a strategy for improving the mental health of refugees. This is in line with psychiatric models of mental health and mental illness. I argue elsewhere (Zarowsky 1998) that individual psychotherapy for survivors of collective violence may be a political act, insofar is it asserts the individuality and separateness that genocidal violence seeks to eliminate along with the collectivity itself. However, to reduce the suffering of refugees or other displaced populations to a question of mental health, seen as fundamentally individual and private, does injury both to the subversive and healing potential of individually oriented therapy itself and, more important, to the individuals and the social networks in which they are inextricably embedded.

Current concern and rhetoric about refugee mental health, including post-traumatic stress disorder (PTSD) and "refugee dependency," express, in part, a desire to see refugees as whole human beings with emotional and psychological lives, rather than as mere numbers. This discourse is also meant to express support for the empowerment of refugees (von Buchwald 1994). One of the advantages of the dominant discourse around refugees as victims is that it facilitates fund-raising for refugee assistance programs. However, this "appeal of experience" (Kleinman and Kleinman 1997) and its expression in graphic images of starving or at least despondent and helpless refugees (Kleinman and Kleinman 1997; see also Malkki 1995, introduction) has consequences rather different from the hoped-for empowerment. Empowerment, if it is indeed a desired condition, seems more likely to arise from the Somali discourse about refugees, which is overtly moral and based on justice.

The discourse of pity erases both the specificity of each refugee situation, and the claims of justice that might be made by one or another party. The further transmogrification of a moral discourse of pity into a purportedly neutral and scientific discourse of psychological distress or illness, whether "dependency" or post-traumatic stress disorder, eliminates even the possibility of identifying the rhetoric *as moral,* and therefore at least implying rights and obligations. Once someone is labeled "sick," the moral dimension of pity, paternalism, and the interests that might be explored in regard to those taking the paternalistic or "helping" role is claimed to have vanished into the unquestionable "facts" of science. This labeling is not new: in the nineteenth century, Irish refugees to the United States were also much more effectively dismissed as rights-holding persons if they were labeled as "mentally ill," rather than as one party among others in a contest for resources (Kraut 1994). Power has been erased—both the real and potential power of the refugee or claimant, and the real and potential power of the donor. Far from leveling the playing field, however, this erasure of the visibility of power tilts the field further in favor of donors, at least until such time as refugees begin, en masse, to claim benefits for their "mental illness."

Although a medicalizing approach to refugee distress—for example, through using a trauma or PTSD model—may at times have a useful place in providing a neutral territory for addressing what are often highly polarized issues, it is critical to examine much more closely the assumptions generally underlying the use of a medicalizing discourse, including the variant around the notion of "refugee dependency." Otherwise, this discourse, which is thought by its agency and medical proponents to express the most benevolent concern for refugee suffering (see, e.g., World Health Organization 1996; de Vries 1998; von Buchwald 1994), will express instead yet another face of colonialism: the appropriation of suffering and the colonization of minds (Kleinman and Kleinman 1997; Nandy 1997; Summerfield 1997). One aspect of this colonialism is that the culturally and historically conditioned Western emphasis on the individual and on the primacy of individual psychology as the "real" core of human nature is attributed to all humanity throughout all time (Summerfield 1996; Young 1995). PTSD and "refugee dependency" are examples of conditions or disorders that are held to be timeless, natural, and subject perhaps to varying cultural window dressing but fundamentally panhuman in their occurrence.

However, the effects of this "colonization of minds" are not limited to a subtle shift in ways of thinking about human nature, which might in any case be argued to be a shift to a better and more humane model (see the exchange between Summerfield 1997, 1998 and de Vries 1998). The globalization of refugee identity in terms of mental (ill) health is important primarily because this discourse obscures the very real political, social, and economic stakes involved in refugee crises and refugee relief. It erases the individual as well as the collectivity, and history, and power.

Notes

1. The office of the United Nations High Commissioner for Refugees (UNHCR) was created by the United Nations in 1951 to deal with the problem of refugee and displaced populations from the Second World War and the postwar partitioning of Europe. The formal definition of "refugee," according to the 1951 Geneva Convention Related to the Status of Refugees, was any individual who

> as a result of events occurring before 1 January 1951, and owing to well-founded fear of being persecuted for reasons of race, religion, nationality, membership of a particular social group or political opinion is outside the country of his nationality and is unable or, owing to such fear, is unwilling to avail himself of the protection of that country; or who, not having a nationality and being outside the country of his former habitual residence as a result of such events, is unable or, owing to such fear, is unwilling to return to it. (United Nations High Commissioner for Refugees 1979:29)

In 1967 the UN agreed on a Protocol Related to the Status of Refugees, which deleted the limitation to events occurring prior to 1951 as well as deleting the option for signatory states to limit their activities to European refugees. In 1969 the "OAU (Organization of African Unity) Convention Governing the Specific Aspects of the Problem of Refugees in Africa" extended the basis on which African states would recognize claims for asylum and refugee status to include

> every person who, owing to external aggression, occupation, foreign domination or events seriously disturbing public order in either part or the whole of his country of origin or nationality is compelled to leave his place of habitual residence in order to seek refuge in another outside his country of origin or nationality (United Nations High Commissioner for Refugees 1979:197).

The refugee determination laws of most European and North American states are based on the narrower, UN definition, and both law and practice seek to limit the admissibility even of persons who could demonstrate "a well-founded fear of persecution" on the grounds specified in the UN definition. However, the practice of UN and nongovernmental agencies, and the common use of "refugee," are more in line with the broader, OAU definition.

2. See Leopold and Harrell-Bond (1994) for an overview of the refugee regime, in particular as it relates to mental health. For a discussion of "political arenas," see Bailey (1969).

3. Apropos of this chapter's discussion of political action and the attribution of mental illness, Mohammed Abdille Hassan was known by the British as the "Mad Mullah"—see Drake-Brockman 1912; Samatar 1982:182–4.

4. Margaret Lock explores this issue with respect to organ transplant (personal communication).

5. I thank Linda Whiteford for drawing my attention to André Gunder Frank's absence from an earlier version of this chapter.

6. The letter *c* in Somali orthography represents the voiced pharyngeal fricative *ayn*.

References

Allen, Tim, and David Turton. 1996. "Introduction: In Search of Cool Ground." In *In Search of Cool Ground: War, Flight and Homecoming in Northeast Africa*, Tim Allen, ed. Trenton: Africa World Press.

Bailey, Fred G. 1969. *Strategems and Spoils: A Social Anthropology of Politics*. Oxford: Blackwell Boltanski.

———. 1993. *La souffrance à distance*, Patrick J. Bracken and Celia Petty, eds. Paris: Metailie.

———. 1998. *Rethinking the Trauma of War*. London: Free Association Books.

Boltanski, Luc. 1993. *La Souffrance à Distance: Morale Humanitaire, Médias et Politique*. Paris: Éditions Metailié.

Bracken, P. J., and C. Petty, eds. 1998. *Rethinking the Trauma of War*. London: Free Association Books.

Cassanelli, Lee. 1982. *The Shaping of Somali Society: Reconstructing the History of a Pastoral People, 1600–1900*. Philadelphia: University of Pennsylvania Press.

Comaroff, John L., and Jean Comaroff. 1997. *Of Revelation and Revolution: The Dialectics of Modernity on a South African Frontier*, vol. 2. Chicago: University of Chicago Press.

Cowen, M. P., and R. W. Shenton. 1996. *Doctrines of Development*. London and New York: Routledge.

Cunningham, Hugh. 1998. "Introduction." In *Charity, Philanthropy and Reform from the 1690s to 1850*, H. Cunningham and J. Innes, eds. London: Macmillan.

Cunningham, Hugh, and Joanna Innes. 1998. *Charity, Philanthropy and Reform from the 1690s to 1850*. London: Macmillan.

de Vries, Fokko. 1998. "To Make a Drama out of Trauma Is Fully Justified," *Lancet* 351: 1579–1580.

Douglas, Mary, and Steven Ney. 1998. *Missing Persons: A Critique of Personhood in the Social Sciences*. Berkeley: University of California Press.

Drake-Brockman, R. E. 1912. *British Somaliland*. London: Hurst and Brackett.

Duffield, Mark. 1992. "Famine, Conflict and Public Welfare." In *Beyond Conflict in the Horn: The Prospects for Peace, Recovery and Development in Ethiopia, Somalia, Eritrea and Sudan*, M. Doornbos et al., eds. Trenton: Red Sea Press.

Foster, George. 1967. "The Dyadic Contract: A Model for the Social Structure of a Mexican Peasant Village." In *Peasant Society: A Reader*, J. M. Potter, M. N. Diaz, and G. M. Foster, eds. Boston: Little, Brown.

Fukui, Katsuyoshi, and John Markakis. 1994. *Ethnicity and Conflict in the Horn of Africa*. London: James Currey.

Gunder Frank, André. 1988. "The Development of Underdevelopment." In *The Political Economy of Development and Underdevelopment*, C. K. Wilbur, ed. New York: Random House.

Hansen, Art. 1990. "Refugee Self-Settlement Versus Settlement on Government Schemes: The Long-Term Consequences for Security, Integration and Economic Development of Angolan Refugees (1966–1989) in Zambia." United Nations Research for Social Development Discussion Paper 17, Geneva.

Harrell-Bond, B. E. 1986. *Imposing Aid: Emergency Assistance to Refugees*. Oxford: Oxford University Press.

Harrell-Bond, B., E. Voutira, and M. Leopold. 1992. "Counting the Refugees: Gifts, Givers, Patrons and Clients," *Journal of Refugee Studies* 5(3/4): 205–225.

Hathaway, James C. 1991. "Reconceiving Refugee Law as Human Rights Protection," *Journal of Refugee Studies* 4(2): 113–131.

Hyndman, Jennifer. 1997. "Managing and Containing Displacement After the Cold War: UNHCR and Somali Refugees in Kenya," *Refuge* 16(5): 6–10.

Kibreab, Gaim. 1987. *Refugees and Development in Africa: The Case of Eritrea*. Trenton, NJ: Red Sea Press.

———. 1993. "The Myth of Dependency Among Camp Refugees in Somalia 1979–1989," *Journal of Refugee Studies* 6(4): 321–149.

Kleinman, Arthur, and Joan Kleinman. 1997. "The Appeal of Experience; The Dismay of Images: Cultural Appropriations of Suffering in Our Times." In *Social Suffering*. A. Kleinman, M. Lock, and V. Das, eds. Berkeley: University of California Press.

Kozlowski, Gregory C. 1998. "Religious Authority, Reform, and Philanthropy in the Contemporary Muslim World." In *Philanthropy in the World's Traditions*, W. F. Ilchman, S. N. Katz, and E. L. Queen II, eds. Bloomington: Indiana University Press.

Kraut, Alan. 1994. "Historical Aspects of Refugee and Immigration Movements." In *Amidst Peril and Pain: The Mental Health and Well-Being of the World's Refugees*, A. Marsella et al., eds. Washington, DC: American Psychological Association.

Lemarchand, René. 1968. "Les relations de clientèle comme agent de contestation: le cas du Rwanda," *Civilisations* 18(4): 553–572.

Leopold, Mark, and B. Harrell-Bond. 1994. "An Overview of the World Refugee Crisis." In *Amidst Peril and Pain: The Mental Health and Well-Being of the World's Refugees*, Anthony J. Marsella et al., eds. Washington, DC: American Psychological Association.

Levine, Donald N. 1974. *Greater Ethiopia: The Evolution of a Multi-ethnic Society*. Chicago: University of Chicago Press.

Lewis, I. M. 1961. *A Pastoral Democracy: A Study of Pastoralism and Politics Among the Northern Somali of the Horn of Africa*. London: Oxford University Press.

———. 1988. *A Modern History of Somalia: Nation and State in the Horn of Africa*. Boulder, CO: Westview Press.

Leys, Colin. 1996. *The Rise and Fall of Development Theory*. London: James Currey.

Malkki, Lisa H. 1995. *Purity and Exile: Violence, Memory and National Cosmology Among Hutu Refugees in Tanzania*. Chicago: University of Chicago Press.

Markakis, John. 1987. *National and Class Conflict in the Horn of Africa*. Cambridge, England: Cambridge University Press.

McBriar, A. M. 1987. *An Edwardian Mixed Doubles: The Bosanquets Versus the Webbs. A Study in British Social Policy 1890–1929.* Oxford: Clarendon Press.

Minear, Larry, and Thomas G. Weiss. 1995. *Mercy Under Fire: War and the Global Humanitarian Community.* Boulder, CO: Westview Press.

Murphy, H. B. M. 1995 [1955]. "The Camps." In *Flight and Resettlement,* H. B. M. Murphy, ed. Montreal: GIRAME, reprint.

Nandy, Ashis. 1997. "Colonization of the Mind." In *The Post-Development Reader,* M. Rahnema, ed. London: Zed Books.

Risse, Guenter B. 1986. *Hospital Life in Enlightenment Scotland: Care and Teaching at the Royal Infirmary of Edinburgh.* Cambridge, England: Cambridge University Press.

Roseberry, William. 1988. "Political Economy," *Annual Reviews in Anthropology* 17: 161–185.

Rosenberg, G., and E. Charles. 1987. *The Care of Strangers: The Rise of America's Hospital System.* New York: Basic Books.

Rostow, Walt W. 1971. *The Stages of Economic Growth: A Non-Communist Manifesto.* Cambridge, England: Cambridge University Press.

Samatar, Said S. 1982. *Oral Poetry and Somali Nationalism: The Case of Sayyid Mahammad Abdille Hassan.* Cambridge, England: Cambridge University Press.

Seligman, M. E. P. 1975. *Helplessness: On Depression, Development, and Death.* San Francisco: Freeman.

Stein, Barry N. 1991. "Slow Progress Since ICARA II." In *Refugee Policy: Canada and the United States,* H. Adelman, ed. New York: York Lanes Press.

Sternberg, Robert J. 1995. *In Search of the Human Mind.* Fort Worth, TX: Harcourt Brace College Publishers.

Summerfield, Derek. 1996. *The Impact of War and Atrocity of Civilian Populations: Basic Principles for NGO Interventions and a Critique of Psychosocial Trauma Projects.* Network Paper 14, Relief and Rehabilitation Network. London: Overseas Development Institute.

———. 1997. "Legacy of War: Beyond 'Trauma' to the Social Fabric," *Lancet* 349: 1568.

———. 1998. "'Trauma' and the Experience of War: A Reply," *Lancet* 351: 1580–1581.

Trimingham, Spencer J. 1965. *Islam in Ethiopia.* London: Frank Cass.

Ulin, Robert C. 1984. *Understanding Cultures.* Austin: University of Texas Press.

UNHCR (United Nations High Commissioner for Refugees). 1979. *Collection of International Instruments Concerning Refugees.* Geneva: UNHCR.

———. 1990. *Guidelines for the Protection of Refugee Women.* Geneva: UNHCR.

———. 1991. *A Manual for People Oriented Planning.* Geneva: UNHCR.

von Buchwald, Ulrike. 1994. "Refugee Dependency: Origins and Consequences." In *Amidst Peril and Pain: The Mental Health and Well-Being of the World's Refugees,* Anthony J. Marsella et al., eds. Washington, DC: American Psychological Association.

Wilson, K. B. 1992. "Enhancing Refugees' Own Food Acquisition Strategies," *Journal of Refugee Studies* 5(3/4): 226–246.

WHO (World Health Organization). 1996. *Mental Health of Refugees.* Geneva: World Health Organization.

Young, Allan. 1995. *The Harmony of Illusions: Inventing Post-Traumatic Stress Disorder.* Princeton: Princeton University Press.

———. 1997. "Suffering and the Origins of Traumatic Memory." In *Social Suffering,* A. Kleinman et al., eds. Berkeley: University of California Press.

Zarowsky, Christina. 1998. "Victimes de choc collectif: visions anthropologique et politique," *Frontières* 10(3): 21–25.

9

Ethical Issues in Human Organ Replacement: A Case Study from India

Patricia A. Marshall and Abdallah Daar

In the international settings of biomedical practice, the human body is transformed and constrained by local context—personal beliefs about human identity and moral agency, conventional forms of healing, and particular technological resources. Taken together, these constitutive elements shape the production of biomedical knowledge regarding organ and tissue replacement therapies. Practices surrounding organ and tissue transplantation elicit profound and compelling questions about human life and the political context of medical practice. What does it mean to be human? What is the nature of death? When is someone "dead enough" or "competent enough" to have his or her organs taken? When resources are scarce, how should society determine who benefits from organ transplant technology? What are the cultural and scientific assumptions that inform procedures for selecting candidates for transplantation? Can marketing approaches for organ donation ever be justified? Is there a place for cultural exceptionalism in determining what is morally correct comportment regarding procurement of organs for transplantation?

Human organ replacement therapies represent a unique articulation of the globalization of biomedicine. Developments in scientific technology, pharmaceuticals, and the legitimation of brain death criteria have encouraged the growth of organ transplantation as an international enterprise. This paper explores local ethical problems associated with the international development of organ transplantation. First, the organization and delivery of transplant technologies are explored briefly, with particular attention to beliefs and practices related to the donation and procurement of human organs in diverse cultural settings. Second, drawing on research conducted in India, the practice of "paid donation" for kidney transplantation with nonrelated living donors is examined. Paid donation refers to the process of financial reimbursement for kidney donation. This practice has been outlawed since the passage of the Human Organs Transplant Act in 1995. Special consideration is given to moral representations of the "self" and "other" and the use of body organs as both "gifts" and "commodities for exchange" in the context of paid donation. Issues associated with obtaining informed consent from individuals vulnerable to exploitation because of poverty are also addressed. Additionally, the local impact of the Human Organs Transplant Act is explored.

Human organ and tissue replacement therapies illustrate the powerful seduction of technological achievements in biomedicine. Scientific technological capabilities, combined with the life-sustaining orientation of biomedicine, reinforce the development of the organ transplantation enterprise. Although ethical debates over organ transplantation question the appropriateness of donation and procurement strategies, rarely have scholars questioned the fundamental issue of whether or not transplantation therapies should be pursued aggressively (Fox and Swazey 1992). Indeed, the literature repeatedly stresses the severe worldwide shortage of organs for transplantation. Despite advances in transplantation technologies, it is likely that this shortage will increase as the demand for organs grows. In this paper, we argue that three factors contribute to ethical concerns in the organization and delivery of organ and tissue replacement therapies: (1) the availability of resources and technologies for organ transplantation; (2) cultural construction of beliefs about the body and personhood; and (3) the articulation of biomedical authority and the negotiation of power relationships in particular social and political contexts. We suggest that separately or together these factors unlevel the playing field.

Organ Procurement and Donation in Diverse Cultural Settings

Since the early successes in the 1950s and 1960s, there have been remarkable scientific advances in the field of human organ and tissue replacement therapies. The result has been a proliferation of transplant centers throughout the world. Although transplant physicians and related health personnel may use similar medical and surgical techniques regardless of where they practice, organ transplantation is enacted in diverse national and cultural worlds that significantly influence the organization and delivery of transplant technologies, and beliefs about appropriate methods for donating and procuring human organs. Religious views and social traditions concerning the treatment of the human body, economic conditions that influence the availability and use of medical resources, and the national political environments of health care delivery impact the development and provision of transplant services in myriad and diverse ways (Lock 1995, 1996a, 1996b; Lock and Honde 1995; Hogle 1995, 1999; Marshall, Thomasma, and Daar 1996; Daar and Marshall 1997; Koenig and Hogle 1995; Joralemon 1995; Sharp 1995; Scheper-Hughes 1996). For example, in her recent critique of the implementation and regulation of science and technology regarding human replacement therapies in Germany, Hogle (1999) illustrates the profound relationship between the therapeutic use of human tissue and organs and the politics of German nationalism.

A range of strategies are employed internationally for consent to obtain organs from living and cadaveric donors (Spital 1997). In a process referred to as *opting-in,* such as we have in the United States, the Uniform Anatomical Gift Act (UAGA) of 1984 requires explicit consent before organs can be removed from someone who has recently died. Adults have a legal right to declare whether or not they wish to donate their organs upon their death, but the number of individuals who indicate a desire to be an organ donor is relatively low. When no advance directive exists, family members must provide consent. Although the UAGA stipulates that the deceased's wishes must be honored, in most cases—even with clear evidence of a wish to donate—family members are approached for consent. In an effort to increase the number of potential organ donors, required request legislation was enacted, and hospital staff are now mandated to approach families of recently deceased individuals about organ donation (Joint Commission on the Accreditation of Healthcare Organizations 1992; Virnig and Caplan 1992). Despite this legislation, the number of donor organs has not increased dramatically (Siminoff et al. 1995). A number of obstacles contribute to the low rate of success with required request, including discomfort experienced by hospital staff who may not want to approach the family and add to their pain, and the reluctance of family members to consent to organ donation if they are not sure what decision the person would have wanted them to make.

Faced with a similar disinclination by family members to consent to donate organs, in Spain transplant professionals devised a highly organized program to encourage donation based on a decentralized network of medical and nursing staff dedicated to the entire process of organ donation from donor identification to organ and/or tissue retrieval (Miranda and Matesanz 1998). The donation rate in Spain has more than doubled since 1989, and the percentage of multiorgan retrieval has risen from 35 percent to 83 percent.

In a system referred to as *opting-out* or *presumed consent,* unless the deceased explicitly stated an objection to donation, organs and tissue may be obtained without consent. Many European countries practice presumed consent for organ donation, including France, Belgium, Finland, Norway,

Portugal, and Austria (Land and Cohen 1992; Roels et al. 1995). In actual practice, opting-out takes different forms. In a weaker version of this strategy, family members maintain the right to refuse donation; in a stronger form, the family has no right to resist donation. One result of the presumed consent approach to organ donation is the routinization of donation procedures in hospital settings. Proponents of this process believe that it increases the supply of organs for transplantation. Indeed, since Belgium adopted this approach in 1986, organ donation has risen substantially (Roels et al. 1991). Critics such as Veatch and Pitt (1995), however, argue that because a significant minority of the public opposes organ donation, it is wrong to presume consent for everyone. Spital (1997) suggests that the true efficacy of presumed consent is not clear. Similarly, Land and Cohen (1992) point out that there is no convincing evidence that presumed consent alone guarantees an increase in cadaveric organ donors.

Another proposal to increase cadaveric donation is referred to as *mandated choice,* also called *required response.* This strategy would require competent adults to make and record their decision about donating organs upon their death. Asking about organ donation on a driver's license or a tax form, and insisting that the question be answered, would accomplish the goal of mandated choice. The decision would be legally binding, although it could be changed at any time. Mandated choice was endorsed by the Council on Ethical and Judicial Affairs of the American Medical Association in 1994, and a recent survey indicates public support for this approach (Spital 1995).

Strategies for optimizing consent for cadaveric organ donation worldwide are a direct response to closing the gap between the voracious demand for human organs and the limited supply available for transplantation. In countries where there are strong cultural or religious considerations that prevent or inhibit cadaveric donation, the shortage of organs is particularly severe. In the Middle East, for example, although there is support from some Islamic religious leaders for organ donation (Hathout 1991), there are strong cultural precepts concerning bodily integrity at burial. Additionally, rejection of the notion of brain death has prohibited the development of cadaveric organ donation in some Middle Eastern and Asian countries. The Iranian parliament, for example, has not accepted the Brain Death Act (Broumand 1997), and in Japan in 1997, after considerable debate and decades of rejecting the concept of brain death, the parliament passed a law permitting the removal of organs from brain-dead patients provided that consent is obtained from the donor before death (Nomoto 1998). This law was applied for the first time on February 28, 1999, when the second heart transplant in Japan's history was performed (WuDunn 1999); the first heart transplant, performed in 1968, resulted in public outrage when the physician was accused of murdering the donor (Lock 1996a, 1996b).

In addition to beliefs about the importance of maintaining the integrity of the human body and concerns over impurities associated with the dead body (Lock and Honde 1995; Lock 1996a, 1996b; Ohnuki-Tierney 1994), the Japanese, in an ongoing public debate, continue to question whether the loss of integrated brain function indicates that a person has actually died. According to Lock (1996b:585), in Japan death is treated as a social event rather than a scientifically defined phenomenon, and it is this understanding of death that reinforces the resistance to cadaveric donation among the Japanese: "because brain death can only be established by the medical profession—because it is *mienai shi* [death which cannot be seen]—it represents a radical departure from a death where the family participates fully in the recognition of the process." The Japanese representation of death stands in sharp contrast to the medicalized death in North America, where physicians play a decisive role in declaring a person dead. Lock (1996b) pointedly questions not why the Japanese have steadfastly opposed brain death, but why North Americans and Europeans have accepted the new definition of death so easily. In the West, attention was placed on the incredible lifesaving heroics of transplantation and importance of donating "the gift of life," not on the source of the organs or the circumstances surrounding their retrieval. Diverse responses to brain-death criteria illustrate the importance of cultural influences on our understanding of the meaning of death, the social context of death, and the timing of death in relation to organ transplantation.

Cultural traditions regarding the proper treatment of the corpse and beliefs about the determination of death have profound implications for the acceptance or rejection of brain-death criteria, which, in turn, has serious ramifications for cadaveric organ donation. Retrieval of organs and tissue from living donors presents other moral challenges, particularly regarding the use of financial incentives for donation.

Marketing strategies to increase the supply of organs from both living donors and cadavers are being debated (Banks 1995; Radcliffe-Richards 1996; Radcliffe-Richards et al. 1998; Rothman et al. 1997; Marshall, Thomasma, and Daar 1996; Murray 1996; Nelkin and Andrews 1998; Mani 1998; Reddy 1993) and, in some cases, have been implemented (Reddy 1993, 1994; Chugh and Jha 1996). Proposals for financial reimbursement vary considerably, and some approaches are more controversial than others. In the United States, the payment of death benefits in the form of tax deductions for the donor's estate and federal reimbursements for burial expenses have been suggested (Schwindt and Vining 1986; Peters 1990); Pennsylvania has now established a state fund to pay the donor's family one thousand dollars for expenses associated with the burial. Cohen (1989) proposed a "futures market" in which individuals would sign a contract with a governmental agency for delivery of specific organs after death. Recently, a committee of the American Medical Association (1995) gave its approval for a "futures market" in organs from deceased individuals. The idea of a prospective sale of organs—individuals would sign contracts that mandate payment to designated beneficiaries after the organs are procured—has also been suggested (Hansmann 1989). Another marketing strategy encourages medical insurance companies to offer a small reduction in health insurance premiums for those who indicate they wish to donate their organs when they die (Hansmann 1989).

In recent years, the direct sale of human organs has been the subject of intense debate (Daar 1992a; Reddy 1993; Radcliffe-Richards 1996; Radcliffe-Richards et al. 1998; Rothman et al. 1997; Marshall, Thomasma, and Daar 1996). The practice has been condemned by national and international governmental organizations such as the British Transplantation Society Working Party (1986), World Medical Association (1985), the World Health Organization (1991, 1992, 1994), and transplantation societies, including the International Council of the Transplantation Society (1985) and the British Transplantation Society Working Party (1986). Commercial trade in organs has been strongly opposed because of concerns about human rights abuses, the inability to obtain informed consent from donors, and the exploitation of the poor by the rich. Despite these arguments against direct trade in human organs, commercial transactions in kidneys for renal transplantation have occurred and continue in a number of places in Middle Eastern, South Asian, and Latin American countries (Chugh and Jha 1996; Santiago-Delpin 1991). Despite legislation banning the sale of organs, it has been estimated that 10–40 percent of the transplants in Brazil and Chile are done using paid donors (Chugh and Jha 1996). In Iran, data published in 1993 indicated that in the 850 renal transplants performed, 70 percent of the kidneys were retrieved from living nonrelated donors, most of whom were reimbursed financially (Broumand 1997). Broumand is very critical of paying donors for their kidneys, noting problems with HIV, HCV, CMV, and tuberculosis, and a reluctance to receive follow-up care among donors. In addition, Broumand sites cases of exploitation:

> A husband, just discharged from the hospital after donating his kidney, brought his wife to donate her kidney as well because the payment for the his kidney was not enough for them to repay their debts. Another person wanted to sell his kidney to be able to buy drugs, and asked if he could sell both of his kidneys and start on maintenance dialysis, as dialysis anyhow was free. (1997:1831)

Similar cases have been reported in India, where commercial trade in kidneys was not illegal before the passage of the Human Organs Transplant Act in 1995. Indeed, the kidney trade in India has received the most attention internationally because of reported scandals associated with the practice of "paid donation."

The Bellagio Task Force, an interdisciplinary group convened by the Columbia University College of Physicians and Surgeons to examine ethical standards for the international practice of organ donation, supports a ban on the sale of living donor organs (Rothman et al. 1997). They conclude that the most vulnerable individuals would be placed at the greatest risk in societies where a significant proportion of the population is impoverished. However, the task force recommends modest payments for cadaver donations. Both legal and illegal commercial transactions in human organs are likely to continue because of the shortage of kidneys for transplantation in areas that do not have well-developed systems for cadaveric donation.

The ravenous appetite for human tissue and organs and the push to move forward the scientific biomedical agenda in transplantation technology have prompted consideration of alternative approaches to alleviate the demand. The use of non-heart-beating cadavers (Arnold et al. 1995; Menikoff 1997; Potts et al. 1998), anencephalic infants (Council on Ethical and Judicial Affairs 1995), and xenotransplantation (Institute of Medicine 1996; Daar and Marshall 1997; Effa 1998) represents strategies involving a redefinition of the donor pool. The creation of artificial limbs and the development of organs from human and nonhuman materials will have a signficant impact on the field of transplantation. Each of these approaches raises serious ethical questions about the boundaries of personhood and the appropriateness of embracing technologies that require continual shifts in definitions of human life and determinations of death. Moral considerations also are associated with the allocation of scarce medical resources in both industrialized and developing countries and the movement of donated organs from poor to rich individuals, from poorer to richer countries. Questions concerning informed consent to donate, human rights abuses, and the potential for exploitation of vulnerable individuals are real and pervasive.

"Paid Donation" in India and the Impact of the Human Organs Transplant Act of 1994

Historically, individuals undergoing a renal transplant in India have relied on both living related donors and living nonrelated donors because cadaver donation has not been available until recently. The practice of "paid donation"—donating a kidney for financial reimbursement—was considered to be a viable alternative for those without relatives who could donate *and* for those who could afford it, regardless of whether a relative was willing or able to donate a kidney.

The Human Organs Transplant Act of 1994, implemented on February 4, 1995, outlawed paid donation for human organs (Kishore 1995).

This act legalized brain-death criteria for cadaver donation and required individual states to set up a committee to oversee and regulate organ donation from nonrelated living donors. The pragmatism of the Indian government is revealed in the existence of provisions in the new law that allow for reimbursement for some expenses such as time off work, hospital and doctor fees, and so on.

Because of the potential for developing heart, lung, and liver transplantation in India, the majority of transplant physicians supported the Human Organs Transplant Act. Not all segments of the Indian population were as enthusiastic, however, particularly those with end-stage renal disease who could afford renal transplantation. When the residents of the state of Tamil Nadu were asked to vote on the new legislation in March 1995, individuals who were waiting for a transplant demonstrated in the streets. They believed—correctly—that passage of this act would seriously diminish the possibility of undergoing a transplant, especially if no relatives could be found to donate (Marshall and Daar 1998).

Social, political, and economic considerations are fundamental issues in the organization and practice of organ transplantation in India. The population of India includes more than 900 million people, and the per capita income is approximately 9,500 rupees (about U.S.$300). In India there are between eighty thousand and one hundred thousand people each year with end-stage renal disease, and prior to the passage of the act, approximately two thousand transplants were performed. Of these, only one-quarter of the donated kidneys came from relatives, the remaining coming from living nonrelated donors. For the most part, it is only middle- or upper-class individuals who can afford the luxury of transplantation combined with the cost of posttransplant immunosuppressive therapies (Mani 1998). The cost of renal transplantation is approximately U.S.$20,000–$25,000, a price afforded only by the financially secure. Moreover, the cost of dialysis for those with end-stage renal failure is approximately 800 rupees a session (about U.S.$26). Even if a person is able to pay for dialysis, uneven water quality and, in some cases, unstable sources of electricity may present other obstacles (Reddy 1993).

Although there have been recent efforts to promote cadaver donation for transplantation, particularly in light of the new act, many problems persist. India does not currently have an infrastructure to support cadaver donation adequately. There is no program such as the United Network for Organ Sharing (UNOS) for organ sharing; and there are few facilities available to handle the harvesting, preservation, and storage of organs. Additionally, just as in the United States and elsewhere, many people are troubled by the idea of removing organs from dead bodies and have fears about the mutilation of human bodies. Moreover, the government is strapped for funds—few resources are available to support the organ transplantation industry, and other priorities such as family planning are considered more important.

Between 1995 and 1998, Marshall visited India three times to explore ethical issues related to kidney transplantation. In 1995 one month was spent in Chennai (Madras) and Bangalore, where fifteen paid donors, fifteen recipients who purchased kidneys for transplantation, and health professionals working in the field of organ transplantation were interviewed. Additionally, information from fifty-two medical case records for paid donors were transcribed. These case reports document what individuals said they would spend their earnings on prior to donation, and how the money was actually spent after donation. In 1997 interviews were conducted in Chennai with four physicians (one woman and three men), six donors (five women and one man), a couple who arranged a paid donor for a family member, their donor (a man), and the cofounder of an organization that provides support for the poor in need of renal transplants. In 1998 interviews were conducted with twelve physicians (six in Chennai—one woman and five men, including the member of a state authorization committee for the approval of nonrelated kidney donors—and six in Delhi, all men), a transplant coordinator, and a recipient and his wife. When necessary, interviews were conducted with the assistance of a translator fluent in Hindi, Tamil, Kanada, and English; most of the interviews were audiotaped and transcribed. Informed consent for the interviews was obtained. Permission to collect material from the case records was granted by the physician in charge of the clinic. The research protocol was approved by the Institutional Review Board for Loyola University of Chicago Medical Center.

Although the practice of selling kidneys has been associated with brokers preying on the vulnerable poor, the majority of the donors interviewed did not use a broker to arrange the sale of their kidney. They received approximately U.S.$1,500 for their kidney. The donors reported using the money to pay off debts incurred for wedding dowries and other types of loans. They also bought equipment to start new businesses (e.g., cycle-rickshaws, sewing machines, food stands) or to purchase land. Most of the donors said they had set aside money in a savings account for children. Finally, donors reported that they were able to redeem family jewelry from pawnshops. There are no systematic investigations of the long-term physical, social, or financial effects of paid donation. However, based on discussions with the donors, financial benefits from paid donation appear to be temporary. For example, one man said that he paid off a dowry debt for one of his three daughters. When asked what he would do about the dowries for the other two daughters, he raised his hands and said, "I do not have to worry now about my first daughter." The cost of a dowry is daunting; it is unlikely that this man will be able to pay for the other dowries without incurring more debt.

Moral Representation of the Self and Other in Paid Donation

Cultural enactments of technological processes such as paid donation reveal the fluid and ambiguous boundaries that separate one individual from another. In her discussion of the management of ambiguity in the classification and regulation of human materials, Hogle (1995, 1999) argues that classifying and standardizing materials removed from the human body gives the appearance of resolving ambiguity in ways that are consistent with social norms. However, as Hogle (1995, 1999) points out, "formal tools and protocols, intended to eliminate variance in medical practice, actually contain or simply shift the variance." According to Hogle, the symbolic order provides an appearance of containment and control, while simultaneously allowing actors and "actants" to function in very different social worlds and very different "regimes of value." Certainly, Indian donors and recipients (and members of the transplant team) who participate in paid donation live in communities separated by a wide range of social markers, including caste membership, educational background, and financial resources.

The application of a property/ownership paradigm to human organs in the act of paid donation calls attention to complex moral issues regarding the value of a human life, the value of a human body. The essentializing force of human identity is obscured by the mechanistic language of organ procurement and transplantation. Organ transplantation technology and discourse surrounding it encourage a view of the person as a disembodied entity—from this perspective persons are at risk of being viewed as marketable objects, rather than as spiritually and socially embodied human beings (Campbell 1992; Childress 1992; Marshall, Thomasma, and Daar 1996). Rabinow (1996:149), in his cultural critique of scientific practices, argues that it is *fragmented body matter* rather than an individual *body* that has potential scientific value:

> The approach to "the body" found in contemporary biotechnology and genetics fragments it into discrete, knowable, and exploitative reservoir of molecular and biochemical products and events. By reason of its commitment to fragmentation, there is literally no conception of the person as a whole underlying these particular technological practices.

Indeed, the narratives of paid donation depict the body as an instrument, an agent, a medium through which morality is lived and expressed. The person becomes an embodied text of social, physical, and political suffering.

In his discussion of the cultural dynamics of organ replacement therapies, Joralemon (1995) has argued that there must be an ideological equivalent of cyclosporine to suppress the "cultural rejection of the view of the body" that transplantation promotes. In the case of paid donation, perhaps the ideological equivalent of cyclosporine is the absolute desperation, the abject poverty, the experience of a life so destitute, that selling a kidney becomes a "way out"—at least for the time being. Experientially, this marginal position in a broader social world, this placement at the edges of community, encourages, facilitates, *and* necessitates a view of the body as objectified commodity, not as a vital part of an integrated whole. Yet individuals have a stake in portraying themselves as moral characters, as agents of relative "goodness." For example, although several donors and recipients alluded to incidents of abuse and exploitation, for the most part they were convinced that, for themselves, it was not a situation of exploitation. When asked about the problem of exploitation, a young married woman who donated her kidney replied, "I have heard of the women being exploited . . . [once] a neighbor had his wife donate a kidney and [when it was done] . . . he spent all the money and finally abandoned his wife. As far as I know, I am not being exploited."

As narrators of their stories, the donors and recipients interviewed presented themselves in a positive light—not as victims or oppressors, but as individuals involved in an altruistic exchange of goods—money for a kidney. A man in need of a kidney who worked with a broker to find an individual willing to donate said pointedly, "As far as I am concerned, there is no problem here. He needs money and I need a kidney. We both want to live and we both are doing right by each other." When asked about her reasons for donating, a young woman replied, "This is one way of saving lives. [Also] in an emergency, if someone needs a kidney, where will they go? [And now there is] money to build a house and thatched roof." Only two of the donors interviewed expressed regret about their decision. For the most part, individuals talked about the chance they saw to reclaim their lives by donating their kidney money (and by reclaiming their own life, they were helping to save someone else's).

The narratives of the donors and recipients demonstrate that individuals are actively involved in creating their stories, imagining their lives transformed by the act of donation and kidney transplantation. Justifications for behavior—in this case, for the buying and selling of kidneys—evolve within this context. Moral representations of paid donation are sanitized in their retrospective reconstructions: recipients hope for redemption in extended lives; donors anticipate redemption in reconstructed lives. There is convergence in the moral representations of intentionality, desire, and suffering; these themes are mirrored in the stories of both the paid donors and the recipients of the purchased kidneys. Illustrating the need to project common values—a social closeness—onto the donor, a recipient describes his perception of the man whose kidney he purchased:

> *[I paid] Re 23,000 for a kidney in 1992 . . . [I put] newspaper ads two months before the transplant . . . 30 people responded . . . the doctors advised against using a broker . . . [I] did not have a relative [who could donate] . . . a lot wanted more money—Re 60,000; one asked for Re 15,000, but he was an alcoholic. The donor was a Jain, also a vegetarian [like me]. I was open enough that if [anyone had come forward] it would not have mattered . . . I feel better that he was a vegetarian. He was a nice fellow . . . good health, middle class family, [he] needed money.*

In this case, the recipient depicts the donor as someone like himself, a "Jain," someone who is not greedy about money, but suffering from the lack of it, someone whose "educated, middle class" background sets him apart from the other prospective donors.

If given a choice, individuals waiting for a transplant, and those who have received a transplant, want the donor—the "Other"—to be someone like them, someone who might share their beliefs and values. In reality, however, this rarely occurs, except perhaps in the imagined projection of a person of "good character." Donors and recipients are positioned very differently in Indian society—and there is considerable disparity in their social power and status. One of the issues discussed in interviews with Indian donors and recipients concerned the influence of caste; specifically, individuals were asked if a person's caste made a difference in their decision to follow through with the renal transplant (time did not allow for an in-depth exploration of this issue). Virtually everyone denied the relevance of caste. One recipient said, "Caste is not a problem, not at all, the donor was a Hindu, [but I] didn't know the caste of the donor. . . . If anyone was concerned, it would have been my sister's husband [because] I don't know what [his] views are about this whole thing [paid donation]." A donor commented, "Caste was not a problem . . . the blood that runs in everybody's veins is the same . . . caste is all man-made." Another donor said, "There was no issue of caste. . . . He [recipient] did not know what caste I was. He never asked." However, a research assistant was more cynical and perhaps more accurate in her portrayal of intentionality: "These are people who would not dream of being seen with or even touching someone of a lower caste [but] when it comes to a situation [like this], when it is life and death, they do not care whose kidney is in them. It could be [a person] from any caste."

The donor represents a stranger, someone foreign to the recipient and his or her family, and once identified becomes an intimate and vital source of life. To say "paid donor" or "donor" is to identify a person in the abstract, a person disconnected, objectified. Familiarity problematizes the distance-keeping mechanisms. To put a name to a face blurs the objectification, and this is where the issues of social reciprocity and moral obligation come into play. One indication of this is the recipient who avoids accepting an organ from his or her own family members. Several recipients, for instance, claimed that their children were too young. One man said, "My son has too much of his life ahead of him." Another said of her daughter, "She still has her children to raise." A fundamental question is this: Why do some people believe that it is morally wrong to ask their own children to consider donation, but approve of asking a stranger to donate—a stranger who may also be young, who may also have children to raise?

Many of the individuals interviewed, including health professionals and lawyers involved in transplantation, commented on the problems that may occur if a family member donates. Their stories often involve family members who donated kidneys and afterward became ruthless in their manipulations to extract payment indefinitely. One narrative concerned a man whose brother-in-law was the donor; after the operation he had to buy his brother-in-law a house and a car, provide him with a job, and pay college tuition for his son. Whether or not this is a "true" story is irrelevant. It is archetypal—a narrative that was repeated to me in different forms. The moral is clear. The respondent who told this story—a recipient of a renal transplant who engaged in paid donation—said, "It's actually cheaper and causes fewer problems to pay a stranger to donate than to ask a relative."

Moral Representations of Kidney Donations as an Altruistic Gift and a Marketable Commodity

There is a paradoxical articulation of organ donation as both a "gift of life" and a "commodity exchange" in the stories told by the donors and recipients. The narratives illustrate the moral conflation of social obligations and property rights. In this way, the "tyranny of the gift," as it has been called by Renee Fox and Judith Swazey (1992), takes on an added dimension that exacerbates the profound implications of being forever "in debt." Thus, expectations about gifting are imposed on the ideology of purchasing a "commodity." Stories of donation, in some cases, become stories about ongoing reciprocity—real, imagined, anticipated, or actualized. In the case previously described involving the Jain donor, for example, the recipient noted that he and his donor "have had no contact since the transplant . . . but [we have each other's] addresses." Another man described his sense of indebtedness in the following way: "[The donor] came by the house one year ago to find out how I was doing. The donor said he was having some pain. I gave him some money—actually if he comes by I have to help him.

Why? Because he saved my life . . . I gave him 200 rupees. I feel like giving him something; if he comes back again, I will give more."

The language of organ procurement reveals deep-seated beliefs about the embodied nature of human existence. The metaphor of a "gift of life" suggests an offering, a tribute, a present that is exchanged between persons outside the realm of a business transaction. In sharp contrast, human body parts signify objects for market contracts when the metaphor of "commodity" is applied to organ donation. In this context, property rights and rules of ownership become instrumental in the process of economic and contractual exchange (Nelkin and Andrews 1998).

Efforts to objectify and disassociate body organs from human identity have been unsuccessful, underscoring the vitality of symbolic representations in relation to our understanding of the person in the "body" and the organ as "gift." The act of gifting sets up moral obligations to repay the gift (Mauss 1954; Fox and Swazey 1992; Sharp 1995). In paid donation, the gift is also a commodity, something purchased in exchange for financial reimbursement. Nevertheless, there is a recognition of the special nature of the offering, that it is not an ordinary "gift" but something that empowers in exceptional ways. The result is an expectation that the gift of a kidney deserves something more, something extra, beyond the money paid for the organ. Indeed, in India it is common for recipients of a renal transplant to offer gifts of food, clothing, money, or medicine to the individuals who have donated their kidneys: "I spoke with the recipient and . . . he gave me two saris. He's a big man in Sri Lanka. We spoke during the blood matching and then after the operation. He was in bed and he kept sending messages through his son, who he would send to visit me." When this does not happen, it may be experienced as an affront. A donor from Madras, for example, expressed dissatisfaction with the man who received her kidney:

> *I never talked to the man. Never met him before or after the operation. The wife came to my room and patted my hand and said, "Are you okay?" but did not offer any other financial help. Everybody else, people came and met them and inquired about them [and brought them gifts]. After all, I've given my kidney and I was quite upset that . . . they did not make any offering.*

The Problem of Social Stigma

Despite the financial pragmatism expressed by many donors, the act of paid donation is imbued with meaning expressed in beliefs about the nature of the human body and how it "ought" to be treated. For some individuals, the stigma attached to the treatment of the body as a commodity implies the potential for social censure:

> *I had a younger sister whose wedding I had to pay for [Re 15,000] so I borrowed money. [Also] I had wanted my children to study. My idea [was] if we do this, we can make some money. . . . Only my husband and I talked about it, he agreed immediately. He was concerned but he agreed. . . . I haven't told anyone in the family. I am worried they would scold me . . . about selling part of my body. "How could you use your body like this?" They would speak unkindly of me.*

More than half of the donors expressed some concern about social judgment and potential stigma. Fear of social rejection is reflected in their statements about those with whom they discussed the decision to donate and those from whom this information was withheld. The woman just quoted indicated she spoke only with her husband about her decision; another woman said:

> *None of my community members are aware of me giving my kidney. People . . . may make bad remarks . . . they would speak ill, and say "How dare you sell a part of your body."' [But] I have no problem. I have done it because I was in dire need and I have no regrets. I don't care what my village would say.*

Comments such as these—made by both donors and recipients—call attention to the fear of being socially stigmatized and the deep-seated ambivalence toward paid donation among many Indians. However, despite the fact that in some Indian communities paid donation has now come to be viewed as a "last resort" for getting out of debt, not everyone in poverty considers paid donation as a source of revenue. The decision to become a paid donor is based on a combination of factors, including (1) the ability to take risks (e.g., a person's willingness to chance rejection from one's family and friends); (2) the level of desperation experienced (only those in desperate straits would consider such an action); and, related to this, (3) the strength of the motive to improve one's life circumstances (e.g., the couple who were able to build a house with a thatched roof after both became donors); and, finally, (4) access to the technological resources that make transplantation possible.

The donors' narratives signify an understanding of the fact that donating a body part—and doing it for money—is not standard practice. In fact, it is something out of the ordinary and not necessarily an act that is sanctioned. Indeed, the stigmatizing properties suggest a metaphor of social scarring consistent with the physical scar left by the removal of the kidney. In Bangalore, during an interview with a young woman who had donated a kidney for money, she lifted her blouse to show her scar and then proudly held up her baby. She was single when she had donated her kidney, and had been afraid that she would never find a husband—that a man would be repulsed by the scar and would not want to marry her. The realization of marriage and a child overcame her fear of stigmatization.

The Challenge of "Informed Consent" in Paid Donation

The question of informed consent is problematic in negotiations between kidney donors, transplant recipients, their physicians, and the brokers who may be involved in the course of transacting the sale of a kidney. Key dimensions of informed consent include the notion that it is voluntary, and that the implications of the request (or the "offer" in the case of paid donation) are understood, including the physical risks associated with donating a kidney. In a commercial transaction between individuals who are not equal in terms of economic and social power, is it ever possible to have "informed" consent?

Proponents of economic incentives such as paid donation balk at the notion that we can or should disallow people to decide freely what they want to do with their bodies (Radcliffe-Richards 1991, 1996; Reddy 1993). Implicit in this criticism is a charge of arrogance and paternalism—arrogance for the judgment implied in laws that ban commercial dealings, and paternalism for presuming that people are not capable of making the right choice if they engage in commercial transactions over body parts. Radcliffe-Richards (1996), for example, argues that it is misguided paternalism to assume that paid donors are incapable of making a rational choice regarding the sale of their kidney. Dossetor and Manickavel (1992:63), in their discussion of the impact of poverty on expressions of personal autonomy, also rejected the idea that financial incentives for donation result in exploitation of the poor: "This argument smacks of hypocrisy. The abject poor are in such a plight that we must protect them from doing themselves harm, yet we don't use state paternalism to relieve their poverty instead." A paid donor mirrors their concern in her comments about her own experience with paid donation: "To those who would condemn us, I say, will you pay my bills? . . . Will the government take care of me?"

Paradoxically, the condition of poverty has been used to justify the arguments of both critics and advocates of the commercial trade in kidneys. Opponents of the practice believe that it is a one-way practice—from the poor to the rich—and is thus inherently exploitative (Sells 1992; Mani 1992; Murray 1996; Chugh and Jha 1996). From this perspective, true informed consent can never be realized. On the other hand, proponents suggest that if someone chooses to better his or her circumstances through selling a kidney, it is that person's autonomous right to do so—the capacity to give informed consent is assumed. Yet only those in desperate circumstances financially would consider donating a kidney for money.

Moreover, it is unlikely that individuals who have been paid donors are able to rise above their conditions of poverty, as indicated in the following remarks made by a woman who donated her kidney:

> *[With earnings] I paid back a Re 15,000 loan, put Re 15,000 in savings for the three children. [The] remaining Re 2,500 went to postoperation expenses. Later, from the savings, [I] took out money and bought a mobile cart for a snack shop [to] sell chicken and beef. Now, [I] only have about Re 2,000 left in savings.... If I [had known]) I would become so weak, I would not have given my kidney. At least I could have worked hard, but now I am not able to do any sort of manual labor.*

However, as the Bellagio Task Force noted in its report on social and ethical issues concerning the international traffic in organs (Rothman et al. 1997:2741), they found no "unarguable ethical principle" that would, *under all circumstances,* justify a ban on the sale of organs. Nevertheless, after considerable discussion, the task force concluded that given the existing social, political, and economic inequities, commercialization places the well-being of disadvantaged populations at risk, particularly in developing countries where they are already jeopardized because of physical hardship, substandard housing, and inadequate nutrition. Representing a slightly different approach to the problem, Radcliffe-Richards and colleagues (1998) argue that there is a need to reopen the debate about the sale of organs with "scrupulous impartiality" and to consider carefully the possibility of strict regulation.

Kopytoff (1986:64) observes in his classic essay on the social life of things, "This conceptual polarity of individualized persons and commoditized things is recent and, culturally speaking, exceptional. People can be and have been commoditized again and again, in innumerable societies throughout history, by way of those widespread institutions known under the blanket term 'slavery.'" Notions of slavery imply a Foucauldian regulation and control of human bodies, human lives. From this perspective, it is possible to depict the impoverished, the destitute, the socially marginalized as "slaves" within any social system in which the poor are disenfranchised and vulnerable to exploitation; this would be true in both industrialized and developing nations. A different form of "slavery" is characterized in the dependency of individuals with end-stage renal disease. These individuals might be viewed as "enslaved" not only to dialysis machines and the biomedical world they are dependent upon, but also to the state, through regulations such as now exist in India, which many view as "condemning" them to death (because paid donation, now outlawed, may be perceived as the only possible route to transplantation).

The situation is complex. The transplantation enterprise is systematically regulated through mechanisms of state and biomedical authority. On one hand, the appropriation of transplantation technology requires the resources—the materials, the skills, the infrastructure, and the patient bodies—to succeed. On the other hand, in a nation like India, concerns about the promotion of family planning and general pubic health are viewed as much more vital to national development than are investments in scientific technologies such as transplantation. There is, however, a strong desire among health professionals involved in transplantation to develop transplantation technologies in India, and to be taken seriously in the global world of transplantation. There are serious constraints, however, in attempts to encourage the widespread development of human organ replacement therapies in a social context that lacks many features basic to the success of organ transplantation—including financial resources, medical facilities, and the existence of mechanisms for procuring and distributing human organs in a systematic fashion.

The Impact of the Human Organ Transplant Act on Paid Donation

Despite the passage of the Human Organ Transplant Act, reports in the public media suggest that paid donation continues to be practiced, particularly in south India, and there have been unproved allegations that some members of the state authorization committees have accepted bribes for approving nonrelated living donors. A number of factors contribute to the ongoing—and now illegal—trade in organs. Historically, the practice of paid donation has been viewed as a viable alternative for those in need of renal transplantation. Moreover, cadaver procurement programs are still in their infancy; there is not yet a well-established infrastructure for cadaver donation and retrieval, and a dialysis transplant registry does not exist. Although recently local hospitals in Delhi, Mumbai (Bombay), and Chennai have cooperated in the development of a system of organ retrieval and allocation, an effort to coordinate transplant activities has not been implemented at the state or national level. The Human Organs Transplant Act was passed in fourteen to fifteen states (Singh, Srivastava, and Kumar 1998), but not yet in the larger states such as Uttar Pradesh and Bihar. This facilitates the operation of kidney transplant centers that may engage in questionable and unregulated activities in those areas.

Some individuals are reluctant to donate the organs of a brain-dead patient because of beliefs about the treatment of the dead and concerns about mutilation of the human body. Additionally, there are no resources for a major public education effort to increase awareness of the potential for organ donation. Finally, the number of individuals in need of a renal transplant remains high, and there is no shortage of individuals willing to be paid donors.

The Human Organs Transplant Act has had several effects on the development of transplantation in India. First, there has been a reduction in the number of renal transplants performed (from an estimated 2,500 to 1,750 per year) and a decrease in the number of transplant centers from sixty to forty in the last four years (Divakar, Thiagarajan, and Reddy 1998). One of the exceptions allowed by the act is the possibility for an "emotionally related donor" approved by the authorization committee at the state level. In Chennai, which had been a major center for unrelated renal transplantation prior to the passage of the act, the authorization committee has permitted more than six hundred "emotionally related" transplants (Singh, Srivastava, and Kumar 1998). This figure represents the annual number of unrelated transplants conducted in Chennai before the act became law. To date, approximately forty kidneys, ten hearts, and eight livers have been transplanted.

The second major impact of the act has been to force the practice of paid donation underground. In 1995, at the time of our first visit to Madras, it was fairly easy to make contact with paid donors, perhaps in part because they were not engaging in illegal activities and neither were their transplant physicians. When Marshall returned in 1997 and 1998, there was greater reluctance among physicians to speak openly about the practice of paid donation, and there was a hesitancy to provide introductions to unrelated donors who were financially reimbursed.

In an interview conducted by Marshall in 1998, a couple discussed their search for a paid donor for the wife's mother. Their narrative suggests the difficulties experienced by potential transplant recipients under the new law. This case, reported by Marshall and Daar (1998), is described as follows.

A fifty-five-year-old woman suffering from end-stage renal disease required a kidney transplant. She had two daughters, both of whom were tested and found to be potential donors for their mother. However, one daughter was pregnant and unable to donate; the other was trying to conceive and her physician advised against it. While their mother waited for a cadaver donor, her eldest daughter and son-in-law considered contacting a kidney broker who would put them in touch with a person willing to be a paid donor. The daughter and her husband were distraught because they were aware of the scarcity of organs from cadavers and the slim chance of their mother's surviving the wait. In India, cadaver donation is a recent phenomenon and donors are rare. The couple realized that they would be breaking the law if they offered to financially reimburse an individual willing to donate a kidney. Moreover, they would need to go before a state authorization committee to seek approval for the kidney donation. They would also have to find physicians willing to perform renal transplants using nonrelated kidney donors. Finally, they wondered if they would be guilty of exploiting a poor person in desperate need of funds. The couple was deeply conflicted about what to do. They did not consider themselves to be criminals. Yet the physicians caring for their mother had indicated it was only a matter of time before dialysis would no longer be an option.

The couple made the decision to work with a broker to find a donor. They described their reasons for choosing the man who became the donor: "He was lighter skinned than the other two people the broker brought to us and he sounded more educated. This made us think he would make a better impression on the authorization committee." They talked about the meetings with the donor to go over what would be said during the interview with the committee. Instead of directly lying to the committee and suggesting the man was a relative, the couple decided the donor would be "a close friend." When asked what they would have done if the authorization committee had not approved the kidney transplant, the couple said they would repeat the process, only the next time simply say that he was a "cousin." Interestingly, one of the transplant physicians interviewed in Chennai suggested that the Human Organs Transplant Act has resulted in a new category of kinship, which he referred to as "kidney cousins."

Cases such as this illustrate one of the ways in which potential transplant recipients and donors work around the system to their advantage. It would be difficult to carry off the deception without some collusion with transplant physicians and, in certain situations, kidney brokers.

The passage of the law making it illegal to sell kidneys for donation serves an underground economy in kidney sales. Although, as we have noted previously, there are compelling reasons to argue against financial reimbursement for kidney donation, effective and stringent regulation of the practice of paid donation might better serve everyone involved in the process. Under the current conditions, it is unlikely that the unregulated traffic in kidneys will end in the near future. For those who are not morally opposed to the practice, or repulsed by the notion of someone donating a kidney—a body part—for money, there appear to be too many incentives to stop the practice outright. Speaking directly to the point, a kidney broker said, "The risks are worth it."

During interviews with donors, recipients, physicians, and a kidney broker, Marshall was reminded of the situation in the United States prior to the legalization of abortion. Women with money had access to physicians who were willing to perform the operation. It was possible to find out through "underground" networks whom to contact to have the procedure done, and the poorest women were the most vulnerable to exploitation and abuse. Similarly, when kidney transplant recipients were asked how they learned about where to find brokers or potential donors, they said they found out through informal discussions with other dialysis patients at the hospital, through friends who had gone through the same process, or through their physicians. Likewise, the donors interviewed said either they were contacted directly by a broker, or they began talking to others in their community who had already donated a kidney for money.

Public acceptance of cadaver donation may increase in the future. Nevertheless, during this transformative period of organ transplantation in India, when the development of a systematic cadaver donation program is in its infancy, the historical legacy of paid donation for renal transplants is still having an important effect.

Conclusion

The international proliferation of human tissue and organ transplantation will continue to challenge our understanding of the uses of human bodies as both gifts and commodities. Assumptions about the meaning of life and death, and beliefs about the fundamental nature of personhood, are embedded in the culturally informed practices of tissue and organ transplantation. The boundaries between what is considered morally correct or ethically reprehensible in transplant therapies will inevitably shift as advances in scientific knowledge present opportunities for new forms of interventions.

Industrialized and developing nations are positioned differently in terms of scientific technological resources, trained professionals, and the priority placed on "high-tech" life-sustaining therapies such as organ transplants. Moreover, diverse cultural and religious traditions have implications for the resolution of moral questions that arise in the development and application of transplantation technology. The negotiation of power—between rich and poor, donors and recipients, transplant specialists and the patients they serve, biotech industries and the researchers who work for them—influences in fundamental ways the possibilities and constraints of human tissue and organ replacement therapies.

Note

We are very grateful to the kidney donors and recipients, and to the physicians and other health providers, who talked with us in Chennai, Bangalore, and Delhi, India. We want to thank especially Dr. Chandra Reddy in Chennai, with whom we have spent many hours discussing the issues surrounding paid donation. We are also deeply appreciative of the technical support provided by Doris Thomasma at the Medical Humanities Program at Loyola University Chicago. Finally, we are grateful for the encouragement and support for the research in India provided by William Stubing through a presidential grant from the Greenwall Foundation.

References

Abouna, G. M. 1993. "Negative Impact of Trading in Human Organs on the Development of Transplantation in the Middle East," *Transplantation Proceedings* 25(3): 2310–2313.

American Medicine Association Council on Ethical and Judicial Affairs. 1995. "Financial Incentives for Organ Procurement," *Archives of Internal Medicine* 155: 581–589.

Arnold, Robert, Stuart Youngner, R. Schapiro, C. M. Spicer. 1995. *Procuring Organs for Transplant.* Baltimore: Johns Hopkins University Press.

Banks, G. J. 1995. "Legal and Ethical Safeguards: Protection of Society's Most Vulnerable Participants in a Commercialized Organ Transplantation System," *American Journal of Law and Medicine* 21: 45.

Blumstein, J. F. 1992a. "The Case for Commerce in Organ Transplantation," *Transplantation Proceedings* 24(5): 2190–2197.

———. 1992b. "The Use of Financial Incentives in Medical Care: The Case of Commerce in Transplantable Organs," *Health Matrix* 3(1): 1–30.

British Transplantation Society Working Party. 1986. "Guidelines on Living Organ Donation," *British Medical Journal* 293: 257–258.

Broumand, B. 1997. "Living Donors: The Iran Experience," *Nephrology, Dialysis, Transplantation* 12(9): 1830–1831.

Campbell, C. S. 1992. "Body, Self, and the Property Paradigm," *Hastings Center Report* 22(5): 34–42.

Childress, James. 1992. "The Body as Property: Some Philosophical Reflections," *Transplantation Proceedings* 24(5): 2143–2148.

Chugh, K. S., and V. Jha. 1996. "Commerce in Transplantation in Third World Countries," *Kidney International* 49(5): 1181–1186.

Cohen, L. R. 1989. "Increasing the Supply of Transplant Organs: The Virtues of a Futures Market," *George Washington Law Review* 58(1): 1–51.

Council on Ethical and Judicial Affairs, American Medical Association. 1994. "Strategies for Cadaveric Organ Procurement: Mandated Choice and Presumed Consent," *Journal of the American Medical Association* 272: 809–812.

———. 1995. "The Use of Anencephalic Neonates as Organ Donors," *Journal of the American Medical Association* 273: 1614–1618.

Daar, Abdallah S. 1992a. "Rewarded Gifting," *Transplantation Proceedings* 24: 2207–2211.

———. 1992b. "Nonrelated Donors and Commercialism: A Historical Perspective," *Transplantation Proceedings* 24(5): 2087–2090.

———. 1997. "Ethics of Xenotransplantation: Animal Issues, Consent, and Likely Transformation of Transplant Ethics," *World Journal of Surgery* 21(9): 975–982.

———. 1998. "Societal Issues in Organ Transplantation," *Annals of Transplantation* 3(2): 5–6.

Daar, A. S., and Patricia Marshall. 1997. "Culture and Psychology in Organ Transplantation," *World Health Forum* 18: 30.

Divakar, D., C. M. Thiagarajan, and K. C. Reddy. 1998. "Ethical Aspects of Renal Transplantation in India," *Transplantation Proceedings* 30(7): 3626.

Dossetor, J. B., and V. Manickavel. 1992. "Commercialization: The Buying or Selling of Kidneys." In *Ethical Problems in Dialysis and Transplantation,* C. M. Kjellstrand and J. B. Dossetor, eds. Dordrecht: Kluwer Academic Publishers.

Effa, P. 1998. "Transplantation and Xenotransplantation: Legal Perspectives for Third World Countries," *Annals of the New York Academy of Sciences* 862: 234–236.
Fox, R. C., and J. P. Swazey. 1992. *Spare Parts: Organ Replacement in American Society.* New York and Oxford: Oxford University Press.
Friese, K., and S. Rai. 1995. "Business as Usual: The Organ's Sales Continue Even as a New Act Takes Effect," *India Today,* March 15, p. 176.
Hansmann, H. 1989. "The Economics and Ethics of Markets for Human Organs," *Journal of Health Politics and Policy Law* 14(1): 57–85.
Hathout, H. 1991. "Islamic Concepts and Bioethics." In *Bioethics Yearbook: Vol. 1, Theological Developments in Bioethics: 1988–1990,* B. Brody, B. A. Lustig, H. T. Engelhardt, and L. B. McCullough, eds. Dordrecht: Kluwer Academic Publishers.
Hogle, Linda A. 1995. "Standardization Across Non-Standard Domains: The Case of Organ Procurement," *Science, Technology, and Human Values* 20: 482–500.
———. 1999. *Recovering the Nation's Body: Cultural Memory, Medicine, and the Politics of Redemption.* New Brunswick, NJ: Rutgers University Press.
Institute of Medicine. 1996. *Xenotransplantation: Science, Ethics, and Public Policy. Committee on Xenograft Transplantation.* Washington, DC: National Academy Press.
The International Council of the Transplantation Society. 1985. "Commercialisation in Transplantation: The Problems and Some Guidelines for Practice," *Lancet* 2: 715–716.
Ivanovski, N., L. Stojkovski, K. Cakalaroski, G. Masin, S. Djikova, and M. Polenakovic. 1995. "Renal Transplantation from Paid, Unrelated Donors in India: It Is Not Only Unethical, It Is Also Medically Unsafe" (letter), *Nephrology, Dialysis, Transplantation* 12(9): 2028–2089.
Joint Commission on the Accreditation of Healthcare Organizations. 1992. *Accreditation for Hospitals, MA 1.3.9, 1.3.10.* Oakbrook Terrace, IL: Joint Commission of Accreditation of Healthcare Organizations.
Joralemon, D. 1995. "Organ Wars: The Battle for Body Parts," *Medical Anthropology Quarterly* 9(3): 336.
Kefalides, P. 1999. "Solid Organ Transplantation: 2. Ethical Considerations," *Annals of Internal Medicine* 130(2): 169–170.
Kishore, R. R. 1995. "The Indian Transplantation Law: Promises and Effects," *World Health Forum* 19(2): 26–31.
Koenig, Barbara, and Linda Hogle. 1995. "Organ Transplantation (Re)examined?" *Medical Anthropology Quarterly* 9(3): 393–397.
Kopytoff, Igor. 1986. "The Cultural Biography of Things: Commoditization as Process." In *The Social Life of Things,* Arjun Appadurai, ed. New York: Cambridge University Press.
Land, W., and B. Cohen. 1992. "Postmortem and Living Organ Donation in Europe: Transplant Laws and Activities," *Transplantation Proceedings* 24: 2165.
Land, W., and J. B. Dossetor. 1991. *Organ Replacement Therapy: Ethics, Justice, Commerce.* Berlin: Springer-Verlag.
Lock, Margaret. 1995. "Transcending Mortality: Organ Transplants and the Practice of Contradictions," *Medical Anthropology Quarterly* 9(3): 391.
———. 1996a. "Displacing Suffering: The Reconstruction of Death in North America and Japan," *Daedulus* 125: 207.
———. 1996b. "Death in Technological Time: Locating the End of Meaningful Life," *Medical Anthropology Quarterly* 10: 575.

Lock, Margaret, and C. Honde. 1995. "Contesting the Natural in Japan: Moral Dilemmas and Technologies of Dying," *Culture, Medicine and Psychiatry* 19(1): 1–38.
Mani, M. K. 1992. "Renal Transplantation in India," *Transplantation Proceedings* 24(5): 1828–1829.
———. 1998. "The Management of End-Stage Renal Disease in India," *Artificial Organs* 22: 182.
Marshall, Patricia, and Barbara Koenig. 1996. "Anthropology and Bioethics: Perspectives on Culture, Medicine and Morality." In *Medical Anthropology: Contemporary Theory and Method,* C. Sargent and T. Johnson, eds. New York: Praeger.
Marshall, P. A., and A. S. Daar. 1998. "Cultural and Psychological Dimensions of Human Organ Transplantation," *Annals of Transplantation* 3(2): 7–12.
Marshall, Patricia, David Thomasma, and A. S. Daar. 1996. "Marketing Human Organs: The Autonomy Paradox," *Theoretical Medicine* 17: 1.
Mauss, M. 1954. *The Gift: Forms and Functions of Exchange in Archaic Societies,* trans. Ian Cunnison. Glencoe, IL: Free Press.
Menikoff, J. 1997. "Doubts About Death: The Silence of the Institute of Medicine," *Journal of Law, Medicine and Ethics* 26: 157–165.
Miranda, B., and R. Matesanz. 1998. "International Issues in Transplantation: Setting the Scene and Flagging the Most Urgent and Controversial Issues," *Annals of the New York Academy of Sciences* 862 (Dec. 30): 129–143.
Murray, T. 1996. "Organ Vendors, Families, and the Gift of Life." In *Meanings and Realities of Organ Transplantation,* R. C. Fox, L. O'Connell, and S. Youngner, eds. Madison: University of Wisconsin Press.
Nelkin, Dorothy, and Lori Andrews. 1998. "Homo Economicus: The Commercialization of Body Tissue in the Age of Biotechnology," *Hastings Center Report* 28(5): 30–39.
Nomoto, K. 1998. "Current Issues in Japan," *Annals of the New York Academy of Sciences* 862: 147–149.
Ohnuki-Tierney, E. 1994. "Brain Death and Organ Transplantation: Cultural Bases of Medical Technology," *Current Anthropology* 35(3): 233–254.
Peters, T. G. 1990. "Life or Death: The Issue of Payment in Cadaveric Organ Donation," *Journal of the American Medical Association* 265(10): 302–305.
Potts, J. T., R. C. Herdman, T. L. Beauchamp, and J. A. Robertson. 1998. "Commentary: Clear Thinking and Open Discussion Guide: IOM's Report on Organ Donation," *Journal of Law, Medicine and Ethics* 26: 166–168.
Prottas, J. M. 1989. "The Organization of Organ Procurement." In *Organ Transplantation Policy: Issues and Prospects,* J. F. Blumstein and F. A. Sloan, eds. Durham, NC: Duke University Press.
Rabinow, Paul. 1996. *Essays on the Anthropology of Reason.* Princeton, NJ: Princeton University Press.
Radcliffe-Richards, J. R. 1991. "From Him That Hath Not." In *Organ Replacement Therapy: Ethics, Justice and Commerce,* W. Land and J. Dosseter, eds. Berlin: Springer Verlag.
———. 1996. "Nefarious Goings On: Kidney Sales and Moral Arguments," *Journal of Medicine and Philosophy* 21(4): 375–416.
Radcliffe-Richards, J., A. S. Daar, R. D. Guttmann, R. Hoffenberg, I. Kennedy, M. Lock, R. A. Sells, and N. Tilney. 1998. "The Case for Allowing Kidney Sales: International Forum for Transplant Ethics," *Lancet* 351(9120): 1950–1952.

Reddy, K. C. 1993. "Should Paid Organ Donation Be Banned in India? To Buy or Let Die!" *National Medical Journal of India* 6(3): 137–139.

———. 1994. "Controversies in Paid Organ Renal Transplantation: An Indian Viewpoint," *Asian Journal of Surgery* 17(4): 326–330.

Roels, L., W. Coosemans, M. R. Christiaens, et al. 1995. "The Relative Impact of Legislative Incentives on Multiorgan Donation Rates in Europe," *Transplantation Proceedings* 27: 795.

Roels, L., Y. Vanreterghm, M. Waer, M. R. Christiaens, et al. 1991. "Three Years of Experience with a 'Presumed Consent' Legislation in Belgium: Its Impact on Multi-organ Donation in Comparison with other European Countries," *Transplantation Proceedings* 23: 903.

Rothman, D. J., E. Rose, T. Awaya, et al. 1997. "The Bellagio Task Force Report on Transplantation, Bodily Integrity, and the International Traffic in Organs," *Transplantation Proceedings* 29(6): 2739–2745.

Santiago-Delpin, E. A. 1991. "Organ Donation and Transplantation in Latin America," *Transplant Proceedings* 23: 2516–2518.

Scheper-Hughes, Nancy. 1996. "Theft of Life: The Globalization of Organ Stealing Rumors," *Anthropology Today* 12(3): 3–11.

Schwindt, R., and A. R. Vining. 1986. "Proposal for a Future Delivery Market for Transplant Organs," *Journal of Health Politics and Policy Law* 11(3): 483–500.

Sells, R. A. 1992. "The Case Against Buying Organs and a Futures Market in Transplants," *Transplantation Proceedings* 24(5): 2198–2202.

Shaikh, R. 1998. "International Issues and Public Perception: Introduction," *Annals of the New York Academy of Sciences* 862: 202–204.

Sharp, L. A. 1995. "Organ Transplantation as a Transformative Experience: Anthropological Insights into the Restructuring of the Self," *Medical Anthropology Quarterly* 9(3): 357–389.

Siminoff, L. A., Robert Arnold, Art Caplan, B. A. Virnig, and D. L. Seltzer. 1995. "Public Policy Governing Organ and Tissue Procurement in the United States: Results from the National Organ and Tissue Procurement Study," *Annals of Internal Medicine* 123: 10–17.

Singh, P., A. Srivastava, and A. Kumar. 1998. "Current Status of Transplant Coordination and Organ Donation in India," *Transplantation Proceedings* 30: 3627–3628.

Spital, A. 1995. "Mandated Choice: A Plan to Increase Public Commitment to Organ Donation," *Journal of the American Medical Association* 273(6): 504–506.

———. 1997. "Ethical and Policy Issues in Altruistic Living and Cadaveric Organ Donation," *Clinical Transplantation* 11(2): 77–87.

Spurr, S. J. 1992. "The Proposed Market for Human Organs," *Journal of Health Politics and Policy Law* 18(1): 196.

Thomasma, D. C. 1997. "Bioethics and International Human Rights," *Journal of Law, Medicine and Ethics* 25: 295–306.

Veatch, Robert, and J. B. Pitt. 1995. "The Myth of Presumed Consent: Ethical Problems in New Organ Procurement Strategies," *Transplantation Proceedings* 27: 2168.

Velasco, N. 1992. "Organ Donation and Kidney Sales," *Lancet* 352(9126): 483.

Virnig, B. A., and Arnold Caplan. 1992. "Required Request: What Difference Has It Made?" *Transplantation Proceedings* 24: 2155–2158.

WHO (World Health Organization). 1991. "Guiding Principles on Human Organ Transplantation," *Lancet* 337: 1470–1471.
———. 1992. *Human Organ Transplantation: A Report on Developments Under the Auspices of WHO (1987–1991)*. Geneva: World Health Organization.
———. 1994. *Legislative Responses to Organ Translplantation*. Dordrecht, Netherlands: Martinus Niojhoff and Kluwer Academic Press.
World Medical Association. 1985. "World Medical Association Statement on Live Organ Trade." Adopted by the 37th Assembly, Brussels, October.
WuDunn, Sheryl. 1999. "Death Taboo Weakening, Japan Sees First Transplant," *New York Times,* Section A.

PART 4
Globalizing Mothering

10

Does Authoritative Knowledge in Infant Nutrition Lead to Successful Breast-Feeding? A Critical Perspective

Arachu Castro and Lauré Marchand-Lucas

Images of children undernourished and dying after inappropriate bottle-feeding with artificial milk flourished worldwide in the 1970s. These images had a powerful impact on consumer organizations and international food policies. As a result, in 1981 the World Health Assembly voted to support the World Health Organization's *International Code of Marketing of Breast-Milk Substitutes* (World Health Organization 1981), and other international agreements were forged to promote, protect, and support breast-feeding.

Some of the wealthiest countries in the world still consider breast-feeding to be "good" for poor countries, but not for themselves (see UNICEF-France 1997 for an example). Despite many years of constant efforts from grassroots organizations and United Nations agencies to implement the code and the subsequent agreements globally, too often breast-feeding is perceived as an important practice in terms of health only when it is bound to poverty and malnutrition. In countries such as France, breast-feeding is perceived as optional: it is a woman's or a couple's feeding choice, which lies outside the scope of institutions such as the Ministry of Health. This attitude disregards the impact that this choice may have in public health terms—increasing evidence exists that the lack of breast-feeding is associated with higher morbidity rates for the mother and for the newborn, both in developing and in industrialized countries (Cunningham, Jelliffe, and Jelliffe 1992; Stuart-Macadam 1995:7–25; AAP 1997).

Even if reasons provided by an objective utilitarian approach—or in "positivist terms" as it has been called elsewhere (Maher 1995:1)—might not constitute a strong enough basis to promote breast-feeding, a second problem related to the lack of informed choice arises. Following the notion that women need to make their own choices, health professionals in France do not provide them with appropriate information on breast-feeding and artificial feeding. Some health professionals fear that if women knew the possible negative health outcomes of infant formula, they would feel guilty if they did not breast-feed. It is in such a context that formula manufacturers justify some of their marketing practices for their own financial benefit. The lack of informed choice raises the question of whether there is a level playing field in the way women and their partners, as well as the whole society, are given appropriate information.

This chapter presents the joint analysis of three different studies. First, we report some of the results of a comparative study, developed in Paris in 1996–1997, on the relationship between discourses on infant nutrition and motherhood in three ethnic groups—those of French, North African, and Southeast Asian descent—living in France (Castro 1998). The study involved open-ended interviews with thirty women before and after giving birth, as well as participant observation in maternity wards and in breast-feeding self-help groups. Second, we present results of a qualitative survey conducted in 1995–1997 on the representations and attitudes of twenty French general practitioners (Marchand-Lucas and Lucas 1998). Finally, we analyze the underlying discourse of current French publications targeted at parents and medical doctors. Results of our combined analysis are clustered into topics: factors that undermine breast-feeding promotion, the medicalization of breast-feeding, the lack of an appropriate model of authoritative knowledge, the role of breast-feeding specialists, and attitudes about individual choices and the socialization of children.

The aim of this chapter is to explain why international recommendations that have proved successful in other countries fail in France. In a context such as France, where a cultural resistance to breast-feeding exists, a woman who wishes to breast-feed is unlikely to receive either technical or emotional support to continue breast-feeding. Technical support is necessary because even though physicians acknowledge the superiority of breast-feeding over artificial feeding, most of the time they lack the appropriate skills to help a mother overcome doubts, pain, or any other physical problems that she may experience when breast-feeding. Where bottle-feeding with artificial milk is the cultural norm, physicians tend to prescribe formula at the first sign of a possible problem. Emotional support is also needed because partners, relatives, or friends might be unfamiliar with the physiology of breast-feeding, and might find formula a socially more acceptable path. Finally, infant formula manufacturers nourish this cultural resistance to breast-feeding by sharply diverting the law and by creating new markets of consumers that would choose formula as the most convenient infant feeding practice.

Reasons for Concern

France has one of the lowest rates of breast-feeding at birth in the world: 59.5 percent of newborns are artificially fed from birth, although 11 percent of them also receive some breast milk (INSERM 1998).[1] This is due, in part, to the fact that health professionals in France are ill trained in the physiology and management of breast-feeding—the curricula of medical schools include only a two-hour lecture on lactation, which consists of the composition of human milk. Even though many medical doctors in France do not have appropriate training to provide informed infant feeding advice, families and institutions look to this body of professionals for reliable information.

The aforementioned data on the rates of breast-feeding at birth are consistent with that derived from health certificates at the eighth day of life, which are established for all French newborns by their physician. In 1995 these certificates indicated that 45.8 percent of newborns were breast-fed—receiving any breast milk—on the eighth day (Direction Générale de la Santé 1996). We can compare the French situation to that in other European countries. Many countries have median breast-feeding figures of more than 90 percent at birth (Denmark, Sweden, Norway, Switzerland, Romania, Poland, Turkey, Croatia). Somewhat lower are Luxembourg (74 percent) and the United Kingdom (63 percent). Only Ireland has a lower figure than France: 34 percent in 1986 (Railhet 1998). Little is known about the duration of breast-feeding in Europe, except for a few countries: Switzerland (three months), United Kingdom (three months), Denmark (six months), and Turkey (twelve months) (Railhet 1998).

Data on the duration of breast-feeding in France have not been gathered. This will probably change in the next few years, as a new item exploring the duration of breast-feeding has been added to the health certificate at nine months. This certificate is to be completed by a physician during the ninth-month visit, which is mandatory for all infants in France if eligible women wish to receive a monthly income from the government. In the meantime we can rely on a few local surveys done in two French regions, which show that figures fall quickly after birth. Figure 10.1 includes figures at birth and at one week from a national study (INSERM 1998; Direction Générale de la Santé 1996), at four weeks from Somme, in the north (Laviolle 1998), and at six and sixteen weeks from Seine Maritime, in the northwest (Lerebours et al. 1991). The graph shows how rapidly weaning takes place for most infants in two regions.

Resuming work is one of the most common explanations women give to wean their infants (Castro 1998). In France 60.2 percent of pregnant women work during their pregnancies (INSERM 1998). As a result of the

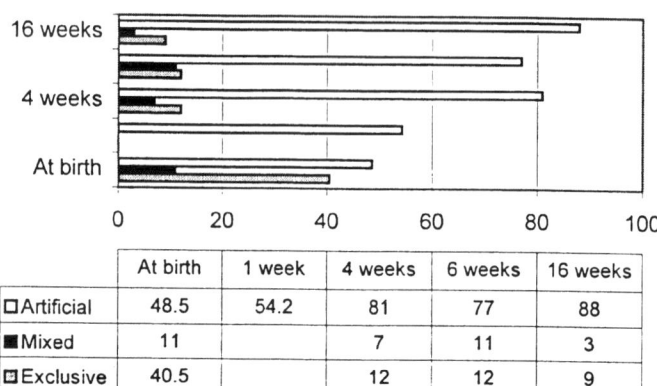

Figure 10.1 Proportion of Infants Breast-Fed and Artificially Fed in France by Age, 1991–1996

	At birth	1 week	4 weeks	6 weeks	16 weeks
☐ Artificial	48.5	54.2	81	77	88
■ Mixed	11		7	11	3
☐ Exclusive	40.5		12	12	9

duration of the legal maternity leave in France—two weeks before the expected date of birth and eight weeks postpartum for singleton deliveries—returning to work does not occur, for the majority of those women, before two months postpartum. Statistics show, however, that most French mothers stop breast-feeding their infants before they return to their job, and at sixteen weeks, only 3 percent to 5 percent of infants are exclusively breast-fed (Lerebours et al. 1991). Moreover, international research indicates that it is not so much that mothers have a job as the characteristics of the job that influence infant feeding practices (Hight-Laukaran et al. 1996).

One of our findings is that two models of knowledge in infant nutrition are held at the same time in France. One is the legitimate and official model, which is practiced by health professionals using the biomedical model or some alternatives—such as the combination of homeopathy with allopathy. This official model can lead to little or no breast-feeding and to the introduction of other foods at two or three months. The other model, which is more empirical, leads to successful breast-feeding, defined as an overall positive breast-feeding experience whereby the child is not forced to stop breast-feeding, and where nursing is perceived as a positive experience for the mother and her nursling.

We suggest that authoritative knowledge of infant nutrition existing in France reproduces itself, not because it is correct, but because it counts culturally and reproduces the dominant paradigm of infant feeding. Jordan defined *authoritative knowledge* as

> the knowledge that participants agree counts in a particular situation, that *they* see as consequential, on the basis of which *they* make decisions and provide justifications for courses of action. It is the knowledge that within

a community is considered legitimate, consequential, official, worthy of discussion, and appropriate for justifying particular actions by people engaged in accomplishing the tasks at hand. (Jordan 1993:154; emphasis in original)

Thus, those who have the authority, such as pediatricians and general practitioners, question the knowledge of experienced mothers because they are not health professionals, and of breast-feeding specialists because they do not reproduce the mainstream values of the French society.

There are many reasons that efforts to implement international breast-feeding agreements and recommendations are hindered in France. Some of those include the low cultural value attributed to colostrum, which is the first milk a mammal secretes during the first three to six days after giving birth (encouraging the use of supplementary liquids); the use of bottles with artificial milk and pacifiers to space breast-feeds (deregulating newborn-driven breast-feeding rhythms and creating nipple confusion between the breast and bottle); and the perception that lack of milk is frequent (justifying the distribution of free samples of artificial milk). The types of beliefs and practices surrounding breast-feeding in France led the authors to analyze why French health professionals maintain a set of assumptions about breast-feeding that differ greatly from the most updated international scientific results.

The Low Cultural Value of Colostrum

In France, even mothers who want to breast-feed are often discouraged from doing so by health professionals, as is illustrated in other European and North American contexts (Dettwyler 1995:174–198; Maher 1995:2). When mothers begin breast-feeding in a context wherein only very young infants are breast-fed, it is likely that breast-feeding will last only a few weeks, as it is perceived as being a maternal sacrifice and an obstacle to modernity.

In 1996, in a public maternity ward in Paris, a woman who had just given birth three hours earlier arrived at her room with her newborn child. A nurse assistant offered to take care of the girl. The woman, who is one of the authors, replied that she preferred to keep the child in her room so that she could breast-feed her as needed. The health worker told her, "It's not worth it, considering what you have!"[2]—referring to colostrum (the milk a mammal secretes during the first three to six days after giving birth). The woman had to justify her request to the health worker—who was not informed about this aspect of lactation physiology—so that she could finally keep the child herself.

In the view of this health professional, colostrum was either not worthy or insufficient to nourish the infant. This low appreciation of colostrum arises more from the cultural values placed on this secretion in some

European regions (Castro 1998) than from scientific knowledge. This last view is also shared in French law: "In any case, the decision to recommend [hypoallergenic formula] *while waiting for the coming in of milk* and/or to complement breast-feeding must be left at the appreciation of the pediatricians (and not of midwives, pediatric nurses or maternity facility administrators); they should not be invited to do so by pressing improper advertising of these products"[3] (NOR: ECO8910166V, Article 2, Paragraph 2.3; italics added). It is thus interesting to note that this law does not reflect the main findings about colostrum supported by research and breast-feeding specialists. First, research shows that colostrum is the only food a newborn needs—except in very rare circumstances. No other product, standard or special, is needed "while waiting for the coming in of milk"— which is in fact the augmentation of the milk supply after the first few hours after birth—because colostrum *is* the first milk.

Second, newborns obtain all the colostrum they need when they nurse efficiently and are offered the breast on cue from birth. However, newborns are likely not to have their colostrum needs met when restricted feeding schedules are recommended. For most newborns and their mothers, a schedule may lead to frustration, especially if the infant wants to suckle outside the timed feeds: the mother might think that her child is hungry because she does not have enough milk, or that this milk is insufficient. Finally, the frequency of early feedings has been shown to have an impact on the timing of what the law names "the coming in of milk." This augmentation occurs earlier and more smoothly when the newborn nurses frequently in the first few days (Righard and Alade 1990; Masse-Raimbault 1992:17; Salle 1993:388).

Systematic Supplementation with Artificial Milk

As we have observed in maternity wards and analyzed in health professionals' and women's discourses, the main justification for giving artificial milk in bottles or pacifiers is, first, to space breast-feeds so that the mother can rest and, second, to prevent the child from being "spoiled." Returning to the case of the aforementioned mother, the next day another nurse assistant brought her bottles with artificial milk and encouraged her to give the child a pacifier in order "to reduce the baby's sucking reflex." However, both of these practices could develop nipple confusion in the child. It is, in fact, expected that full-term newborns should not ask to be fed more than six or seven times per twenty-four hours, which is the usual pattern for bottle-fed newborns. Therefore, the feeding patterns of an exclusively breast-fed newborn—who frequently nurses eight to twelve times per day—are interpreted as a sign of "spoiling" or as an indication that the mother's milk production is insufficient.

Inaccurate advice about the need for supplementary bottle feeding, in contrast to international standards, is also frequently seen in the media. One example is the information contained in a magazine given free of charge to all pregnant women at their first prenatal visit in France. The section on the first days postpartum reads:

> It is however important to know that if you are tired or worried your milk can suddenly diminish and your baby will be hungry and will cry. . . . The remedy is simple: rest, drink a lot, and your milk will come back. Of course, in the meantime, if baby is very hungry, it is always possible *to offer a supplementary bottle,* in the most simple way in the world. (Comité National de l'Enfance 1997:121)

On the same page, short feeds of not more than ten minutes on each breast are recommended. However, research shows that the restriction of duration of the feed, together with the restriction of the number of feeds, will impair a mother's ability to produce milk (Tully and Dewey 1985; Van Esterik 1988; Masse-Raimbault 1992:17).

Perception of Lack of Milk as a Frequent Occurrence

On the day of the mother's hospital discharge, two midwives offered her a can of infant formula "to help out in case she experiences a lack of breast-milk production."[4] It is important to note that for most health professionals a can of infant formula is considered a "gift" to the mother, and only few health professionals are aware that this gift could undermine the mother's breast-feeding plans (Bergevin, Dougherty, and Kramer 1983).

Since February 8, 1999, formula manufacturers have not been allowed by law to have financial agreements with public and private maternity wards. Such agreements are called *tours de lait,* that is, turns to distribute free samples of milk. The formula company provides free formula cans, ready-to-use bottles with artificial milk, plus a fixed fee for every child—the fee varying from one hospital to another. In exchange, the ward agrees to use that company's products exclusively (Walter 1999:3–4; Brisset 1997:27). These agreements were promoted by companies because research shows that parents who buy formula tend to rely on the same brand as the one used in the maternity ward (Reiff and Essock-Vitale 1985).

The *insufficient milk syndrome* is in fact a biological manifestation created by behavioral factors that vary as a function of the sociocultural context, in particular the family structure, gender roles, and motherhood (Obermeyer, Makhlouf, and Castle 1997:40). The syndrome relates to the perception of a lack of the mother's milk and to cultural factors contributing to the insufficient production of milk. These factors include, for example, the positioning at the breast that renders the sucking reflex inefficient (the infant's body facing the ceiling and head turned to the side for sucking as if for a bottle, instead of being in a face-to-face position). In fact, signs of good positioning and attachment have been described as "the baby is close to the breast and facing it, his mouth is quite wide open, his lower lip is turned outwards, his chin is almost touching the breast, his cheeks are round, and there is more areola above the baby's mouth than below it" (UNICEF/World Health Organization 1993). Equally, the cultural norm of determining the spacing of feeds by the clock instead of by the infant's demand can inhibit milk production. Third, in some instances, the advice to press upon the breast with the fingers—to separate the breast from the infant's nostrils—can in fact displace the nipple and risk rendering the sucking painful and/or ineffective (the infant's nostrils are designed for breathing to the side).

Finally, a mother's perception of insufficient milk production can itself create an anxiety that inhibits her release of milk (Tully and Dewey 1985; Van Esterik 1988). Sometimes fatigue, stress, and depression can cause a temporary lack of milk, but that can be sustained by the mother's lack of confidence in her ability to feed her child. Introducing artificial milk when the mother thinks she does not have enough milk generates a vicious circle that can result in a complete cessation of lactation. When the infant is fed with supplements, they satisfy the child, who therefore has less desire to breast-feed, which correspondingly results in a reduction in the mother's milk production. The existence of this syndrome therefore reflects the downfall of a traditional system of support for breast-feeding, and is in part a consequence—and cause—of the lack of confidence on the part of some mothers in their ability to feed their children.

International and French Agreements to Support Breast-Feeding

Three main international agreements and a set of initiatives are being implemented worldwide to promote breast-feeding. Each of them constitutes a landmark in the battle to avoid unethical marketing strategies of breast-milk substitutes. Nonetheless, their implementation is far from being automatic.

The WHO International Code (1981)

The WHO *International Code of Marketing of Breast Milk Substitutes,* adopted in 1981 by the Thirty-fourth World Health Assembly (WHA), was signed by France along with all other countries except the United States. Its aim is "to contribute to the provision of safe and adequate nutrition for infants, by the protection and promotion of breast-feeding, and by ensuring the proper use of breastmilk substitutes, when these are necessary, on the basis of adequate information and through appropriate marketing and distribution" (World Health Organization 1981, Article 1). Since 1981 subsequent World Health Assemblies have adopted motions to end the distribution of free supplies of breast-milk substitutes—including formula given free of charge or at low cost at maternity wards. One such motion was also signed by France in 1994, although the application of the decree started in 1999.

The WHO/UNICEF Joint Statement (1989)

Second, the 1989 WHO/UNICEF *Joint Statement Protecting, Promoting and Supporting Breastfeeding: The Special Role of Maternity Services* was targeted at maternity wards. This statement is twofold: "to increase awareness of the critical role health services play in protecting and promoting breast-feeding, and to describe what should be done to provide mothers with appropriate information and support" (World Health Organization/UNICEF 1989:5). This statement is summarized in the *Ten Steps to Successful Breastfeeding*, which state that all healthcare facilities where childbirth is undertaken should:

- Have a written breastfeeding policy that is routinely communicated to all health care staff.
- Train all health care staff in skills necessary to implement this policy.
- Inform all pregnant women about the benefits and management of breastfeeding.
- Help mothers initiate breastfeeding within half-hour of birth.
- Show mothers how to breastfeed, and how to maintain lactation even if they should be separated from their infants.
- Give newborn infants no food and drink other than breast milk unless *medically* indicated.
- Practice rooming-in—allow mothers and infants to remain together—24 hours a day.
- Encourage breastfeeding on demand.
- Give no artificial teats or pacifiers (also called dummies or soothers) to breastfeeding infants.
- Foster the establishment of breastfeeding support groups and refer mothers to them on discharge from the hospital or clinic. (World Health Organization/UNICEF 1989:iv)

The Innocenti Declaration (1990)

The third key international agreement is the *Innocenti Declaration on the Protection, Promotion and Support of Breastfeeding*, which was adopted in 1990 by the secretaries of health of thirty countries. Although France was not present and thus did not sign the agreement at that time, it later voted for the 1991 World Health Assembly resolutions, whose purpose was to implement the objectives of the *Innocenti Declaration* (World Health Assembly 1991). This declaration establishes the following objectives designed to protect, promote, and support breast-feeding: each government should (1) create a national multisector committee for the promotion of breast-feeding with a national coordinator; (2) ensure that services provided by maternity wards respect the *Ten Steps to Successful Breastfeeding*; (3) take measures to put into practice the principles and goals of the International Code of Marketing of Breast Milk Substitutes; and (4) enact imaginative legislation protecting the breast-feeding rights of working women and established means for its enforcement (World Health Organization/UNICEF 1990).

Initiatives and Recommendations

A series of initiatives and recommendations have followed these agreements (see Van Esterik 1989 and 1995 for a detailed international political background of these events). The UNICEF/WHO *Baby Friendly Hospital Initiative* was first launched in 1991. Its objectives are "to transform hospitals and maternity facilities into baby friendly institutions, comply to the Ten Steps according to the global criteria, and to end free and low cost supplies of breastmilk substitutes" (UNICEF/World Health Organization 1991). Until 1995 the WHO recommended exclusive breast-feeding for all children for four to six months, with continued breast-feeding, along with progressive introduction of the family's food, for up to two years and beyond (WHO 1995:117–20). In 1995, the WHO continued to recommend exclusive breast-feeding for all children four to six months old with continued breast-feeding along with progressive introduction of the family's food for up to two years and beyond (WHO 1995: 117–120). Other influential professional associations, such as the American Association of Pediatrics, recommend a minimum breast-feeding period of one year (American Association of Pediatrics 1997).

In France, as of January 1999, no such National Committee for the Promotion of Breast-Feeding has been created. In 1994, the authors participated in the first meeting, sponsored by UNICEF-France, on the creation of a national breast-feeding committee, held at the International Children's Center. A second meeting took place in 1996 at UNICEF-France headquarters, to which one of the authors was invited. However, the results of this last meeting were discouraging; even among people making efforts to promote breast-feeding there was no consensus, and UNICEF-France made no efforts to follow up on the tasks proposed at the meeting. Instead, the president of UNICEF-France, a lawyer appointed by the French government in

1996, was instructed by the secretary of health not to promote breast-feeding, with the justification that women need to decide for themselves (Bernadette Puiseux 1997, personal communication; Puiseux is the UNICEF breast-feeding coordinator in France). Among breast-feeding advocates, there is a growing suspicion that infant formula manufacturers are lobbying the Ministry of Health (some evidence is suggested in Walter 1999). This lobbying may be done indirectly through the French Society of Pediatrics, which is financed by the infant formula manufacturers (Société Française de Pédiatrie 1998).

To date in France, implementation of the international objectives include the law on Competition, Consumption, and Repression of Fraud (NOR:ECO8910166V of February 2, 1990) and the law on the Marketing of Breast Milk Substitutes (number 94–442, NOR:ECOX9300172L of June 3, 1994). Although the latter was voted on in 1994, the application decree finalizing this law was not published by the French government until August 8, 1998, just in time to comply with directives coming from the European Union. Therefore, its application could not begin until February 8, 1999. However, maternity wards and health professionals, supported by infant formula manufacturers, have already made statements about some strategies to subvert the law (Walter 1999).

Everything Against Breast-Feeding

The French government emphasizes the idea that breast-feeding does not need to be promoted. Instead, it argues that breast-feeding information must be provided, and that women will decide what is best for them. This approach, which uses a subjective utilitarian framework, is based on the assumption that information provided through official institutions and health professionals is scientifically grounded and free from any conflict of interest. The assumption is incorrect, however, first, because the government does not seem to use information produced by reliable sources, and, second, because media are flooded with misinformed and misleading information sponsored often by infant formula manufacturers.

No Governmental Goodwill

As we stated earlier, the great proportion of general practitioners and medical specialists as well as the Division of Health within the Ministry of Work and Social Affairs do not consider the low incidence and prevalence of breast-feeding in France a public health concern. The fact that France is currently the only country in the European Union without a national committee on breast-feeding, even though the proportion of children breast-fed at birth is the second-lowest in the European Union, reflects this lack of concern. In a letter written in April 1997, the vice director of the government's Population Health Office states: "Concerning the Baby-Friendly Hospital Initiative—which consists in 'labeling' maternity hospitals that follow the ten steps recommended by the WHO and UNICEF—it is not the government's intention to create a National Committee on Breastfeeding that would enable the implementation of the protocol. In a country like France, it seems better to act directly on women through information, while respecting their individual choices, instead of relying on institutional labeling"[5] (Direction Générale de la Santé 1997:1).

However, the French Committee of Public Health prepared a perinatal report in 1994 that stated at several points the importance of promoting breast-feeding for all pregnant women. It even suggested that information on how to breast-feed and work should be provided (Haut Comité de la Santé Publique 1994:73). In fact, the only breast-feeding protocol that the Division of Health has since recommended is that obstetricians and midwives encourage pregnant women who want to breast-feed to take a second HIV test at the end of their pregnancy (Régine Schirrer 1996, personal communication). Although HIV testing during pregnancy is not mandatory in France, 87.8 percent of pregnant women have at least one test (INSERM 1998). It is given to most women after the mandatory prenatal visit at six months, and is paid for by the social security system, which covers the great majority of the population. After birth, if a newborn cannot be directly breast-fed—such as a tube-fed newborn hospitalized for medical reasons—the mother is not allowed to feed the child with her own milk unless she has recent results of various tests. (These are HIV 1 + 2, HB antigen, HCV and, sometimes, HTLV 1 + 2 [Direction Générale de la Santé 1997]). The costs of these tests are entirely reimbursed by social security if performed during the last trimester of pregnancy.

These protocols, designed to prevent health workers from being sued for iatrogenic viral transmission, rather than to protect mothers and newborns, illustrate how the perception of risk of viral contamination through breast milk is very strong in France (Firtion 1995). This fear had spread especially after HIV-contaminated blood was used in that country without proper treatment at blood banks in the late 1980s. Although these regulations do not prevent mothers from breast-feeding, breast-feeding rates are likely to suffer even more as a result of the HIV pandemic in settings such as France, where even health professionals regard formula as a "good or very good product" (Marchand-Lucas and Lucas 1998).

Two major reasons explain the gap between the lack of breast-feeding practice in France and the lack of interest from the Ministry of Health in promoting breast-feeding despite recommendations from the Committee of Public Health. The first reason is the lobbying by formula manufacturers at official health institutions, as well as their marketing strategies, which target newborns as their youngest consumers. A second reason lies in the cultural domain of a medicalized society in which the medical discourse is "constructed in ways which produce only conventional meanings, i.e., ones resonant with the dominant ideology" (Young 1980:134). In the predominant French culture, where fewer than 50 percent of mothers breast-feed and where breast-feeding duration is short, women's breast-feeding knowledge, know-how, and attitudes have not been transmitted from mother to mother during social interactions. In this situation, the inexperience and lack of support from partners, friends, and relatives are at the same time cause and effect of cultural representations that are inappropriate for successful breast-feeding. Thus, the process that leads to little breast-feeding is continually maintained or even made worse.

Misinformed and Misleading Information

Popular magazines addressed to parents frequently publish papers on infant feeding. IPA (Information pour l'Allaitement), a French breast-feeding information organization, reported on the representation of breast-feeding in the three most frequently read monthly magazines for prospective and new parents (*Famili, Enfants Magazine*, and *Parents*), in a study conducted during four months in 1997. The report states that 93 percent of pictures of infants being fed depict bottle feeding. Breast-feeding is always presented as the unusual case, if presented at all. In the few instances in which information on breast-feeding is provided, it is incomplete (Roques 1998). As a result, readers obtain, at best, misleading information on infant feeding. In some instances one wonders whether misinformation is purposely printed to mislead readers.

In another magazine, published by the National Committee on Children (Comité National de l'Enfance 1997) and given free of charge to all pregnant women at the time of their first prenatal visit, most illustrations include a bottle. There are also many advertisements for bottles and follow-up formula. Next to one of these ads there is an article on "Feeding Your Baby" that reads: "Feeding a baby, at the breast or with the bottle, what is it? Two very simple but equally fundamental things: providing the baby with the energy and the elements necessary for growth, development, immune protection, and body functioning; providing the baby, day after day, with a wonderful proof of love" (Comité National de l'Enfance 1997:112–113). The text is illustrated with the drawing of a smiling baby reaching for a bottle. Pregnant women in France learn, through this widely distributed text, that breast-feeding and bottle-feeding artificial milk are both "very simple" and "equally fundamental." Yet this information is misleading and unethical, as it creates the impression that both types of feeding are equivalent in all regards—including antibodies, which do not exist in formula.

Even the adult milk industry in France promotes the idea that breast-feeding women require supplemental nutrition. This milk industry is currently targeting pregnant and lactating mothers as potential purchasers of their products; "enriched" milks are sometimes recommended by physicians as the only way to get enough of all the nutrients a breast-feeding mother needs, and are also marketed to pregnant women. At the National Day of French Milk Banks one such milk was presented by a nutritional pediatrician as "an only product containing all the supplements that a breast-feeding mother with an average balanced nutrition would need" (cited in Boutry and Marchand-Lucas 1998).

In this context, the health professional's knowledge of breast-feeding has been shown to be strongly determined by cultural trends. Thus, even though breast-feeding is viewed as good for the child's physical and psychological health, it is often hindered by various circumstances (including complications) leading, after a few weeks, to its replacement by artificial feeding (Marchand-Lucas and Lucas 1998).

The Medicalization of Breast-Feeding

The nutritional role of women's breasts has been decreased by an emphasis on hygiene and substitutes for breast milk. Although, historically, most French mothers who have not breast-fed their children have resorted to wet nurses (Badinter 1980; Le Roy Ladurie 1979), the use of the bottle and complementary feeding actually date back quite far in history (Le Roy Ladurie 1979:15; Levenstein 1983:76). More recently, this practice means that the control of the child's nourishment has been transferred from women (mothers, midwives, and wet nurses) to other medical specialists and industry.

Feminism or Sexism

According to certain feminist discourses, both essentialist (La Leche League 1997) and poststructuralist (Altergott 1991),[6] a whole series of the benefits of breast-feeding have been neglected, including control of one's own body and the self-esteem that it affords some mothers. Certain earlier feminist discourses (Raphael 1985), however, laid claim to the right to bottle feeding with artificial milk as the only solution allowing productive and reproductive lives for women who wish to become mothers. This is in contrast to the more recent international studies mentioned previously.

At the beginning of the twentieth century, French feminists fought to ensure that women could have maternity leaves to protect their pregnancies from overwork and to breast-feed their infants (Cova 1997). This civil movement led in 1920 to the right of working mothers with an infant (that is, a child younger than one year) to interrupt their shifts twice daily for half an hour to feed their children (Articles L 224-2 and L 224-3 of the *Labor Code*). Currently, however, these laws, which have not been modified, are most often interpreted by working women and employers who are aware of them as the right either to start the shift one hour later or to finish one hour earlier, thus disregarding the reasons for which they were created.

Current feminism in France is a legacy of Simone de Beauvoir, one of the most prominent French feminists in the 1960s. She wrote in *The Second Sex*: "Mammary glands have no role in a woman's economy, and we could get rid of them at any time"[7] (Beauvoir 1961). According to Beauvoir, breast-feeding would be "an exhausting servitude,"[8] which reflects the perception of an association between sacrifice and breast-feeding. More recently, Elisabeth Badinter, an influential writer and philosopher in current France, stated that "when women start to breastfeed and nurture their children, all they do is to comply devotedly to the combined ideas of physicians and philosophers"[9] (Badinter 1980). This perspective of women, largely shared in France, privileges a woman's productive role in the economy and undermines certain aspects of her reproductive functions, such as breast-feeding, especially if, from a sexual perspective, those functions represent no benefit to men. Many women fear that their breasts will be deformed by breast-feeding. This anxiety is a consequence of the expectation that women need to please men. French women are usually expected to remain attractive and sexually active, and, within the family, this role is often more important than that of nurturing children through breast-feeding.

By contrast, representation of breast-feeding is, for most women and health professionals, an "almost sacred" activity: the breast-feeding mother is pictured in an intimate setting, dressed in a gown, looking intensely into the eyes of her newborn. It is commonly perceived that if the mother is not totally concentrated on her baby while breast-feeding, she might as well bottle-feed (Laviolle 1998). This contemplative perception of a nursing mother leaves little room for representing her as an active person who might be willing and able to perform other tasks while breast-feeding—such as eating, reading, or walking. It also induces some fathers to think that their partners are devoting more time to the child than to themselves. Some women refrain from breast-feeding as a result of their expected role to please men.

Decision and Implicit Choice

Studies on the symbolism of breast-feeding and its relationship to cultural discourse on motherhood remain rare in France (see Jodelet and Ohana 1996 for one recent exception). Research on the chosen method of feeding often focuses on its relationship to the information a woman receives during her pregnancy or childbirth in the hospital setting, to her resumption of work after maternity leave, or to her membership in a given socioeconomic group (see Branger et al. 1998 for an example). Little is known about sociocultural constructions on breast-feeding and weaning.

It has been suggested (Castro 1998) that the social mechanism of cessation and resumption of breast-feeding begins with the society's elite, similar to other sociological processes (Bourdieu 1979). The elite groups differentiate themselves from other social classes by adopting new and expensive practices. Other classes attempt to imitate the elite; then, once all groups are in a position where they can adopt such practices, these are abandoned by the elite, as they are no longer useful as a means of distinction. This is one of the factors that explain why, in many of the poorest African, Asian, and Latin American countries, the wealthiest classes use infant formulas as substitutes for breast-feeding, and why in industrialized countries the lowest socioeconomic classes allocate a significant portion of their budget to the purchase of infant formula.

It is important to establish the distinction between implicit choice and conscious decision in order to better understand the sociocultural construction of breast-feeding and weaning. This distinction is particularly important where alternatives to breast-feeding do exist and, above all, in contexts where those alternatives constitute the norm, as in France. Based on previous research (Castro 1998), when these alternatives to breast-feeding do not exist, or when they exist but do not represent the cultural norm because of problems with access, most pregnant women have no need to make a decision; they simply breast-feed. As alternatives become more accessible, some women enter a conscious decisionmaking process and thus actively consider reasons for and against breast-feeding. When strategies for avoiding breast-feeding become common in a culture, they end up becoming the norm, as has happened in France—at least since the widespread practice of hiring wet nurses.

In such a context, mothers breast-feed under two possible circumstances. The success of breast-feeding promotion efforts can, in fact, depend upon the type of circumstances that make women breast-feed. First, women breast-feed when they do not consciously make a decision because they have no need to justify breast-feeding, even if they can rationalize their behavior later. Second, women breast-feed after they initially question the practice and thus look for supporting arguments. For example, the reasoning "I will breast-feed to give my child antibodies, but I will wean him/her so that I can go back to work" is quite common among French women who decide to breast-feed. Among this second group, the duration of nursing is also usually determined before birth (Lerebours et al. 1991; Castro 1998). This leaves little possibility for prolonging breast-feeding beyond the preestablished period.

On the other hand, in the case where a mother breast-feeds (as a result of an implicit choice) without having made a conscious decision (or even when the decision to breast-feed has been made very early in her life), she rarely decides on the duration of breast-feeding; rather, she follows a cultural norm (Castro 1998). Mothers in this category can also often be encouraged to continue nursing longer, especially when they see children who are older than their own child still being breast-fed, for example, during meetings of support groups for breast-feeding mothers such as La Leche League (see Radius and Joffe 1988 for stimulation among adolescent mothers). Such social stimulation does not seem to be as effective among women who have established their intended duration of breast-feeding before the birth of the child.

During the interviews conducted in Paris (Castro 1998), when a woman related that she decided to breast-feed her child until the end of her maternity leave, she was asked by the interviewer if she had information on how to continue breast-feeding after returning to work, and if she was interested in having that information. In all cases, these women replied that their decision had already been made and that they would not change it, in part because it would be "too complicated" (Castro 1998). It is noteworthy that mothers in this group, often of French origin, breast-feed because they are conscious of the fact that it is better for the child (and/or for themselves), yet they do not wish to do something (to breast-feed) that they perceive as involving constraints on their own behavior. In reality, they do not want to act against their social assumptions, which imply that breast-feeding beyond three months is considered an egocentric means of "keeping the child for themselves," and thus preventing the child's socialization by intermediaries other than the mother, as we explain later in this chapter.

Both French medical literature and practice, as much in pediatrics as in child care, reinforce the idea that medical intervention is necessary in infant health, including infant feeding and infant care, and at the same time disregard international recommendations. Even though a theoretical consensus exists regarding the advantages of breast-feeding among French physicians, in practice their lack of information based on internationally recognized authoritative knowledge prevents them from offering successful advice and support (Marchand-Lucas and Lucas 1998). Instead, they rely on complementary feeding with formula at the least suggestion that the child is not sufficiently nourished through breast milk, or when the mother wants to resume work.

Health Professionals Feeling Guilty

The dominant medical discourse in France considers it inevitable that the mother makes a decision regarding breast-feeding and that this decision involves a conscious choice, which includes the intended duration of breast-feeding (Castro 1998). This discourse is based on the assumption that making such a decision needs to be explicit, and does not consider that breast-feeding could be quite simply a choice without conscious logic. Furthermore, this dominant discourse takes for granted that each woman must evaluate reasons for and against breast-feeding; if the woman says she does not wish to breast-feed, the vast majority of professionals will not offer information on breast-feeding, often for fear of making her feel guilty. Only after a woman explicitly says that she wants to breast-feed will she receive some help to position the newborn correctly at the breast.

For instance, during a breast-feeding training session for midwives in a public hospital in France—led by one of the authors—one of the midwives shared how guilty she felt. A woman expecting her second child had recently moved into town and anticipated a repeat cesarean section for medical reasons. She was discussing the issue of separation from her baby at birth and was adamant about the importance of being able to bond and stay close to her child. The midwife learned that with the woman's first child, hospital routines had prevented contact with her healthy newborn for two days, despite repeated requests to have the baby with her. The midwife reassured the woman that in her ward all mothers had their babies nearby. She even mentioned that newborns under special care also had their mothers with them because the obstetric and pediatric wards worked to keep mothers and newborns together.

The midwife, instead of asking the usual question about feeding method (How are you planning to feed this baby?), said, "I can see that you regard bonding and contact with your baby as so important, I imagine that you breast-feed your babies." The woman responded, after a few seconds of silence, "Well, no, I bottle-fed my first child. But do you think that breast-feeding would help the bonding and contact better than bottle feeding?" The midwife recalls that she felt very embarrassed. When the mother finally said she was going to breast-feed, the midwife felt guilty that she had interfered in this woman's choice. At the time of the training session, that mother was happily breast-feeding her two-month-old and had thanked the midwife for letting her know about the possibility of breast-feeding. Despite this mother's positive outcome, the midwife said she would never do that again.

Medical magazines also reflect this guilt. In 1995 a medical journal, *Impact Médecin Hebdo,* quoted a pediatrician working in a public maternity hospital in Paris: "The choice should be enlightened, but we are not supposed to blame mothers when they do not want to breast-feed, *and we do not have to let them think that they are taking risks for their infants*" (Grandsenne 1995:27; italics added). The journal published this quote to make general practitioners and specialists aware that if they promote breast-feeding, they could be suggesting that bottle feeding with artificial milk has certain risks, which most health professionals do not want to believe.

This reluctance to be critical of artificial milk and bottles is partly due to the fact that they have been promoting formula for most of their careers. However, it is also true that most of the information they read on breast-feeding differs from the international scientific consensus: pediatricians and general practitioners read mostly publications from French medical magazines that have not been peer-reviewed internationally. The infant formula manufacturers lobby these medical magazines through biased papers, such as the articles in the general press about the presence of dioxin in breast milk (*Sciences et Vie,* May 1998, and *Que Choisir,* June 1998).

The medicalization of infant feeding, like techniques of antenatal prediction, is a new phase for the human species, one that not only has implications for women's perceptions of their own identity, including their physical identity, but also one that will undoubtedly play a role in the future of human reproduction. This medicalization obscures the fact that even those women who make a conscious decision about breast-feeding do not do so as freely as they think—their decision is rarely based on an informed choice. Their decision rests directly on the information provided by the medical establishment, which is often poorly informed on the issue of breast-feeding (Marchand-Lucas and Lucas 1998; Chauvard 1995), as well as by the infant formula industry, which elaborates and provides most of the information that physicians, including pediatricians, read about breast-feeding.

Scientific Knowledge Versus Authoritative Knowledge

The knowledge of breast-feeding specialists comes mainly from a global and multidisciplinary approach: global, because breast-feeding specialists from all parts of the world tend to share experiences, views, and scientific knowledge, and multidisciplinary because they are either parents or professionals coming from many different fields, such as the human sciences and health professions. This knowledge contains embodied knowledge, which has been defined as the "subjective knowledge derived from a woman's perceptions of her body and its natural processes as these change throughout a pregnancy's course" (Belenky et al. 1986). We argue that such a definition should include menstruation, birth,[10] lactation, and menopause experiences as well, as they can all provide further perceptions about women's bodies. The aim of breast-feeding specialists is to transmit ideas and practices that improve women's ability and confidence to breast-feed by overcoming the obstacles of their suffering.

Contents of the Authoritative Knowledge

In contrast, French physicians perceive feeding as an uncertain subject that needs to be measured, by the clock or by the bottle. Most French general practitioners and medical specialists who deal with lactating mothers or with their infants refer to the biomedical model. The only set of knowledge available is the one taught in medical schools, which deals only with the composition of breast milk and its superiority as compared to artificial milk. As a result, French health professionals are not aware of any negative effects of formula use. Research shows that the majority of them consider that there are advantages to breast-feeding (Marchand-Lucas and Lucas 1998), but they have no training on how to counsel and support lactating mothers who experience difficulties. Moreover, the notion of "advantages" implies that bottle feeding with artificial milk is the norm and, thus, breast-feeding is an improvement over the norm.

However, this authoritative knowledge also assumes that breast-feeding is incompatible with most prescribed drugs (instead of the converse)—that substituting breast milk with formula is safer than taking the risk that the child ingests any amount of drugs through breast milk. Second, it assumes that insufficient milk supply is a common problem, an idea especially nourished by the aforementioned practices and by infant formula producers (Aublin 1990; Thirion 1993; Wong 1998). Even though only about 1–5 percent of mothers worldwide are unable to produce enough milk (Ageitos 1995; La Leche League [France] 1996), the infant formula manufacturers market their products with the statement "for mothers who do not produce enough milk." Furthermore, their marketing suggests that insufficient milk is a very frequent situation.

Third, the assumption of the biomedical model is that the *painful* engorgement that takes place a few hours (or a few days) after birth is unavoidable. A recent study carried out among multiparous women in Paris shows how this pain is more frequent among French mothers than among mothers from Northern Africa or some countries of Southeast Asia (Castro 1998). One explanation is that pain is created by infrequent and restricted early feeds. Engorgement, defined as an inflammatory process of the whole breast (or often both breasts), takes place three to six days after birth due to the increase of milk volume. It is well-known among breast-feeding specialists that engorgement can be avoided or minimized by early and frequent suckling (Evans, Evans, and Simmer 1995).

The biomedical model appears to encourage breast-feeding on demand, but actually includes some scheduling. "Feeds should be at least two hours apart and four hours at the most" is a frequent recommendation from health professionals (see Comité National de l'Enfance 1997:115 for an example). Very short feeds are also encouraged in the belief that all babies, even newborns, get all the food that they need in the first few minutes of a feed, and that a longer time at the breast leads to cracked nipples.

Through our reseach we have observed that maternity hospitals in France often encourage the use of bottles with artificial milk during the first days after birth, especially at night. The importance of rooming-in at night is countered by the belief that the mother needs to get rest, and that this is best achieved if the infant is in a nursery. Health professionals also encourage practices that are in contradiction to successful breast-feeding management, such as breast washing before and after each feed, the use of creams and disinfectants "to prevent cracked nipples," and the use of pacifiers to fulfill the infant's suckling instinct.

Pediatricians and general practitioners often tend to base decisions on their own experience, both professional and personal (Marchand-Lucas and Lucas 1998), instead of referring to evidence-based health research. This situation has been described in a study carried out in the United States:

> The significant effect of prior personal breast-feeding experience—improved clinical treatment and increased frequency of breast-feeding promotion activity—was disappointing. It is reasonable to expect that prior personal experience would enhance physician confidence, but it should not be a major determinant of the amount or effectiveness of breast-feeding promotion. Instead, prior professional experience is the most appropriate correlate of pediatrician knowledge, attitudes, and activity related to breast-feeding promotion. (Freed et al. 1995:494)

In France, when physicians talk about breast-feeding they seldom refer to the scientific literature, but to their own—or their partner's—experience: If they breast-fed for one month only and their child is healthy, they tend to extrapolate to claim that one month is sufficient (Marchand-Lucas and Lucas 1998).

General practitioners tend to infer that if they did not find a solution to a problem encountered in their personal experience, there is no solution in general to that problem. For instance, having hypogalactia (the medical term for deficiency of milk secretion) after a few weeks of giving birth is regarded as unavoidable for some. This happens especially after practitioners have seen their own infants unsatisfied at the breast—probably due to an infant's growth spurt, and hence an increased demand for milk, which was not recognized as such. As a result they tend to prescribe supplements to infants when consulted by their mothers (Marchand-Lucas and Lucas 1998). This results in less milk intake and, thus, in less milk production. As digestion time for artificial milk is about twice as long as for breast milk, supplements result in a decrease in the stimulation of the breast, which might in turn inhibit the production of milk.

Barriers to Breast-Feeding Specialists in France

In 1956, to counsel and support women interested in breast-feeding their children, seven women living in the Chicago, Illinois, area, who were also the mothers of breast-fed children, decided to meet with a few pregnant and breast-feeding friends. La Leche League (LLL) was then created, working as a self-help group, to share breast-feeding and parenting experiences (La Leche League 1997). These women did not expect the tremendous impact they would later have. In forty years the organization had moved from the founders' kitchen table to a large office in Schaumburg, Illinois. The organization includes about 8,000 leaders (trained volunteers) in sixty-six countries, including around 170 in France. The mission of the organization remains the same as at the time of the foundation: "To help mothers worldwide to breastfeed through mother-to-mother support, encouragement, information, and education and to promote a better understanding of breastfeeding as an important element in the healthy development of the baby and the mother" (La Leche League 1997:34).

In 1982 La Leche League International established a Lactation Consultant Department. Lactation consultation emerged to provide supportive care for breast-feeding mothers. In 1985 lactation consultants established an independent organization to assess competency through certification by the International Board of Lactation Consultant Examiners (IBLCE). Professional organizations now exist throughout the world. The International Lactation Consultant Association represents more than four thousand members (individuals and organizations) and publishes the *Journal of Human Lactation*. In France there are fewer than twenty-five lactation consultants, many of whom are also voluntary LLL leaders of self-help groups, or medical associates. A medical associate in France is a medical professional who has voluntarily chosen to support La Leche League. Requirements for these positions, as stated in the letter of commitment signed and returned to LLL France, are as follows:

> These professionals are interested by breastfeeding, [and] wish to inform themselves on the practical and theoretical aspects of lactation and breastfeeding. These professionals commit to support the breastfeeding mothers in their practice if they choose to start solids by the middle of the first year of their child (unless there is a medical contraindication) and if these mothers want to continue breastfeeding after that. If needed, they can offer conservative solutions to breastfeeding difficulties.

The French law and social security system prevent lactation consultants from developing some aspects of their practice. Lactation consultation involves dealing both with other health care providers in related professions and with the mothers directly. The French government has not yet recognized the profession, and government officials and health care professional bodies show extreme caution in doing so. In general, many health professions such as chiropractors as well as lactation consultants are illegal in France. Therefore, it is illegal for a nonmedical professional, even when a medical doctor is present, to participate in the diagnosis or treatment for any illness or surgical procedure. Physicians are illegally practicing medicine if they assist someone not authorized to practice by law, or if they advertise their practice as a "lactation consultant." However, it is not illegal to offer information or more technical, albeit general, counseling with regard to breast-feeding.

When the lactation consultant is not a physician and is presented with a pathological case, he or she needs to refer the woman to avoid being guilty of illegal practice. The course of action recommended by breast-feeding specialists usually differs drastically from the course of action recommended by physicians, who would often prescribe formula feeding. In these circumstances, a lactation consultant sharing his or her observations and discussing treatment plans with the patient might be considered by some physicians as illegally practicing medicine.

Due to the legal limits of their profession, most French lactation consultants now, therefore, have to work as trainers for other health care professionals in maternity wards, as well as in neonatology services and pediatrics divisions in hospitals. Some who are medical doctors or midwives working in a hospital setting or in the community can practice their lactation consultation "art" from time to time, but it is unlikely that they make a living by opening a clinic. Honoraria of midwives and medical doctors are fixed by the government's social security system. For most professionals, opening this kind of practice would cost more money than it could generate. The fixed consultation price for a general practitioner is about U.S.$20 per consultation, whatever the time spent. A general practitioner who is also a lactation consultant is therefore not allowed to charge more than $20 for a lactation consultation, even though an average lactation consultation takes about two hours. It is important to know that about half of this amount is paid either as professional charges or as taxes. As a result, the net income for such a consultation is reduced to about $5 per hour (which is the usual rate for a baby-sitter). When the child is present, the general practitioner and lactation consultant can make, after taxes, about $10 per hour by charging two visits (which is the usual rate for a cleaning person).

Some health professionals label lactation specialists as breast-feeding fanatics (Ferragu 1993:24). They are criticized because their understanding of infant nutrition and motherhood is contrary to current pediatricians' recommendations and is sometimes considered dangerous and unhelpful. When a health professional seeks information from a lactation specialist, it seems that what is expected is knowledge that would provide solutions to breast-feeding difficulties without changing current practices. Moreover, although health professionals paradoxically state that "breast is best," feeding infants with breast milk substitutes is considered a valuable option, especially after a few weeks (Marchand-Lucas and Lucas 1998).

After fieldwork in different French hospitals, we have observed that in most maternity wards mothers are seldom referred by health professionals to breast-feeding self-help groups, due in part to the lack of awareness of those self-help groups. This happens particularly when those groups advocate and encourage breast-feeding for more than a few weeks, such as LLL. Many professionals tend to believe that what they do for the mother is sufficient to inform and help her, and that their clients (new mothers) do not need support groups. Some are suspicious of what is said in a non-medical setting; in these instances, not referring the mothers to a self-help group is seen as a way of "protecting" her.

La Leche League and many lactation consultants utilize another paradigm, which could be defined through the moral philosophical term of "universal communitarianism," as opposed to dominant cultural trends in France. Breast-feeding is represented as beneficial for both mother and child, for the family and the society in general. In turn, because of the presumed value of strong family ties, breast-feeding is thought to prevent such things as domestic violence, environmental pollution, and dependence on consumer products. This alternative framework of lactation consultants, which goes beyond the breast-feeding domain, is seen by some as a dangerous, bothersome ideology. It is a paradigm of collectivization—breast-feeding is not only beneficial, but essentially good for humanity—that questions the prevailing values of a capitalist society.

The Need for a Rapid Socialization of Infants

Health professionals often refer to nutritional and psychological reasons for weaning children (Ferragu 1993:24). In 1996 an obstetrician explained a recent consultation in a letter published in the French medical journal *Le Concours Médical*. His patient was a thirty-year-old woman, nine weeks pregnant and breast-feeding a twelve-month-old child. Her general practitioner had recommended that she wean her child, and she wanted a second opinion from the obstetrician. The obstetrician states in the medical journal that, although the woman is in good health, she has a psychological problem because she does not want to stop breast-feeding. He asks for recommendations from colleagues, and the journal publishes one answer that includes: "The other drawback, which is on the psychic domain, is not less important. Wanting to feed a child and a fetus at the same time raises a challenge that can have an effect on the mother's balance and on the complex future relationship between the mother and her child. There is an all-powerful issue from the mother that disturbs" (Allart 1996:2842). Those comments, which come from a male physician, reflect fear; they construct the lactating woman as a danger to the medical establishment and to the social order, because of the psychological relationship of mother and child that breast-feeding is seen to symbolize, a relationship that prevents the early socialization of children.

Dominant French culture supports the early separation of mother and child for successful socialization of infants. After hospital discharge, it is considered normal to put the child to sleep in a room of its own, or leave a child for a few hours or even a few days in the first weeks after birth. Early weaning to a nonhuman milk (wet weaning) and the early introduction of solids (dry weaning) have been highly valued in France since at least the Renaissance (Badinter 1980). Although most physicians agree that milk is sufficient for the first four months of life, breast-feeding for that long is rarely encouraged. Therefore, complements and infant formula are introduced at two or three months after birth, following pediatric advice.

We have observed that from the birth of the child, mothers are taught not to feel sad, bad, or guilty about separation and not to respond to their embodied knowledge in relation to it. One of our informants, mother of a second child, said, "It feels so good when my [two-month old] baby is in contact with my body, but I don't do it often because I don't want him to be so dependent on me." Mothers who do not feel good about separation are faced with a dilemma; either they comply with the norm against their own perceptions, or they live their own way. Those who go against the norm would be judged as unacceptable, overanxious, overprotective, or selfish mothers and partners, and are seen as keeping the child for themselves. They may even be regarded as giving priority to the child over their partner. Separation is seen as something good for the child, but also good for the mother, as a corollary for family unit.

Breast-feeding for more than three months may be considered to be a way of preventing the infant's maturity. Because the child, in essence, belongs to his or her mother, the infant's access to "real food" and to broader socialization is impeded. Socialization through association with other children is highly valued, even more than through the family (Ferragu 1993:27). When the child's behavior is considered unacceptable—such as when he or she wakes up at night, or does not accept a few hours' separation—breast-feeding is often blamed, more so when the child gets older, by those who carry the current authoritative knowledge on infant nutrition in France.

Deepening Conversations: From Theory to Policy

The main argument put forward in this chapter is that the low incidence and prevalence of breast-feeding in France cannot be sufficiently explained by saying that the individual choice of most French women is not to breast-feed, or to breast-feed for just a few weeks. To understand the issue of individual choice more completely requires a wider framework, explored, as is the case here, from a political-anthropological perspective, which moves back and forth between the political arena and individual women, which locates the power of the private sector and health professionals, and which includes the analysis of the cultural construction of breast-feeding. It analyzes how the actors involved channel and receive their knowledge, and how the government maintains the fallacy of a level playing field in the access to information and resources. The applied aim of such anthropological analysis is to seek a strategy based on public health recommendations, which can be built on a new reorganization of power.

Although France has legislation to promote breast-feeding (due to mandates from the European Union and international agreements), the French government remains silent about the rules of the game and lets the infant formula manufacturers manipulate those rules. As a consequence, the underpromotion of breast-feeding by French decisionmakers and health professionals is not justified by scientific evidence, but by vested interests of the private sector. Some less-than-optimal practices, such as bottle feeding with artificial milk and with other products, are presented as positive and controlled technological advances that are part of the dominant biomedical paradigm. Data suggests that infant formula manufacturers manipulate parents and health professionals and that, as a result, women's decisions do not follow the standards of informed choice. This local context needs to be addressed to promote breast-feeding successfully in France. Although local initiatives carried by self-help groups and a minority of health professionals do have an impact in providing counseling and support to pregnant and breast-feeding women, their scope is limited due to the barriers set around breast-feeding and breast-feeding specialists.

The French Ministry of Health should acknowledge the current vested interests in the underpromotion of breast-feeding and organize multilateral conversations gathering together women's groups, medically and nonmedically trained breast-feeding specialists, and other health professionals, such as midwives and pediatricians, in order to change the current authoritative knowledge in infant feeding. This dialogue would be aimed at developing strategies to guarantee informed choice and to provide a supportive sociocultural context for breast-feeding mothers, including the workplace, as well as appropriate counseling for parents. Changes could be achieved by monitoring the implementation of the law on the Marketing of Breast Milk Substitutes, legalizing the profession of breast-feeding specialists, revising the current curricula of medical schools, and convincing women's groups to include breast-feeding promotion in their agendas.

As the data from France suggest, the distance between an internationally generated policy and local programs is great. This distance, which unlevels the playing field, extends the social suffering of those caught in the liminal area in between. As Kleinman suggests, to understand the implications of the causes and consequences of increased social suffering requires an analysis of variables drawn from a wide range of domains such as history, politics, economics, and cultural traditions (Kleinman, Das, and Lock 1996). Mothers in France want the best for their children and suffer from the lack of consistent information provided to them. To understand why they are not provided with information and programs reflective of the international guidelines, one must study the history, contemporary culture, and politics of France, as this study has attempted to do.

Notes

We would like to thank Dora Gutiérrez for her helpful technical revision, Debbie Sabin, Andrea Ledward, and Michael Reich for their thoughtful insights, and Linda Whiteford and Lenore Manderson for their comments and encouragement.

1. These data do not include incidence of breast-feeding at birth from overseas departments and territories.

2. "Cela ne vaut pas la peine, pour ce que vous avez!"

3. "En tout état de cause il faut laisser à l'appréciation des pédiatres (et non des sages-femmes, des puéricultrices ou des gestionnaires des établissements d'accouchement) de les recommander ou non en attendant la montée laiteuse et/ou en complément de l'allaitement maternel, sans qu'une publicité abusive ne les y invite de manière pressante."

4. "Pour la dépanner en cas de manque de lait."

5. "En ce qui concerne l'initiative "Amis des Bébés" qui consiste à labelliser les maternités qui obéissent aux dix recommandations préconisées par l'OMS et l'UNICEF, il n'est pas dans les intentions du Gouvernement de créer un Comité National d'Allaitement pour mettre en place ce protocole. Dans un pays comme la France, il paraît en effet préférable d'agir directement auprès des femmes par le biais de l'information tout en respectant leurs choix individuels, plutôt que de s'appuyer sur une labellisation des établissements."

6. For essentialist feminists the woman's inner self is different in essence from that of men, whereas for poststructuralist feminists a woman's specificity is built through her relationship with other human beings, and there is no such thing as a basic feminine nature.

7. "Les glandes mammaires n'ont aucun rôle dans l'économie de la femme, et on pourrait en faire l'ablation n'importe quand."

8. "Une servitude épuisante."

9. "Lorsque les femmes se mettent à allaiter et à materner leurs enfants, elles ne font qu'obéir béatement aux incitations conjuguées des médecins et des philosophes."

10. Please note that the French word *accouchement*—literally meaning lying down—is the process lived by the woman since the first contractions until the delivery of the placenta. *Naissance* is the process of being born—it relates thus to the

newborn and not to the mother. In English, "birth" is used for both *accouchement* and *naissance*.

References

AAP (American Association of Pediatrics). 1997. "Breastfeeding and the Use of Human Milk," *Pediatrics* 100(6): 1035–1039.
Action pour l'Allaitement. 1995. *L'allaitement maternel et la commercialisation des substituts du lait maternel en France.* Strasbourg: Rapport d'enquête IBFAN/APA.
Ageitos, María Luisa. 1995. "Conocimientos actuales sobre la lactancia materna." In *Reunión del Comité Nacional de Lactancia.* Córdoba: Sociedad Argentina de Pediatría.
Allart, J. P. 1996. "Allaiter pendant une grossesse," *Le Concours Médical* 118(39): 2842.
Altergott, Marjorie. 1991. "Artificial Infant Feeding: Women's Loss, Men's Gain," *Issues in Reproductive and Genetic Engineering* 4(2): 129–141.
Aublin, P. C. 1990. "Comment conduire un allaitement maternel," *Le Concours Médical* (June 6): 2052–2056.
Badinter, Elisabeth. 1980. *L'amour en plus: Histoire de l'amour maternel (XIIe siècle–XXe siècle).* Paris: Flammarion.
Beauvoir, Simone de. 1961. *Le deuxième sexe.* Paris: Gallimard.
Belenky, Mary Field, et al. 1986. *Women's Ways of Knowing: The Development of Self, Voice, and Mind.* New York: Basic Books.
Bergevin, Y., C. Dougherty, and M. S. Kramer. 1983. "Do Infant Formula Samples Shorten the Duration of Breast-Feeding?" *Lancet* 21(8334): 1148–1151.
Blondel, B., G. Bréart, C. du Mazauburn, G. Badeyan, M. Wcislo, A. Lordier, et al. 1997. "La situation périnatale en France: Évolution de 1981 à 1995," *Journal de Gynécologie, Obstétrique et Biologie Reproductive* 26: 770–780.
Bourdieu, Pierre. 1979. *La distinction: Critique sociale du jugement.* Paris: Minuit.
Boutry, B., and L. Marchand-Lucas. 1998. "Report Summarizing the Presentations." Unpublished report, *Journée Nationale des Lactariums,* Bordeaux.
Branger, B., et al. 1998. "Facteurs influant la durée de l'allaitement. Une étude de 150 femmes," *Archives de Pédiatrie* 5(5): 489–496.
Brisset, Claire. 1997. "Ces biberons qui tuent," *Le Monde Diplomatique,* December 1997, p. 27.
Castro, Arachu. 1998. "Costruzioni socioculturali sull'allattamento al seno e lo svezzamento: Uno studio comparativo tra donne francesi, magrebine e del sudest asiatico che vivono in Francia," *PRAE, Quaderni del Centro Scientifico Regionale di Prevenzione Sanitaria* 1: 3 (Milan).
Chauvard, Sandrine. 1995. "Allaitement maternel. La France à la traîne," *Impace Médicin Hebdo* (294): 26–27.
Comité National de l'Enfance, ed. 1997. *L'enfant du premier âge. La grossesse. L'accouchement. Le bébé de sa naissance à 2 ans.* Paris: Comité National de l'Enfance.
Cova, A. 1997. *Maternité et droits des femmes en France: XIXème–XXème siècles.* Paris: Anthropos.
Cunningham, Allan S., Derrick B. Jelliffe, and E. F. Patrice Jelliffe. 1992. *Breastfeeding, Growth and Illness: An Annotated Bibliography.* New York: UNICEF.

Dettwyler, Katherine A. 1995. "Beauty and the Breast: The Cultural Context of Breastfeeding in the United States." In *Breastfeeding: Biocultural Perspectives,* P. Stuart-Macadam and K. A. Dettwyler, eds. New York: Aldine de Gruyter.

Direction Générale de la Santé. 1996. *Certificats du 8ème jour.* Paris: Ministry of Health.

———. 1997. Letter number DGS/SP2-247 (April 2).

Evans, K., R. Evans, and K. Simmer. 1995. "Effect of the Method of Breast Feeding on Breast Engorgement, Mastitis and Infantile Colic," *Acta Paediatrica* 84(8): 849–852.

Ferragu, Christiane Cormier. 1993. *Lorsque l'enfant tète, relation de proximité et autonomie: Un image de la petite enfance.* Rennes: University of Rennes.

Firtion, Ghislaine. 1995. "L'allaitement maternel à l'heure des virus," *Dossiers de l'Allaitement* 24: 8.

Freed, Gary L., Sarah J. Clark, Jacob A. Lohr, and James R. Sorenson. 1995."Pediatrician Involvement in Breast-Feeding Promotion: A National Study of Residents and Practitioners," *Pediatrics* 96(3): 490–494.

Grandsenne, Philippe. 1995. "Allaitement maternel: La France à la traîne," *Impact Médecin Hebdo* 294(October 6): 27.

Haut Comité de la Santé Publique. 1994. *La sécurité et la qualité de la grossesse et de la naissance: Pour un nouveau plan périnatalité.* Paris: Ministry of Welfare and Health.

Hight-Laukaran, Virginia, et al. 1996. "The Use of Breast Milk Substitutes in Developing Countries: The Impact of Women's Employment," *American Journal of Public Health* 86(9): 1235–1240.

INSERM (Institut National de la Santé et de la Recherche Médicale). 1997. "Résultats de l'enqête périnatale faite dans quatre départements pilotes en France," *Journal de Gynécologie, Obstétrique et Biologie Reproductive* 26(8): 770–780.

Jodelet, Denise, and Jocelyne Ohana. 1996. "Rappresentazioni sociali dell'allattamento materno: Una pratica sanitaria tra natura e cultura." In *Psicologia sociale della salute,* Giovanna Petrillo, ed. Naples: Liguori.

Jordan, Brigitte. 1993. *Birth in Four Cultures: A Cross-Cultural Investigation of Childbirth in Yucatan, Holland, Sweden and the United States.* Prospect Heights, IL: Waveland Press.

Kleinman, Arthur, Veena Das, and Margaret Lock. 1996. "Preface to the Issue 'Social Suffering,'" *Daedalus* 125(1): xi–xx.

Kleinman, Arthur, and Joan Kleinman. 1996. "The Appeal of Experience; The Dismay of Images: Cultural Appropriations of Suffering in Our Times," *Daedalus* 125(1): 1–23.

La Leche League. 1997. *The Womanly Art of Breastfeeding.* New York: New American Library.

La Leche League (France). 1996. "Le manque de lait: Mythes et réalités," *Allaiter Aujourd'hui* (janvier/février/mars): 7–9.

Laviolle, G. 1998. "L'allaitement en France aujourd'hui. Quelques pistes de réflexion," *Dossiers de l'allaitement* 35: 12–13.

Le Roy Ladurie, Emmanuel. 1979. "L'allaitement mercenaire en France au XVIIIe siècle," *Communications* 31: 15–21.

Lerebours B., P. Czernichow, A. Pellerin, L. Froment, and T. Laroche. 1991. "L'alimentation du nourrisson jusqu'à 4 mois en Seine-Maritime," *Archives Français de Pédiatrie* 48: 391–395.

Levenstein, Harvey. 1983. "'Best for Babies' or 'Preventable Infanticide'? The Controversy over Artificial Feeding of Infants in America, 1880–1920," *The Journal of American History* 70(1): 75–94.

Maher, Vanessa. 1995. "Breast-Feeding in Cross-Cultural Perspective: Paradoxes and Proposals." In *The Anthropology of Breast-Feeding: Natural Law or Construct,* Vanessa Maher, ed. Oxford: Berg.

Marchand-Lucas, L., and E. Lucas. 1998. *Le Généraliste face aux déterminants de la conduite d'allaitement maternel.* Paris: Faculté de Médecine Paris VI.

Marchand-Lucas, Laure. 1990. "L'insuffisance de la lactation," *Les dossiers de l'obstétrique* 169: 16–17.

Masse-Raimbault, Anne-Marie. 1992. "Du lait maternel . . . au plat familial," *L'Enfant en Milieu Tropical* 202–203: 73 pages.

Obermeyer, Makhlou, Carla Castle, and Sandra Castle. 1997. "Back to Nature? Historical and Cross-Cultural Perspectives on Barriers to Optimal Breastfeeding," *Medical Anthropology* 17: 39–63.

Radius, S. M., and A. Joffe. 1988. "Understanding Adolescent Mothers' Feelings About Breast-Feeding," *Journal of Adolescent Health Care* 9: 156–160.

Railhet, F. 1998. "L'allaitement en chiffres," *Dossiers de l'Allaitement* 35: 9–11.

Raphael, D. 1985. *Only Mothers Know.* Westport, CT: Greenwood Press.

Reiff, M. I., and S. M. Essock-Vitale. 1985. "Hospital Influences on Early Infant-Feeding Practices," *Pediatrics* 76(6): 872–879.

Righard, L., and M. O. Alade. 1990. "Effect of Delivery Routines on Success of First Breast-Feed," *Lancet* 336: 1105–1107.

Roques, Nathalie. 1998. "Initiative Hôpitaux Amis des Bébés. La triste exception française," *Les Dossiers de l'Obstétrique* (260): 12–16.

Saadeh, Randa J., et al. 1993. *Breastfeeding: The Technical Basis and Recommendations for Action.* Geneva: World Health Organization.

Salle, B. L. 1993. "Le lait de femme." In *Traité de nutrition pédiatrique,* C. Ricour et al., eds. Paris: Maloine.

Société Française de Pédiatrie. 1998. "Nos Partenaires." Online at http://www.societefrancaisepediatrie.asso.fr/.

Stuart-Macadam, Patricia. 1995. "Biocultural Perspectives on Breastfeeding." In *Breastfeeding: Biocultural Perspectives,* P. Stuart-Macadam and K. A. Dettwyler, eds. New York: Aldine de Gruyter.

Thirion, M. 1993. "L'allaitement maternel. Des données nouvelles pour tordre le cou aux idées reçues," *La Revue du Praticien* 7(226): 29–38.

Tully, Julia, and Kathryn G. Dewey. 1985. "Private Fears, Global Loss: A Cross-Cultural Study of the Insufficient Milk Syndrome," *Medical Anthropology* 9(3): 225–243.

UNICEF. 1995. *The Baby-Friendly Hospital Initiative in Europe: Progress Report 1994.* Geneva: UNICEF.

UNICEF-France. 1997. "Favoriser l'allaitement maternel," *La Lettre de l'UNICEF,* October 1997, pp. 1–4.

UNICEF/World Health Organization. 1991. *The Baby-Friendly Hospital Initiative.* Geneva: World Health Organization.

———. 1993. *Breastfeeding Counseling: A Training Course.* Geneva: World Health Organization.

Van Esterik, Penny. 1988. "The Insufficient Milk Syndrome: Biological Epidemic or Cultural Construction?" In *Women and Health: Cross Cultural Perspectives,* Patricia Whelehan, ed. South Hadley, MA: Bergin and Garvey.

———. 1989. *Beyond the Breast-Bottle Controversy.* New Brunswick, NJ: Rutgers University Press.

———. 1995. "The Politics of Breastfeeding: An Advocacy Perspective." In *Breastfeeding: Biocultural Perspectives,* Patricia Stuart-Macadam and Katherine A. Dettwyler, eds. New York: Aldine de Gruyter.
Walter, Pascale Camus. 1999. "Quel avenir pour le décret?" *Dossier de l'Allaitement* 38: 3–4.
World Health Assembly. 1991. Report WHA44.33, *World Summit for Children: Follow-up Action.* Hbk Res., Vol. III (2d. ed.), 1.12.1; 7.1.3.
WHO (World Health Organization). 1981. *International Code of Marketing of Breast-Milk Substitutes.* Geneva: World Health Organization.
———. 1995. *Weekly Epidemiological Report* 17, pp. 117–120.
WHO/UNICEF. 1989. *Joint Declaration on the Protection, Promotion and Support of Breastfeeding.* Geneva: World Health Organization.
———. 1990. *The Innocenti Declaration on the Protection, Promotion and Support of Breastfeeding.* Florence: United Nations. (The article is also in *Ecology of Food and Nutrition* 26[1991]: 271–173.)
Wong, C. 1998. "Allaitement maternel. La meilleure façon de téter" and "Les pathologies maternelles de l'allaitement," *Le Généraliste FMC* 1847 (March 27): 6–14.
Young, A. 1980. "The Discourse on Stress and the Reproduction of Conventional Knowledge," *Social Science and Medicine* 14B: 133–146.

11

Reforming Routines: A Baby-Friendly Hospital in Urban China

Suzanne Zhang Gottschang

It is impossible to enter any neighborhood food store in Beijing and ignore the counters and shelves of infant formula products graced with pictures of chubby, smiling babies. The domain of infant feeding in China has not escaped the integration of foreign economic and social forces that are changing urban Chinese society. Indeed, the baby food sector is rapidly expanding in China. In 1995 total Chinese sales for baby food in China reached 37.1 million yuan (U.S.$4.5 million at 8.3 yuan = 1 U.S. dollar) and were expected to increase to U.S. $27 billion (224.7 billion yuan) by the year 2000, with foreign companies such as Nestlé and Borden the market leaders in this industry (*Eurofood* 1996:3). The influx of baby food products and their companies' promotional efforts are readily apparent not only in stores but also in urban hospitals that distribute informational pamphlets on pregnancy, breast-feeding, and infant care and, most important, also distribute promotional material on infant formula products.

Interestingly, this dissemination of information about breast-milk substitutes contradicts the Chinese government's recent laws that aim to promote breast-feeding. To this end, in the 1990s China renovated and reorganized more than 4,957 urban hospitals into "baby-friendly hospitals" to promote breast-feeding (Xinhua News Agency 1996b). These hospitals constitute one aspect of the Chinese government's response to a dramatic decrease in the rate of breast-feeding in urban areas. In spite of policies supporting breast-feeding that were implemented prior to the economic reforms and the appearance of Western brands of infant formulas in 1985, the number of urban mothers who breast-feed declined from 81 percent in 1950 to less than 11 percent who breast-fed for six months in 1992 (Ministry of Public Health, in *China Daily* 1992). In collaboration with the

World Health Organization (WHO) and the United Nations Children's Fund (UNICEF), the Chinese government developed policies and laws to increase the rate of breast-feeding as part of an overall program to improve child health by the year 2000.

The goal of the Baby Friendly Hospital Initiative (hereafter BFHI), as defined by UNICEF and WHO, is to promote the practice of breast-feeding by reorganizing hospital routines, spaces, and knowledge in maternity wards and obstetrics clinics (BFHI brochure, UNICEF 1992). Thus, outside international agencies are working within a Chinese context that is fraught with ambivalence about infant feeding practices. This ambivalence in turn has produced conflicting ideals about the natural and medical aspects of infant feeding and mothering.

The data for this paper are based on sixteen months of fieldwork in the obstetrics clinic at the Number 385 Hospital[1] in Beijing from 1994 to 1996, where I followed a group of thirty women from four to six months' pregnancy to four to six months postpartum, and worked with the nurses and physicians charged with implementing the BFHI. Although the women in my study sample form the core of my research focus, the staff at the Number 385 Hospital's obstetrics and gynecology department added their insights and ideas to my understanding of the process of becoming a mother. Indeed, as representatives of the hospital's baby-friendly initiative, they were invested in women's decisions about infant feeding. Their positions as providers of care during pregnancy, childbirth, and the early days of motherhood form a nexus from which we can better understand the ways that institutions are in reality a network of individuals with sometimes separate identities and interests (Cohen 1994). I consider here how the promotion of breast-feeding works at the level of international ideologies, Chinese state-level policies, local hospital practices, and women's individual choices (Barlow 1994; de Lauretis 1987:ix). Specifically, I focus on the recent law protecting women and children (Xinhua News Agency 1995), the one-child policy, and the UNICEF/WHO Baby Friendly Hospital Initiative in an urban Chinese hospital to illuminate the intersection of national and transnational ideologies of motherhood. I also document the increasing importance of foreign infant formula in the Chinese market and the ways that it represents modernity, consumerism, and participation in a global milieu for Chinese mothers and health care workers alike (Manderson 1984). The framework suggested by Kleinman and Kleinman (1991) that focuses on individual experience as interpersonal mediation between local and larger political and social processes in which individuals have interests and personal stakes (1991:227) leads me to examine how a nurse, in her role as breast-feeding educator in a baby-friendly hospital in Beijing, used her medical authority and the ideals of infant feeding practices to cope with the rules of the baby-friendly hospital in relation to other external demands of postreform urban China's increasingly pervasive baby food market and consumer culture. My larger goal in presenting this case study is to contribute to our understanding of how health professionals stand at the intersection of international and state policies, medical institutions, and local and global economic forces.

Economic Reform and Women's Status in 1990s China

To better understand the social and cultural context in which all urban women live and work in 1990s China, we must begin with the social and economic milieu brought about by the economic reforms and the opening of China's markets. In the scholarly literature, much pessimism has been expressed about whether urban Chinese women are benefiting or suffering as a result of the economic reforms that began in 1978 (see, for example, Wolf 1985). Indeed, the new challenges that urban women workers face, as China's state-owned enterprises dismantle cradle-to-grave benefits, are concerns that were shared by many women in my study.

With 90 percent of urban women of working age in the labor force, China ranks as one of the leaders in women's labor-force participation (Riley 1996:22). Official rhetoric maintains that women's rights and roles remain central to governmental efforts to modernize the Chinese economy. Yet urban Chinese women face discrimination in employment that results in underemployment, lower salaries, fewer opportunities for managerial positions, and discriminatory hiring practices. Not surprisingly, the reasons that women are discriminated against centers in part on the perception that their primary responsibilities and roles are to their families. Riley (1996: 23) notes that both women themselves and their managers cite these familial responsibilities as a negative influence on work performance and on opportunities for women to advance in the workplace. Ironically, recent labor reforms—such as the 1995 labor law's expansion of earlier laws that granted a fifty-six-day maternity leave to one that entitles women to a minimum ninety-day leave, and a recent law promoting maternal and child welfare mandating that nursing women be allowed two half-hour breaks in addition to a lunch break to breast-feed their children—have produced a reluctance among firms to hire women. In an era of increasing competition, women workers are thus viewed as less desirable because these enterprises must maintain a productive workforce. As a result, women who are married or at an age when they are likely to desire children are perceived by employers as less productive workers and are often not hired or not assigned to positions of authority. Thus, the economic reforms and government policies designed to modernize China have increasingly destabilized women's position in the workforce. Factories and work units that need to make a profit in the market economy now view female employees as more costly than men because women's maternal roles require that companies provide maternity leaves and other benefits that limit profits (Honig and Hershatter 1988).

The conflict between work and motherhood has also been affected by the implementation of the one-child policy. Many scholars have investigated the effects of the one-child policy on women and their health, the strategies rural women use to bear more than one child, and other ways the Chinese citizenry subvert the regulations that limit family size (see, for example, Croll, Davin, and Kane 1985; Greenhalgh 1993). For the purposes of my research I found that the hospital, as an institution that promotes the one-child policy and the importance of family planning, is only one site in a web of institutions that enforce and elaborate the policy. Indeed, the importance of the single-child policy does not end after a woman becomes pregnant, because the policy emphasizes the necessity of producing a healthy, normal future citizen and ultimately creating a strong, healthy, physically able population. Furthermore, the notion of the ideal family as a small family is often equated with modernization. Several women in my study reflected that China's one-child policy was necessary not only for the well-being of future generations but also for helping China to become more like modern, developed nations such as the United States.

For the women in my study, it seems that once a woman became pregnant, she felt the pressure to bear an intelligent, healthy future citizen and worker from a variety of sources. In addition to literature women received from family planning workers, they were often reminded during checkups and at other critical junctures that it was their duty to produce a healthy child. For example, the nurses in the Number 385 Hospital often informed women who were not gaining enough weight during their pregnancy that poor nutrition would affect the baby's brain and might result in a less intelligent child. Moreover, the infant formula industry has incorporated the state's rhetoric about producing the perfect baby in its advertising literature to sell nutritional drinks to pregnant women.

In addition to being affected by these state-level policies, urban Chinese women are becoming mothers in a period when China has witnessed phenomenal economic growth. The economic reforms since 1978 have moved China from a centrally planned economy to a socialist market economy, and its rapid economic development has brought improved living standards and increased disposable income and earning opportunities for many people in rural and urban areas. These changes have transformed the entire country in numerous ways, but in particular they have created unprecedented opportunities for foreign companies to enter the Chinese market and have encouraged the development of enterprises that provide the Chinese consumer with an unending array of foreign and locally produced goods. Beijing's street billboards, formerly used to promote the central government's latest policy campaign, now advertise Japanese televisions, automobiles, and Gerber baby food products. Retail sales in China have increased more than fivefold between 1980 and 1992, and retail outlets have grown from two million in 1979 to over twelve million in 1993 (Tong 1994). This consumerism and increased prosperity have led to the proliferation of products and expectations that are new to socialist China (Zha 1995).

International Ideologies of Mothering and Infant Feeding

As I suggest earlier, institutions that affect reproduction, such as government policies to promote breast-feeding, the one-child policy, and the consumer culture of 1990s China, are subject to national and global interests guided by assumptions that are in turn shaped by international and national leaders and institutions. Women as reproducers are linked to these larger forces. Health care professionals who facilitate reproductive health in hospitals and clinics are also connected to these broader interests. The Chinese government's goal of maintaining a position in the world economy, and the international norms generated by multilateral organizations such as the United Nations Children's Fund and the World Health Organization, which are interested in rescuing women and children from poor health, impact women's choices and the kind of care they receive in medical settings.

One area of concern for Chinese health officials centers on the decline in breast-feeding that has occurred in China, and which has been quite remarkable and rather sudden relative to other countries' experiences. As I mentioned previously, in spite of supportive policies for breast-feeding implemented before the economic reforms, the number of urban Beijing mothers who breast-fed their infants for six months declined from 81 percent in 1950 to 10.4 percent in 1985 (Zhu 1994; Yuan 1997). Nationwide, the breast-feeding rate was 30 percent in 1990 (Chen Ya 1996:15). In 1992 China, with assistance from the United Nations Children's Fund and the World Health Organization, sought to remedy the dramatic decline in breast-feeding occurring in urban areas by reorganizing the ways that obstetrics clinics and wards delivered care to women and their infants. In the Chinese baby-friendly hospital, women are no longer separated from their infants immediately after birth; babies are roomed with their mothers for the duration of their hospital stay; and all pregnant women must attend three prenatal breast-feeding classes. Women receive a variety of written materials on breast-feeding during the class sessions, a nurse meets with each woman individually to discuss preparation and techniques to ensure successful breast-feeding, and all participants watch a Chinese-produced video on the benefits and techniques of breast-feeding. The BFHI provides women with a number of informational sources about the benefits of breast-feeding. It also marks a significant change in the hospital's role in defining and disseminating the ideals of motherhood, so that being a "good" mother now requires that one must breast-feed.

Promoting breast-feeding, however, creates one of "the most difficult dilemmas in feminist thought and action—the sexual division of labor and the fit between women's productive and reproductive activities" (Van Esterik 1989:68). Ideologies and practices related to breast-feeding provide a lens for exploring the construction of motherhood in twentieth-century global and national contexts. Breast-feeding, like pregnancy and birth, represents a contradiction between "both the cultural and natural mother; that is the socially constructed and the biological are inextricably intertwined" (Blum 1993:291). Here I want to discuss the consequences of this contradiction and how it results in two layers of representation about breast-feeding: First, women through their reproductive capabilities are tied to nature, and second, proper, adequate mothering in terms of breast-feeding requires medical intervention. The UNICEF/WHO Baby Friendly Hospital Initiative's efforts to promote breast-feeding articulate these contradictions in the rhetoric they use to justify their program and policies. Later, I discuss how the Chinese government also uses these notions to articulate and implement its vision of a modern, scientifically advanced nation.

The ideologies of such multilateral organizations as the WHO and UNICEF tend to follow from Western cultural assumptions that view breast-feeding as a "natural" aspect of maternal nurturance (Scheper-Hughes and Lock 1987). The assumption that breast-feeding is natural obscures the importance of the cultural and social contexts of motherhood, including, in a place like 1990s urban China, forces of modernization that regulate, mediate, and define women's experiences as mothers (Scheper-Hughes 1984). The arguments and supposition made by these international organizations thus need to be "read" in ways that highlight the partial, mediated, and culturally constructed knowledge of nature and biology (Laqueur 1990). In the course of explicating constructions of motherhood and infant feeding in the following discussion, I do not mean to deny biological dimensions of breast-feeding or the health benefits associated with it. Rather, I wish to demonstrate the ways that nature, breast-feeding, and good mothering are constructed in the interests of promoting breast-feeding globally. Unraveling the rhetoric and assumptions underlying the BFHI indicates the ways that such initiatives, in their efforts to promote the interests of children, obscure the social, cultural, and economic power structure surrounding women as they become mothers.

The opening section of an English-language pamphlet promoting the UNICEF/WHO Baby Friendly Hospital Initiative naturalizes breast-feeding and links the use of bottle feeding to the forces of modernization and industrialization. The section is entitled "The Challenge to Nature" (United Nations 1996). This pamphlet argues that it is only recently that "humans have tried to replace the natural means of feeding newborns which is given to every mammalian species on Earth" (1996:7). The naturalizing of breast-feeding in this passage ignores the important fact that breast-feeding among humans is learned behavior for both mothers and infants (Jelliffe and Jelliffe 1978). There are certainly innate aspects of the process, but much trial and error is necessary for successful breast-feeding for many women. This statement links humans to the animal world and implies that breast-feeding is a simple (natural) process, much like the unthinking act of a cat nursing her kittens.

The corollary to this assumption, one that is suggested throughout the various documents published by WHO/UNICEF, is that mothering is natural. Ultimately, the decline in breast-feeding, then, is linked to the interference of industrialization and modernization, which have taken women outside their homes to work and forced them to use infant formula to feed their babies. Specifically the pamphlet states:

> The challenge to Nature took hold in the industrialized countries in the 20th century and especially after the Second World War, which had brought many more women into the workforce. Technological advances in packaged foods made it possible to offer breast milk substitutes to women trying to balance the pressures of their work both in and outside the home. . . . Hospitals tied to the rigorous schedules of industrialized societies encouraged the switch to regular bottle-feed. "Baby's bottle" became a typical advertising image of modern "progress." (1996:7)

This passage reveals a number of important cultural assumptions about women's reproduction in relation to industrialization. First, there is the assumption that "nature" is best. Nature, in the sense used in this passage, can be read as opposed to "culture" or, as it is defined in the passage, to "industrialization." The assumption here is that the universal physiological capability to breast-feed is hindered by external forces such as work outside the home, increased availability of commercial infant formulas, and hospital routines that separate mothers and infants in the interests of efficiency.[2] In this view, natural maternal nurturance through breast-feeding is thwarted by women's encounters with the modernizing world (Scheper-Hughes 1987).

The solution proposed by UNICEF/WHO is to promote the baby-friendly hospitals, which can counter these impediments to good mothering and breast-feeding. These organizations suggest that hospitals must change their policies and practices and "put infants and children first . . . [and this] will lead the world's return to breast-feeding and put an end to thousands of infant deaths" (United Nations 1996:3). However, these statements also contain a submerged message—that good mothering and even infant survival are incompatible with women's participation in the workforce (Maher 1994; Nerlove 1974). They thus validate the idea that women are best relegated to the traditional spheres of home and family (Blum 1993:302). Ironically, however, as our knowledge about breast-feeding cross-culturally increases, many researchers are finding that even women in "traditional" agrarian societies confront situations where breast-feeding is incompatible with their work. For example, Levine suggests that the increasing use of breast-milk substitutes illuminates just how long-standing are practices of supplementation when women's work is incompatible with the breast-feeding demands of infants. She finds that traditional supplementary foods are introduced early in infancy because demands for women's agricultural labor are incompatible with their additional responsibilities for child care and breast-feeding (Levine 1988:247).

Therefore, linking the loss of traditional lifeways and non-breast-feeding women's distance from nature as articulated in the BFHI pamphlets suggests a simplistic interpretation of the reasons for the worldwide decline in breast-feeding. In addition, the solutions it proposes reflect an ideology of motherhood that ties women to the traditional roles of mother and home-worker. This view, however, does not reflect the reality of most women's lives. And paradoxically, the modern, international Baby Friendly Hospital Initiative inadvertently advocates a patriarchal view against which many women have fought in the interests of their autonomy.

"They should make mother-friendly hospitals, since we are the ones who care for babies!" Mrs. Wang, one of the thirty women who participated in my research, was one of several women who remarked to me that the idea of a baby-friendly hospital was problematic. Mrs. Wang and others believed that as mothers, *they* needed a supportive and nurturing environment so that they could be good mothers to their infants. The stated goal of the BFHI initiative and others like it is, first, to create an environment more conducive to breast-feeding by changing practices in urban hospitals and, second, to educate women about the benefits of breast milk for their infants.[3] The problem raised by Mrs. Wang, however, indicates an important tension inherent in the concept of creating a baby-friendly world through the baby-friendly hospital. On the one hand, it argues that mothers are naturally suited to rear children because of their physiological characteristics, and on the other it suggests that mothers need the regulation and surveillance of institutions in order to be "good mothers." This contradiction outlines the ways that the rubric of mother and child protection carries multiple meanings and ideologies. The interests of individual mothers are relegated to larger institutional concerns with protecting the future generation. Reproduction then becomes an international and national concern and one that must be controlled and monitored in the interests of maintaining a healthy nation and world (see, for example, Ginsburg and Rapp 1996). Such policies also assume that women must be rescued from situations that contribute to their poor health, high infant mortality, and low child survival, and that women's experiences in all third-world countries is universal. In so doing, these policies remove agency from women in their local context. Finally, they ignore the underlying assumption that "ostensibly neutral political processes and concepts such as nationalism, citizenship and the state are fundamentally gendered" (Waylen 1994:10).

National Ideologies of Motherhood

Protective policies such as the Baby Friendly Hospital Initiative and laws that regulate women's reproductive health also offer a productive way to examine the link between nationalism, politics, and gender relations. Furthermore, these relationships create important social structures in which individuals mediate their own and others' experiences. These policies are not necessarily designed to intentionally oppress or discriminate against women, but are developed according to prevailing assumptions and ideologies about the role of women, the nature of the family, and the proper relations between men and women (Moore 1988:128). In this section I will look at the Chinese government's adoption of the UNICEF/WHO Baby Friendly Hospital Initiative as it intersects with the recent law protecting women and children (1995) and the one-child policy in terms of women's narratives about mothering and motherhood. The adoption of the UNICEF/WHO recommendations to increase the rate and duration of breast-feeding in urban China meshes closely with these policies and with the state's aim to produce healthy future citizens and a healthy nation. Moreover, just as multilateral agencies' policies reflect assumptions about gender roles, women's relationship to the state in terms of creating ideologies of motherhood and mothering also reveal important concepts about gender (Yuval-Davis and Anthias 1989). These concepts, in turn, create implications for the roles and concerns of health care professionals charged with implementing programs such as the BFHI. Here I want to briefly describe how the Chinese government's adoption and implementation of United Nations conventions on women's health and child welfare reveal some of the specific ideological definitions of women's reproductive relationships with the state. Indeed, the formulation and adoption in the 1990s of the Law on Health Protection of Mothers and Infants and the Law on Protection of Women's Rights and Interests echo deeper worries in China about the role of mothers as reproducers of the nation, transmitters of Chinese "spiritual civilization," and productive workers in China's modernizing economy (Anagnost 1995).

China's premier, Li Peng, signed the World Declaration on the Survival, Protection and Development of Children as well as the Plan of Action for Implementing the World Declaration on the Survival, Protection, and Development of Children in the 1990s. These two documents were adopted by countries participating in the United Nations World Summit for Children in 1990. In addition, China cosponsored the draft resolution for the United Nations Convention on the Rights of Children, which was formally approved in 1991 and adopted by the Chinese government in 1992 (Xinhua News Agency 1996b). The active participation by the Chinese government in the development of these United Nations documents and its subsequent implementation of the policies and plans associated with them marks an important instance of the Chinese government's role in the development of international standards and goals for maternal and child well-being. In part, China's participation signifies its recent international economic importance, and the success of the economic reforms. Moreover, China's interest in participating in international legal realms, including the ratification of the Convention to Eliminate all Forms of Discrimination Against Women (CEDAW),[4] its bid for a seat in the World Trade Organization, and its strategic placement as a potential leader in the world order are linked to the nation's overall interest in becoming a "world player." However, to be considered on par with other developed countries, China must raise its living standards and improve the health and well-being of its citizens. In my view, the Chinese government's interest in supporting and adopting protective policies toward reproduction, however, can be attributed to more than an objective of becoming a "global player." In fact, the stated goals and plans to protect women's and children's health and wellbeing mesh closely with policies like the one-child policy and broader goals of the Chinese state: the reproduction of a strong, modern, and healthy nation.

As Yuval-Davis notes, "The inclusion of a new baby in a national collectivity is far from being only a biological issue" (1996:17). The nationalist project of the Chinese government entails the modernization and development of the nation through a variety of means. Since the late 1970s, however, population growth has been defined as one of the largest impediments to China's modernization project (Greenhalgh 1993). The concern with excessive population growth in China is predicated on Malthusian assumptions. The fear is that uncontrolled population growth will bring about national or international disaster and hinder further attempts to modernize (Hartmann 1987). China's one-child policy, initiated in the late 1970s, aimed to limit population growth by allowing each married couple one child. Much attention has been devoted to the one-child policy in China and the ways that it has enabled the state to intervene directly in

Chinese women's reproductive decisions. Indeed, some argue that the state has replaced the "private patriarchy" of the traditional family with a "public patriarchy" of the government (Stacey 1983: 235).[5]

In fact, national concerns about producing physiologically sound children as an outgrowth of the one-child policy goal has created an increased interest in regulating pregnancy and maternity. The 1992 Law Protecting the Rights of Women and Children exemplifies this new interest (Xinhua News Agency 1996b). Examining the rhetoric of the 1992 laws pertaining to women, public health laws, and other family law illuminates how the state regards, regulates, and responds to the needs of women as mothers. Moreover, such an analysis illuminates the state's actions toward the goal of modernization and its interests in taking its place as a developed nation in the world (Anagnost 1995:39)

What can the "rules" surrounding the protection of child welfare through the promotion of breast-feeding tell us about the assumptions that the Chinese state makes about motherhood? And how do these assumptions fit with women's productive roles in the modernization of China? It is difficult to ignore Foucault's notion of bio-power in addressing these two questions. It is true that Foucault's analysis of the development of bio-power rests on his historical reading of developments in the early modern West. Yet many aspects of his ideas resonate with the project of modernization in China. As he states: "The body [is] imbued with the mechanics of life and serves as the basis of the biological processes: propagations, births, mortality, the level of health, life expectancy. . . . Their supervision was effected through an entire series of interventions and *regulatory controls: a bio-politics of the population*" (Foucault 1990:139).[6] With the looming problem of overpopulation, the socialist state has deemed it necessary to intervene directly in reproductive life. In fact, it is the intersection of common interests, as articulated by multilateral organizations such as UNICEF or the WHO, and China's participation in promoting their policies that makes Foucault's notion of bio-power a useful tool for analyzing the current policies to promote maternal and child well-being.

A policy paper issued by China's state council in 1996 outlines the situation of children and notes many advances in the well-being and health of children (Xinhua News Agency 1996b). However, it is difficult to ignore the clear link made between the importance of children in the state's plans to improve the overall population and, ultimately, the "health" of the nation. For example, the paper states: "Children's survival, protection and development, which are the basis for improving the quality of the population and the prerequisite conditions for the advance of mankind, directly concern a country and a nation's future and destiny" (Xinhua News Agency 1996b). This passage indicates in explicit terms the Chinese state's assumptions about the link between children and the well-being, strength, and longevity of the nation. The importance of improving child nutrition through breast-feeding is clearly stated in the new law protecting maternal and child health (Xinhua News Agency 1995).

The first statement of the document directly links state concerns with improving the quality of births in relation to maternal health: "This law is formulated according to the Constitution to guarantee the health of mothers and infants to improve the quality of births" (Xinhua News Agency 1996b: 1). The importance of the mother is signified only as the means to produce an infant, and the subsequent quality of potential children is emphasized most clearly in the extensive sections of the law addressing health care during pregnancy and childbirth. In essence, the law requires the supervision of conception, pregnancy, and postpartum practices by medical personnel in the interests of producing healthy, physically normal infants. The law specifies that in any situation where the potential for abnormality of the fetus exists as the result of hereditary conditions, lifestyle, or other disease, health care providers may intervene and determine the necessity of terminating the pregnancy. The stated goal is the production of healthy children through the monitoring and control of women's bodies. Mothers are invisible as agents in these state-produced documents and at least at this level of discourse are relegated to physical bodies through which the nation can reproduce and develop. This is not surprising. Jaggar notes that in most cultures, pregnant women "are viewed less as individuals than as the 'raw material' from which the 'product' is extracted. In modern circumstances, it is possible to understand then how the physician rather than the mother comes to be seen as having produced the baby" (Jagger 1989: 311). In the case of Chinese policy and law, however, the state and its representatives in the form of health care workers act as the ultimate authority and define the terms and conditions under which women may reproduce, and the standards of the quality of the product (the child).

The laws protecting child and maternal health attempt to eliminate women's authority over their bodies and define the ways that the state, in the collective interests of the nation, can legitimately regulate and control reproduction. Mothers in Chinese law and policy are thus vehicles for reproduction, and their autonomy and interests are subsumed by the state's authority. As a result of China's adoption of the WHO/UNICEF initiative to increase breast-feeding, women's postpartum decisions and autonomy are now circumscribed by the state's interest in producing healthy citizens. Moreover, such protectionist policies have helped to reshape the nature of health care professionals' roles in promoting and enacting the policies designed to produce these healthy infant citizens.[7]

Marketing Infant Formula

The National Provisions on Marketing of Breast-Milk Substitutes was passed in 1995 in China. This law limits the marketing and selling of infant formulas to women in hospitals. The law and the international code that it is based on represent a multilateral response to the marketing practices of infant formula companies in developing countries. The "infant formula scandal" of the late 1970s brought to light the fact that feeding artificial formulas to babies in developing countries where mothers had no access to clean water, or sufficient money to purchase adequate amounts of formula, resulted in large numbers of infant deaths (Maher 1994). Mothers in hospitals were often given free samples of formula by medical workers or formula company representatives. Researchers found that mothers perceived infant formula as more "modern" because it was associated with the hospitals that distributed free samples, and thus medically superior to breast milk (Popkin et al. 1986). However, as scientific knowledge has increased about the protective benefits of breast milk, such as the immune properties that it transmits, as well as the link between diarrheal diseases in small children as the result of drinking formulas made with contaminated water, researchers and activists advocated restrictions to be placed on the aggressive marketing tactics of formula companies. Consequently the World Health Assembly through the United Nations developed an international code for the marketing and promotion of infant formula in developing countries. This was ratified by over 118 countries in 1981.

This code contains ten provisions to limit the marketing of breast-milk substitutes, cereals, teas, and bottles: no advertising of any products to the public; no free samples to mothers; no promotion of products, including the distribution of free or low-cost supplies, in health care facilities; no company sales representatives to advise mothers; no gifts or personal samples to health workers; no words or pictures idealizing artificial feeding or pictures of infants on labels of infant milk containers. They state that information given to health workers should be scientific and factual; all information on artificial infant feeding should explain the benefits of breast-feeding and the costs and hazards associated with artificial feeding; and unsuitable products such as sweetened condensed milk should not be promoted for babies (World Health Organization 1981).

China, as I have mentioned, has adopted its own version of this code and has publicly made several statements that it seeks to limit the sale and promotion of infant formulas in its efforts to increase breast-feeding. However, the attractions of foreign investment and profit seeking have overcome the state's reluctance to produce and promote infant formula. The formula industry in China is dominated by three foreign companies and a myriad of Chinese firms.[8] Breast-milk substitutes are also profit-making products as indicated by Mead Johnson's annual report, where Enfamil (a breast-milk substitute) was listed as one of the "high growth products," with a 24 percent increase in sales worldwide, and was the company's third-best-selling product (Mead Johnson Company 1996). China, with its vast population and nearly twenty million births every year (China Statistical Yearbook 1994), represents a huge potential market for infant formula.[9] In fact, a recent report notes that Mead Johnson recently formed the Mead Johnson (Guangzhou) Company joint venture to produce and package infant milk products, with a total investment of U.S.$30 million, 85 percent of which is provided by the U.S. company (Zhao 1996).

The contradiction between the state's adoption of the international code to limit the sale and marketing of breast-milk substitutes as a means to promote breast-feeding on the one hand, and the development of joint ventures to produce infant formula on the other, speaks to the paradoxical realities of the problem of infant feeding. Although the state promotes the idea that breast milk is the best means to feed an infant, it also has an interest in providing high-quality alternatives that also bring profit and investment to China. This contradiction and tension between interests in promoting child health through increasing breast-feeding and the realities of economic development that faced China in the 1990s reflected, at a macro level, the contradictions inherent in conceptions of contemporary motherhood. In addition, the promotion of nutritional drinks for pregnant and nursing women creates an additional structure of authority for defining ideals of motherhood and mothering. Using the rhetoric and concerns articulated by state policies and authorities, these types of products medicalize maternal nutrition as a condition that requires intervention. These contradictory approaches are played out in the hospital setting and ultimately are confronted by health professionals and mothers as they make decisions about how to feed their infants.

Through the Back Door

Zuo hou men (use the back door) is a phrase commonly heard in China when individuals seek to obtain access, services, or goods that are not readily available through normal bureaucratic channels. I discovered during my sixteen months of research at the Number 385 Hospital that the back door of the Number 385 Hospital's obstetrics clinic was literally an opening through which foreign infant formula representatives entered into the breast-feeding education classroom supervised by Nurse Bai. These salespeople were technically not allowed by Chinese law to promote their products in hospitals (Xinhua News Agency 1996c). As we shall see in the following, Nurse Bai circumvented this law in specific ways in her role as the breast-feeding educator for the Number 385 Hospital.

I had worked almost daily with Nurse Bai, and after about six months, one day after we had eaten lunch, she went into the corridor, unlocked the back door of the clinic, returned to the room, and sat chatting with me. We were waiting for a group of pregnant women to arrive so that I could observe Nurse Bai teaching a breast-feeding class. I assumed that she had unlocked the door so that the women could use the more conveniently located back door to enter the clinic, and thus the classroom. I was wrong.

The women arrived, and the class began. As I sat taking notes, Mrs. Zhou and four other women who were in their ninth month of pregnancy practiced the different ways of holding an infant for breast-feeding after observing Nurse Bai's demonstration with a model of a breast and a plastic doll. As the class was ending, a young-looking, well-dressed woman with two large briefcases entered the classroom. Nurse Bai introduced her to us and explained that she wanted to share some information with us. Candy (her English name) greeted the group and asked if she could talk to us about some nutritional information and products for pregnant women and nursing mothers. Nurse Bai told everyone to move down on the benches to give Candy some room to sit. Candy opened her briefcase and handed out several colorful brochures about nutritional drinks for pregnant and nursing women. As she did so, she told us that she was also a doctor (a cardiologist) but had decided to work for this company to expand her opportunities. Then she began a rapid sales pitch to the women and Nurse Bai. Leaning toward them, she began by saying:

> *I am a mother too, my son is two years old. . . . But we all know how busy we can get and sometimes you don't have enough time or energy to make or eat a balanced meal. Especially when you are a new mother, your baby needs a lot of attention. Research studies have shown that many women do not get enough vitamins during or after pregnancy when their bodies need them most. Our drinks provide a convenient way to make sure you receive all the good nutrition you need.*

One woman interrupted Candy and asked why she would need this if she ate vegetables, fruits, and meat. Candy replied that it was possible to do this, but it may be more difficult when one is busy or too tired to cook a meal. The women all looked at the pamphlets Candy had passed out, and no one said anything for a few minutes. Finally, one woman asked her if her company also made formula for infants. Candy replied that, yes, they did, and that these were the most scientific types of infant formula on the market. At this point, Nurse Bai interrupted Candy and told her that this was not a topic that she could talk about. She suggested that it was time to resume the class. As Candy prepared to leave, she dug out some more pamphlets from her bag and handed Nurse Bai some samples of the nutritional drinks and infant formula. As Candy was leaving, Nurse Bai moved to a cabinet at the back of the room, unlocked it, and put the samples and pamphlets in it. Nurse Bai, as she returned to the group of women, told them that they all were very healthy and that there was no need to buy any special products.

After the class meeting, I did not have an opportunity to talk with Nurse Bai about the sales representative's visit, but I knew that this sort of solicitation was not allowed according to the rules of the Baby Friendly Hospital Initiative. The rules were in Chinese, posted prominently in the breast-feeding classroom. Soon after the class was over a young man appeared at the classroom door looking for Nurse Bai. She invited him in and introduced us. She explained to me that his wife had just returned home after giving birth to a baby girl in the hospital. As she talked, she unlocked the same cabinet and removed a number of packets of both a nutritional drink for women and infant formula produced by a foreign company. She wrapped the packets in a bag and instructed the young man to return when his wife needed more. Once we were alone, I felt this was an opening for me to ask her why she was handing out infant formula in direct violation of the rules of the hospital. When I asked why she had given the husband the infant formula, she said:

> *This young couple owns a small store in the neighborhood and they are very poor. Mrs. Wu, the mother, has been sick since she returned home from the hospital. I am worried that she is not eating well and is weak. Her husband came to see me to ask my advice about feeding the baby. Mrs. Wu's health is not good and she is having a difficult time breastfeeding. She wanted to give the infant cow's milk, but her husband was worried that this might upset the baby's stomach. So, she sent him to me for advice. I keep these samples so I can give them to women like Mrs. Wu. Foreign formulas are more nutritionally complete, they are more scientifically produced. Mrs. Wu doesn't have enough money to buy this formula, but I can get it free. You wouldn't believe how much I get from the salespeople who visit me. I don't have too many patients like Mrs. Wu, but some people are having a difficult time with the changes in our society. Not everyone is making a lot of money and living in new apartments.*

When I asked Nurse Bai whether the director of the obstetrics clinic had any problems with Nurse Bai doing this, she responded:

> *This is complicated. The other people in the clinic know that I get these free samples because I meet with the representatives, but they don't like it. Partly because they often give me small gifts for accepting their samples! But what is a key chain, or a calendar—nothing too important. They know I don't sell the samples the way I have heard that other hospitals do. They sell them at a discount, but they keep the money for themselves!*

> This is corruption. I am trying to help people that need something that I can get for nothing. In the past, before the economic reforms, people were able to get these things or extra money for them from their work unit. Now, everyone must take care of themselves; the government does not help us.

Nurse Bai also told me that the sales representatives wanted to meet with women during pregnancy to promote their products. She said:

> I let them talk to women in my classroom but only about the maternal drinks that they sell. They are not allowed to talk about infant formula. This way, they are doing their job and I am not letting them influence women's ideas about breast-feeding too much. Then they give me as many free samples as I want.

Nurse Bai's actions reflect her awareness of individual women's circumstances outside the hospital that might discourage breast-feeding. She knew that Mrs. Wu was not going to breast-feed. She also knew that Mrs. Wu's family was too poor to purchase the more expensive foreign formula.[10] She believed that under such conditions, the best alternative for Mrs. Wu's infant was the more "scientific" foreign infant formula. Nurse Bai used her position and resources in this situation to mediate between the goals and ideals of the program to promote breast-feeding in her hospital and the realities of individual women's lives.

An additional dimension of Nurse Bai's narrative that warrants further examination is her comment regarding the ways that social and economic support for individuals in urban China has been undermined by the economic reforms. As she stated, the Chinese urban work unit no longer offers support to individuals in need. The social and economic problems facing the average person (including herself) in the era of economic reform were ones that we frequently discussed during breaks between classes. It is through these discussions that I learned how Nurse Bai was a stakeholder in the complex transactions she negotiated to help new mothers feed their infants, using the best means possible. Moreover, her personal history and age operate as important dimensions of her subjective experience in relation to the BFHI and infant feeding.

During my research, I followed Nurse Bai through her days as the nurse in charge of breast-feeding education. A fifty-year-old nurse who has specialized in obstetrics and gynecological nursing for most of her twenty-six-year career, Nurse Bai spent every morning conducting classes on breast-feeding for expectant mothers in the obstetrics clinic and worked in the afternoon among the women patients in the obstetrics unit who had recently given birth, helping them learn to breast-feed and answering nutrition questions.

Nurse Bai had one child and had continued with her professional life. We often discussed the tensions and struggles she experienced as a young mother, and she frequently reflected on how young women in contemporary China face a much different set of expectations than she had. Nurse Bai had become a mother during the Cultural Revolution, and she described the logistical hardships of trying to mother her child and continue to work at a time of social upheaval. She graduated from nursing school in 1964 and immediately found employment at the Number 385 Hospital, where she worked in general surgery for almost thirteen years. She was able to work during the Cultural Revolution, but she said that it was a chaotic time at the hospital. She gave birth to her son at age twenty-three in 1967 and took only a brief maternity leave of thirty days before returning to work full-time. She frequently talked to me about how she would have to ride a neighbor's bicycle one half hour each way in the middle of the day to feed her son. There was no day care provided by the hospital, so she left her son at home with her mother-in-law. Despite the past hardships she described on many occasions, Nurse Bai was apprehensive about the changes that the economic reforms were bringing to people's lives. As is the case with most health care workers, her salary of 500 yuan (about U.S.$60) a month was not adequate even when combined with her husband's income. Her son, who was twenty-eight years old, had been employed part-time for several years at a municipal government job and had not yet married. She believes that he has had difficulty competing with more economically successful young men in the marriage market.

Nurse Bai's decisions and interests in subverting the rules and regulations designed to promote breast-feeding, and her personal history and position in the hospital, reveal the essential connection that creates a local moral world in which she feels her provision of infant formula to some new mothers is justified.

The Uneven Playing Field of Infant Feeding in Postreform China

Nurse Bai's actions clearly contradicted the goals and implementation of the Baby Friendly Hospital Initiative. She was handing out free formula samples to a woman who was not breast-feeding. However, her decisions about when to provide women with the formula were based on her understanding of women's lives outside the hospital environment. Nurse Bai's assessment of Mrs. Wu's situation provides us with an insight into the complexities of negotiating between international policies that assume breast-feeding is a universal capability of all women, and the personal, social, and economic realities that mothers face as they make decisions about feeding their infants. Nurse Bai believed that, in spite of her mandate to uphold the ideals of breast-feeding, larger social and economic circumstances created an "uneven playing field" for individual women. Most interesting, however, is that the policy designed to promote breast-feeding placed Nurse Bai in a critical position as the medical authority on infant feeding practices in the Number 385 Hospital.

The authority she holds in her position as breast-feeding educator is based on the notion that breast-feeding is the most "scientific" means to feed infants. The medical authority invested in Nurse Bai by the hospital structure is implicated in any understanding we have about the transmission of representations of the scientific aspects of infant feeding. The fact that a class on breast-feeding is a required part of women's prenatal care in the hospital imparts the idea that medical knowledge and authority are essential to breast-feed successfully. Furthermore, it suggests that the most qualified individuals for imparting this information are medical professionals. The importance of the medical professional as an authority on breast-feeding is also apparent in the way Candy, the formula representative, presented herself to the group of women in the class. She tells them that she used to be a cardiologist as a way of conveying to them that she is a member of the professional medical community rather than a salesperson with no special background in medicine or health. Ironically, the medical authority vested by the baby-friendly hospital program in individuals like Nurse Bai also positions her to use this authority to assist women who make the decision to use formula rather than breast milk to feed their infants.

Other researchers have frequently noted that the urban hospital operates as an important location for influencing women's decisions about breast-feeding (see, for example, Hull et al. 1989; Popkin et al. 1986). Generally, urban hospital practices in developing countries are viewed as discouraging breast-feeding, because the routines and practices of the maternity ward often separate mother and child and thus limit opportunities for breast-feeding (Van Esterik 1989). These problems have been addressed with the reorganization of the Number 385 Hospital into one where babies are roomed with their mothers, are put to the breast within a half hour of birth, and are provided with breast-feeding support. However, in addition to issues of hospital practices, Popkin et al. (1986) note that:

> Health professionals' lack of knowledge of infants' nutritional needs, the transmission to mothers of negative attitudes towards breastfeeding, patients' use of health professionals as role models, and the implicit or explicit influence of the infant food industry . . . have all been cited as having potentially negative effects on the practice of breastfeeding. (Popkin et al. 1986: 99)

One can conclude that the Number 385 Hospital's breast-feeding program has fallen prey to a number of these negative forces. Yet the complexities that underlie such forces are revealed, if only briefly, in the preceding descriptions. The example of Nurse Bai, with her access to free foreign formula, her authority to help women make infant feeding decisions, and her awareness of the complexities of individual women's lives, requires that we seek more in-depth understandings of the nature of the relationships between medical workers, international health policies, and the globalization of the economy.

Notes

1. A pseudonym, as are all names of individuals in my study.
2. See Greiner, Van Esterik, and Latham 1981, Gussler and Briesemeister 1980.
3. See also the Innocenti Declaration ratified by thirty-two governments (including China) in 1990 that calls for support for global breast-feeding.
4. The United Nations Convention on the Elimination of All Forms of Discrimination Against Women was ratified in 1980 in China with some modifications. See Paul McKenzie 1993.
5. See, for example, Croll, Davin, and Kane 1985, Greenhalgh 1990, 1993.
6. Emphasis in original.
7. See Molony (1995) for discussions on motherhood protection in Japan.
8. Interview with Mead-Johnson sales representative 1995.
9. I wrote to the three formula companies with a prominent presence in the Beijing area and have received no information regarding their sales, or production information.
10. Locally produced formulas are perceived by many as inferior to foreign products. This perception partly results from the numerous scandals about food products that were contaminated, of poor quality, or labeled in misleading ways.

References

Anagnost, Ann. 1995. "A Surfeit of Bodies: Population and the Rationality of the State in Post-Mao China. In *Conceiving the New World Order: The Global Politics of Reproduction,* Faye Ginsburg and Rayna Rapp, eds. Berkeley: University of California Press.

Barlow, Tani. 1994. "Theorizing Woman: Funu, Guojia, Jiating." In *Body, Subject and Power in China,* T. Barlow and A. Zito, eds. Chicago: University of Chicago Press.

Blum, Linda. 1993. "Mothers, Babies, and Breastfeeding in Late Capitalist America: The Shifting Contexts of Feminist Theory," *Feminist Studies* 19(2): 291–311.

Chen Ya. 1996. "Breastfeeding Promotion in China," *Beijing Review* (August 25): 15–16.

China Daily. 1992. "Ministry of Public Health Announces Breast-Feeding Decline," August 8, p. 10.
Cohen, Anthony P. 1994. *Self Consciousness: An Alternative Anthropology of Identity.* New York: Routledge.
Croll, Elizabeth, Delia Davin, and Penny Kane, eds. 1985. *China's One-Child Policy.* Basingstoke, UK: Macmillan.
de Lauretis, Teresa. 1987. *Technologies of Gender: Essays on Theory, Film and Fiction.* Bloomington: Indiana University Press.
―――. 1994. "Potential for Growth in Chinese Baby Food Sector," *Eurofood* 1 (May 22): 3.
Eurofood. 1996. "Potential for Growth in Chinese Baby Food Sector," May 22, p. 3.
Foucault, Michel. 1990. *The History of Sexuality: An Introduction.* New York: Vintage Books.
Ginsburg, Faye, and Rayna Rapp, eds. 1996. *Conceiving the New World Order: The Global Politics of Reproduction.* Berkeley: University of California Press.
Greenhalgh, Susan. 1990. "Evolution of the One-Child Policy in Shaanxi 1979–1988," *China Quarterly* 122: 191–234.
―――. 1993. "Controlling Births and Bodies in Village China," *American Ethnologist* 21(1): 233–256.
Greiner, T., P. Van Esterik, and M. Latham. 1981. "The Insufficient Milk Syndrome: An Alternative Explanation," *Medical Anthropology* 5(3): 233–247.
Gussler, J., and L. Briesemeister. 1980. "The Insufficient Milk Syndrome: A Biocultural Explanation," *Medical Anthropology* 4(2): 145–174.
Hartmann, Betsy. 1987. *Reproductive Rights and Wrongs.* Boston: South End Press.
Honig, Emily, and Gail Hershatter. 1988. *Personal Voices: Chinese Women in the 1980s.* Stanford: Stanford University Press.
Hull, Valerie J., Shyam Thapa, and Gulardi Wiknjosastro. 1989. "Breastfeeding and Health Professionals: A Study in Hospitals in Indonesia," *Social Science and Medicine* 20(4): 355–364.
Jaggar, Alison. 1989. "Introduction." In *Gender/Body/Knowledge: Feminist Reconstructions of Being and Knowing,* A. Jaggar and S. Bordo, eds. New Brunswick, NJ: Rutgers University Press.
Jelliffe, D. B., and E. F. P. Jelliffe. 1978. *Human Milk in the Modern World.* Oxford: Oxford University Press.
Kleinman, Arthur, and Joan Kleinman. 1991. "Suffering and Its Professional Transformation: Toward an Ethnography of Interpersonal Experience," *Culture, Medicine and Psychiatry* 15(3): 275–301.
Laqueur, Thomas. 1990. *Making Sex: Body and Gender from the Greeks to Freud.* Cambridge, MA.: Harvard University Press.
Levine, N. 1988. "Women's Work and Infant Feeding: A Case from Nepal," *Ethnology* 27(3): 231–251.
Maher, Vanessa, ed. 1994. *The Anthropology of Breastfeeding: Natural Law or Social Construct.* Oxford: Berg.
Manderson, Lenore. 1984. "'These Are Modern Times': Infant Feeding Practice in Peninsular Malaysia," *Social Science and Medicine* 18(1): 47–57.
Marcus, George, and Michael Fischer. 1986. *Anthropology as Cultural Critique: An Experimental Moment in the Human Sciences.* Chicago: University of Chicago Press.
McKenzie, Paul. 1993. "Women's Rights in China: An Update," *China Law Reporter* 7(1): 7–11.

Mead Johnson Company. 1996. *Annual Report.*
Molony, Barbara. 1995. "Japan's 1986 Equal Employment Opportunity Law and the Changing Discourse on Gender," *Sings* 20(2): 268–287.
Moore, Henrietta. 1988. *Feminism and Anthropology.* Minneapolis: University of Minnesota Press.
Nerlove, Sara B. 1974. "Women's Workload and Infant Feeding Practices: A Relationship with Demographic Implications," *Ethnology* 13: 207–214.
Popkin, B., R. Bilsborrow, J. Akin, and M. Yamamato. 1986. "Breastfeeding Determinants in Low Income Countries," *Family Planning* 9: 1–31.
Riley, Nancy. 1996. "Holding Up Half the Economy," *China Business Review* 23(1): 8–17.
Scheper-Hughes, Nancy. 1984. "Infant Mortality and Infant Care: Cultural and Economic Constraints on Nurturing in Northeast Brazil," *Social Science and Medicine* 19(5): 535–546.
———. 1987. *Child Survival: Anthropological Perspectives on the Treatment and Maltreatment of Children.* Dordrecht: Kluwer.
Scheper-Hughes, N., and M. Lock. 1987. "The Mindful Body: A Prolegomenon to Future Work in Medical Anthropology," *Medical Anthropology Quarterly* 1(1): 6–41.
Stacey, Judith. 1983. *Patriarchy and the Socialist Revolution in China.* Berkeley: University of California Press.
———. 1994. *Statistical Yearbook of China.* China Statistical Publishing House: Beijing.
Tong, Louis. 1994. "The 'Consumer Society' Comes to China," *Business Korea* 12(6): 38–41.
UNICEF (United Nations Children's Fund). 1992. *Baby Friendly Hospital Initiative Brochure.* New York: United Nations, p. 1.
United Nations. 1992. *Baby Friendly Hospital Brochure.*
———. 1995. *Baby Friendly Hospital Initiative Newsletter* 5: 1.
———. 1996. *Baby Friendly Hospital Initiative Newsletter* 7: 3.
Van Esterik, Penny. 1989. *Beyond the Breast-Bottle Controversy.* New Brunswick, NJ: Rutgers University Press.
Waylen, G. 1994. Women and Democratization: Conceptualizing Gender Relations in Transition Politics," *World Politics* 46(3): 327–354.
WHO (World Health Organization). 1981. *Contemporary Patterns on Breast-feeding: Report on the WHO Collaborative Study on Breast-Feeding.* Geneva: World Health Organization.
Wolf, Margery. 1985. *Revolution Postponed: Women in Contemporary China.* Stanford: Stanford University Press.
Xinhua News Agency. 1995. "Maternal and Infant Welfare Law," *Foreign Broadcast Information Services,* November 21.
———. 1996a. "China Adopts the Convention on the Rights of Children," *Foreign Broadcast Information Services,* March 14.
———. 1996b. "Adoption of Convention on the Rights of Children," *Foreign Broadcast Information Services,* April 3.
———. 1996c. "China Leads in Baby-Friendly Hospital Initiative," *Foreign Broadcast Information Services,* April 13.
Yuan, Xiaohong. 1997. "Baby-Friendly Action in China: Protection, Promotion, and Support of Breastfeeding." In *1997 Asian Conference of Pediatricians Abstracts.* Hong Kong: Association of Asian Pediatrics.
Yuval-Davis, Nira. 1996. *Gender and Nation.* London: Sage.

Yuval-Davis, Nira, and Floya Anthias. 1989. *Woman, Nation, State.* New York: St. Martins Press.

Zha, Jianying. 1995. *China Pop.* New York: New Press.

Zhao, Olivia. 1996. "China Business: Sales and Investments," *China Business News* (July-August): 48–52.

Zhu, Baoxia. 1994. "Breast-Feed Babies, Says Conference," *China Daily,* July 30.

PART 5

Conclusion

12

International Health Research: The Rules of the Game

James Trostle

Publication as an International Health Policy Issue

This book has shown that local data (statistics, perceptions, laws, rules, knowledge) often fail to guide or even to influence international policies. Prior chapters have described case studies of contradictions between local and international concepts and definitions of disease, between local idiom and global communication, between local expectation and multinational marketing, between local nuance and state discourse. Why, then, is it appropriate to conclude these case studies with a comparative analysis of rules about publication?

Publishing is still a fundamental way to disseminate biomedical advances, impose and announce policies, and communicate across local and international boundaries. Even though metaphors of global networks, information superhighways, and cyberspace are proliferating with the expansion of the Internet, people still speak of "publishing," or even "e-publishing," their scholarship on the Net. This book is one among millions of examples of scholars' continuing interest in printing and distributing their analyses. But even this fundamental commitment to sharing information suffers from the contradictions mentioned in prior chapters.

So in part this chapter is a warning or corrective to the weight of this book: The types of challenges described here are being presented in a form capable of reaching the international planners we critique, but are quite unlikely to reach many of the local people and movements we support. Our scholarly tendency to publish these critiques may not be—and often is not—tied to any local system of information distribution. We are distanced from the local even in a publication championing the local.

This chapter illustrates another dimension of global-local strain. To maximize their applicability and appropriateness, international policies must mediate among and respond to all relevant local sources of knowledge, data, and political pressure. Prior chapters have discussed the global eddies and flows of technology, products, laws, bodies, organs, knowledge, and various other services and commodities. This one looks at obstructions to the free circulation of research and information about all these areas. Such obstructions are critical impediments to effective policies.

Finally, this chapter poses a sobering challenge and potential corrective. International providers of health research funds have systematically studied barriers to publication and broad circulation of information. The challenge is that even these well-intentioned donors tend to miss some critical barriers hindering local scientists from participating in global science and policymaking. As I show in this chapter, their analyses have focused on the quality of the playing field, and not on the fact that they have made up the rules of the game.

Problem Statement

When I was a graduate student, I read that science could be defined as a form of communication (Kaplan and Manners 1972). I like that definition now because it exhorts scientists to disseminate their results and helps justify my teaching my students about one possible role of science in society. But although science can be defined as a structured form of communication, it can also be defined as an industrial form of knowledge production, accompanied by a set of cultural rules about how best to present evidence and establish authority. These cultural rules about evidence and authority pass as natural, or at least inevitable, rules about the importance to science of peer review, publishing, and the free flow of ideas.

To trace the process through which publication in peer-reviewed journals became equated with dissemination and quality in science, we would need to refer to a full historical review (see, e.g., Altbach 1987; Cronin 1984). I will instead adopt a more anthropological approach, focused on actors and institutions, to explore differences in contemporary publication incentives among institutions primarily outside the United States. These differences highlight the impact of local incentives on publication strategies, and expose the arbitrariness of some of the rules of science as practiced in the United States. Extensive citation lists, multiple publications from single research projects, and lengthy lists of authors are not inevitable parts of science; they are, however, predictable outcomes of certain specific incentives.

International development agencies focused on research often acknowledge the absence of a level playing field for health researchers in developing countries: libraries without current journals; outdated computers or unreliable electricity; low wages; researchers holding multiple full-time jobs. The international Commission on Health Research for Development helped bring these disparities to public attention in its 1990 report. It stated that about 93 percent of the world's burden of premature mortality lies in developing countries, whereas only about 5 percent of the world's health research funding is spent on the health problems of developing countries (Commission on Health Research for Development 1990:30, figure 3.1). In the case of health research, then, rather than describing a playing field that is not level, we might better note that one side has Astroturf and lights for night play, while the other side is dark and rocky.

My experience as a donor and as a consultant to international health development agencies has caused me to conclude that donors are studying and learning important facts about the pitch and quality of the playing fields, but are still neglecting the rules of the game. Many national and international agencies eager to improve health research in developing countries assume that such research should develop and be disseminated according to models used in industrialized countries. Their local (industrialized) systems of professional prestige and ranking help to define who has expertise and who does not. Local expectations about public discourse also influence what types of scientific writing and analysis are valued. Some sites and disciplines value highly theoretical presentations; others value more applied and issue-oriented work. Some value research relevant to an international audience, others to a national or local one. Paying attention to what this chapter calls "rules" may help donors distinguish between two rationales for supporting research: because it is valued, and because it is labeled high quality.

The choice of specific indicators of research quality is guided by various influences. Staff in organizations providing financial support for research are usually educated at elite universities in industrialized countries, and almost invariably are trained in the Western scientific tradition. They face few incentives to experiment with other models of research support, because the existing system successfully produces millions of research papers, and new systems would be expensive to create and evaluate. Consistent application of a single model of research development also brings benefits to donors: they can standardize methods of support and evaluation; and their reliance on a university-based research model allows them to continue their patronage of university researchers and policy advisers, historically influential players in deciding what work donors should support. But these assumptions about what constitutes good work are rarely stated and hardly questioned, even as the sustainability of these research models becomes doubtful in industrialized countries.

This chapter reviews some of what is known about publication of health research, points out some differences in institutional rules promoting different types of publications, and describes how researchers from a few developing countries rank different types of dissemination products. It argues that these rules foster the differential growth of types of scientific products in different countries and limit the flow of information across national borders. More important, and less noticeably, these rules themselves impede the career opportunities of researchers in developing countries, because they allow researchers in industrialized countries to continue to dominate and control scientific literature. The chapter, therefore, concludes with a plea to choose and justify research dissemination strategies according to the purpose of the research and its relevance to specific audiences such as the public, other researchers, and policymakers. This is better than choosing and justifying dissemination strategies based on culture-specific definitions of what constitutes scientific quality.

Tools for Disseminating Health Research

Beginning in the 1960s, facilitated by the growth of computerized databases, two different tools helped measure scientific production worldwide. An indexing or abstracting service is required to find, or simply to count, research articles. The oldest of these is the *Index Medicus,* started in the United States in 1879, a compilation of journals in the National Library of Medicine. The computerized version of the *Index Medicus,* called *MedLine,* began in 1966. There is some prestige, and sometimes some effort, in having a journal included in the major computerized indices. Failure to be listed is akin to failure to be consulted by many scientists, for these databases are the primary sources for finding others' work.

The second tool for measuring influence is the citation index, which takes the further step of both indexing *and linking* not only titles of articles but also all the citations contained in those articles. The primary source for estimating scientific productivity and scientific authority (as measured by citation counts) is the Science Citation Index (SCI), produced since 1963 by the Institute for Scientific Information (ISI), a private company based in Philadelphia.[1] The SCI is an expensive research tool: in 1998 a subscription to the CD-ROM version of the SCI costs a small liberal arts college in the United States more than $20,000 per year.

These indices should theoretically give access to the breadth of scientific literature. But they do not. Looking at worldwide production of publications in science, engineering, and medicine from 1981 to 1994, a recent study found that more than 81 percent of papers listed in the SCI were published from just fifteen countries (May 1997). The United States produced most, with almost 35 percent of the total, whereas the rest of the "top ten" (United Kingdom, Japan, Germany, France, Canada, Italy, India, Australia, and the Netherlands, in order of decreasing proportional contribution) together accounted for an additional 41 percent. Concerning production of papers per capita, the order changed somewhat: Switzerland was the most productive country measured in terms of papers per capita, with the rest of the top producers (in decreasing order) being Israel, Sweden, Denmark, Canada, the Netherlands, Finland, the United Kingdom, the United States, and New Zealand.

A slightly different ranking was obtained by looking at papers listed in the SCI just in 1994 (Gibbs 1995:92). The same group of "top ten" countries produced 73 percent of papers in the SCI in that year. In contrast, for example, Brazil produced 0.6 percent, Mexico 0.3 percent, Thailand 0.09 percent, Pakistan 0.06 percent, the Philippines 0.04 percent, and Indonesia 0.01 percent of the science literature in the SCI in that year. Countries thus differ greatly in their levels of scientific productivity as measured by numbers of scientific articles included in computerized databases, with developing countries drastically underrepresented.

The ISI states that its "basic mission as a database publishing company is to provide comprehensive coverage of the world's most important and influential research conducted throughout the world" (Testa 1997:1). But the phrase "most important and influential" hides a multitude of limits to comprehensive coverage, because most published literature does not make it into the international indices at all. Looking specifically at the international medical literature, for example, of 715 medical journals published in Latin America in 1975, only 52 were included in the *Index Medicus* (Arends 1975:506). In the 1980s, there were more than 70,000 scientific journals in the world. The ISI covered about 4,500 of these journals, with only about 90 of them, or 2 percent, coming from developing countries (Gaillard 1992:58). In 1981 the Science Citation Index listed 80 journals from developing countries, but by 1993 this had declined to 50 (Gibbs 1995: 94). In 1977 the Science Citation Index listed 829 journals with "above average" impact, but only one of these (the *Revista Mexicana de Astronomía*) was on the list of journals from developing countries. In 1984 Latin American authors produced a little over 1 percent of articles listed in the ISI (Pellegrini 1992:22).

Computerized indices, the primary points of access to the international scientific literature, filter out many more journals than they include. Some of that filtering is appropriate, because indexing is expensive, science journals have widely varying levels of criticism in their review processes, and not all information is of equal value. But some of that filtering is based not on quality or value but on language, with a clear preference in most databases—and most international journals—for articles published in English (Bottiger 1983; Haiqi et al. 1997; Nylenna et al. 1994; Sanberg et al. 1996).

Some of the filtering is also based on estimates of the needs of the primary consumers of the databases. Describing its customized dataset services group, the ISI website (http://www.isinet.com/prodserv/rsg/rsghp.html) states it provides information to "science policy agencies, government laboratories, universities, libraries, independent research institutes, industrial firms, venture capital groups, investment advisory groups, and other research organizations." The ISI also states that "the ISI editorial team's mission is to identify and evaluate promising new journals that will be useful to ISI subscribers" (Testa 1997:1) and that "high journal publishing standards, especially timeliness, and English language bibliographic elements remain essential" (Testa 1997:3). Thus, developing country researchers are in a bind: it is difficult for them to build international reputations unless their work appears in the bibliographic or citation indices, and they are likeliest to make it into these indices if they publish in English.

But even publication in English may not be enough. As citation practices garner increasing research attention (in the journal *Scientometrics,* for example, published since 1979), some evidence is emerging that the absence of developing country research in the English-language (so-called "international") literature cannot be attributed to language alone. For example, studies of health research and of psychological research concluded that professionals in the United States and the United Kingdom primarily cited material produced in their own countries and rarely cited that produced outside their countries (Campbell 1990). Moreover, despite the common language in these two countries, "both studies demonstrated that U.K. authors cited U.S. material much more than the U.S. authors cited U.K. material" (Campbell 1990:381). This has also been described as an "intellectual imbalance of trade in favor of the United States, with Britain running a large deficit" (Klein 1991:276). Some of the reasons for this preference to cite locally include "proximity or sense of loyalty to local colleagues; institutional affiliation; ease of access to home-produced literature; vague political or cultural pressures; linguistic isolation" (Cronin 1984:71). These selective factors limit the usefulness of the standard electronic databases for estimating the productivity, not to mention finding the science, of researchers in developing countries (Gaillard 1992; Gibbs 1995; Sanz et al. 1995).

For these reasons the World Health Organization and other organizations have started their own supplemental databases, such as *ExtraMED,* the *African Index Medicus,* or the *BIBLAT* or *PERIÓDICA* for Latin America, to cover research literature in developing countries. But these sources still do not offer any citation-based tool to assess connections among the information in these journals. In contrast, the ISI's Web page advertises its "National Science Indicators on Diskette, 1981–1996" as offering "the most up-to-date measures on national performance in the sciences and social sciences based on the Institute for Scientific Information's unique and authoritative publication and citation statistics. The database contains the number of ISI-indexed papers from each nation and the number of times the papers were cited through 1996" (November 8, 1997, http://www.isinet.com/prodserv/rsg/natsciin.html). The ISI openly describes its English-language preference, yet it also advertises its services to nations eager to assess and compare the size of their national scientific publication record. To date, its services face no competition from others offering more complete or accurate citation-based coverage of the scientific output from developing countries.

Rules About the Production of Health Research

International, institutional, and cross-cultural influences shape how scientific research is organized, practiced, and presented. International differences emerge from varying levels of social and financial support for research, and different types of occupational opportunities for research scientists. Institutional differences stem from different leadership styles, work habits, and types of institutional resources. Cross-cultural differences emerge from different ideas about the relative value of "open criticism" and "saving face." The rest of this chapter will focus on the dissemination of health research through publication.[2]

Some basic Western assumptions about the production of science include the rules of scientific evidence (that methods be reproducible, hypotheses clear, propositions testable) and extend to the dissemination of that evidence. This organized evidence, or knowledge, should be reviewed by peers and disseminated publicly in journals. Writing papers and citing others' ideas are important components of this process. The sociologist Robert Merton wrote that peer recognition through publication, citation, and attribution is a central part of the incentive system for any scientist. According to Merton, "Once we understand that the sole property right of scientists in their discoveries has long resided in peer recognition of it and in derivative collegial esteem, we begin to understand better the concern of scientists to get there first and to establish their priority" (1988:623). These comments about the symbolic power of citations come from an article entitled "The Matthew Effect," after the biblical phrase from the Gospel according to Matthew: "For unto everyone that hath shall be given, and he shall have abundance; but from him that hath not shall be taken away even that which he hath" (Merton 1988:608–609). Merton's point was that famous scientists get more opportunity to produce research and are given more recognition for whatever they publish. There is also a Matthew effect in international science: productive institutions and productive nations get more recognition and greater opportunity to create more science, whereas the production of undeveloped countries must be ratified by "legitimate" scientists and indexing systems before it will be accepted.

Scientists in the United States, and some other industrialized countries, have a particular vision of health research as best circulating through journals, and best judged, at least in part, through citation counts. Scientific institutions in the United States have created a system that values quantity of production just as much, if not more, than quality. Consequently, we see university-based researchers resorting to "salami publishing": dividing their results into the thinnest possible slices for maximum distribution. This pressure to find publication outlets is met by a proliferation of journals, leading to what has been called "journal pollution" (Susser and Yankauer 1993).

Almost seventy-four thousand scientific journals are published in the world today, with most coming from the United States. If these journals were being used, their existence might be justified, yet a survey of the four thousand Science Citation Index journals found that 55 percent of papers published in these journals between 1981 and 1985 received no citations at all in the five years following their publication (Hamilton 1990). In the social sciences, almost 75 percent of papers in the Social Science Citation Index (SSCI) remained uncited within five years (Hamilton 1991). Although citation is an imperfect measure of influence, complete absence of citation on this scale suggests that "the literature" in many fields has become too large to absorb and use. Should emerging communities of researchers be urged to emulate this system of communication? To put the problem closer to home: Is the problem only that "they" don't publish enough, or is it also that "we" publish too much?

Merton views science as a quest for knowledge and esteem, but others adopt metaphors of science as a set of stratagems (Cronin 1984:4). The evidence discussed so far supports an analysis of publication as a response to a particular set of institutional incentives and a particular set of national and cultural expectations about the primacy of peer review, rather than as a component of participation in an "invisible college" of scholars. This helps explain why a university dean from a Southeast Asian country told me in 1990 that there were fundamental problems with getting scientific manuscripts reviewed in his country: Reviewers were happy to praise the good parts of papers, but reluctant to criticize the bad. Reviewers who did not like papers tended not to return any comments to the journal at all. At about the same time, the president of this university was publicly urging his staff to make greater efforts to publish in English-language journals, to increase institutional prestige and visibility.

North American academics tend to assume that researchers in other countries can, should, and do practice science as they do. The premiums and spoils of doing science in the United States include membership on review panels at the National Institutes of Health or the National Science Foundation; federal and foundation grants for one's department; invitations to international meetings; tenure; and perhaps limited fame (though usually not fortune). But how much do we know about the incentive structures, career options, and perceived audiences of scientists in developing countries?

The answer, predictably enough, is "not much." Between 1988 and 1995 I worked in the Applied Diarrheal Disease Research Project (ADDR) at the Harvard Institute for International Development. This project was designed to provide financial and technical assistance to researchers in developing countries. One of our goals was to increase the number and quality of researchers and research institutions in developing countries. (And one of the most important measures of our own project's success was the number of articles published by scientists we had funded.)

In the course of my work with ADDR I compiled information about research organization and incentives from three sources: first, from my experiences consulting with researchers and organizing proposal development and data analysis workshops; second, from texts describing institutional rules for career advancement in developing countries; and third, from questionnaire data from eighty-nine ADDR-funded investigators in eight countries.

ADDR funded approximately 150 research studies in fourteen countries. (See Trostle and Simon 1992 for a more detailed description of ADDR's objectives and challenges.) In some of these countries (Mexico, Peru, Pakistan), scientists were eager to publish in international journals and able to devote significant proportions of their time to research. Their research was published in prestigious national and international journals. In other countries (e.g., Indonesia and Thailand), many scientists were less able to publish internationally and more consumed by clinical practice and administrative tasks. Researchers from these countries tended to submit final documents to us as long research reports, bound and distributed by the investigator's institution.

Many of these differences can be highlighted by comparing incentives for research production in Indonesia and Mexico. Both countries evaluate scientists according to clearly specified and objective criteria, namely, highly structured point systems at the national level. These point systems are designed to be objective indicators of merit and quality (perhaps to counter earlier problems with promotion based on patronage rather than merit). Whether they are successful measures, and how they are used in practice, needs to be debated. I offer them here only as records that can be evaluated for their intent, not as evidence that they have been implemented or had influence.

The Indonesian system rewards investigators for publishing *nationally,* whereas the Mexican system rewards investigators for publishing *internationally.* I will describe here only the publication-based part of these systems, though points are also awarded for various types of teaching, service, and educational experiences.

Research for Local Consumption: The Case of Indonesia

The career and salary steps of Indonesian researchers are evaluated through a complex point system. The system promotes biomedical research for local consumption: for example, Indonesian researchers commonly disseminate their research results through lengthy reports, each of which carries an International Standard Serial Number (ISSN), published and distributed by their institutions. They rarely send scientific papers to be published in international journals. As seen in Table 12.1, different point totals are required to advance to new ranks.

Points can be collected through various activities, ranging from acquiring an advanced degree to serving on professional organizations to completing classroom materials. Table 12.2 presents the credit points awarded for various written works.

As Table 12.2 shows, an Indonesian researcher receives ten points for a research review in a journal acknowledged by the Ministry of Education, ten points for a scientific chapter in a book, and only fifteen points for a piece of original research published in a scientific journal. Obviously, few researchers will invest the considerable effort required to translate a paper into English, put it into the necessary format, wait several months for reviewers' comments, decipher reviewers' comments, resubmit, and wait several more months for publication. A researcher who goes through these steps will receive ten credit points fewer than if the researcher had written a book-length report in the Indonesian language and distributed it to other universities in Indonesia. This point system helps explain the Indonesian practice of obtaining ISSN numbers for paperbound reports issued by local universities and other organizations: these numbers almost magically transform reports into books or monographs, worth more credit points for promotion and salary increases.

Other disincentives to publishing international health research in Indonesia include poor and fragmented library resources, limited maintenance and replacement of computer resources, and lack of fundamental

Table 12.1 Categories of Faculty in Indonesia, and Points Needed to Attain Each Rank

Title	No. of Points
Middle expert assistant	100
Expert assistant	150
Junior lecturer	200
Middle lecturer	300
Lecturer	400
Middle head lecturer	550
Head lecturer	700
Middle professor	850
Professor	1,000

Source: Ministry of Education, Jakarta, No. 2492/D/C/88, December 20, 1988.

Table 12.2 Points Awarded for Diffusion of Scientific Products in Indonesia

Product	No. of Points
Original research	
Publish book with national distribution (with ISSN number)	25
Research paper acknowledged by Ministry of Education (without ISSN number)	15
Scientific paper in book	10
Unpublished scientific paper	5
Nonresearch publication (e.g., literature review)	
Edited book or journal with national distribution (with ISSN number)	20
Paper in journal acknowledged by Ministry of Education (with ISSN number)	10
Write textbook, tutorials, curricula	5
Popular scientific article	2

Source: "Credit Points for Faculty in Higher Educational Institutions," Ministry of Education, Jakarta, Circular #61395/MPK/1987, September 28, 1987.

curricular support for research (Hull 1994). Indonesian researchers based in universities are rarely paid enough to subsist, so they must supplement their salaries with extra jobs. One analysis stated that "the low pay of the civil service [in Indonesia] means that universities cannot compete for the time of their staff" (Clark and Oey-Gardiner 1991:138–139). This need for double or triple job responsibility manifests the government's lack of commitment to research as a public career. The regulations concerning credit points for publications manifest the government's lack of commitment to publishing research in peer-reviewed international journals.

Government policy in Indonesia rewards local distribution of applied research. If the Indonesian government seeks to support the production and dissemination of research *within Indonesia*, its credit point policies can be seen as justifiable and potentially effective. Researchers have documented that national journals in Spain play an important role in disseminating applied research inside the country (Sanz et al. 1995), whereas international journals are chosen by Spanish authors to publish their basic research. A similar argument could be made for this Indonesian incentive system, though I do not have data to corroborate whether applied research is published locally while basic research is sent overseas. The Indonesian point system rewards scientists for disseminating their scientific work in the local language, and to a national rather than an international audience. But if external (international) indicators of relevance and impact are chosen, or if Indonesian policies were designed to promote basic research of broad international relevance, then the incentives do not appear to match the objectives.

The case of Indonesia represents incentives for local dissemination and consumption; the case of Mexico provides the opposite example, with its own unique set of outcomes.

Research for International Consumption: The Case of Mexico

The Mexican system of evaluating scientific performance is just as complex as the Indonesian one. The publication incentives of the Mexican Social Security Institute (Instituto Mexicano del Seguro Social [IMSS]) cover most of the medical researchers in the country. As in Indonesia, the IMSS also has a published point system for determining career progress, seen in Table 12.3.

This evaluation system requires points to be distributed across three different categories (see Table 12.4), with research productivity measured by number of articles published and number as first author, and research impact measured by citations. The system expects research associates to increase their responsibility for original ideas over time, as manifested in increasing numbers of first-authored publications. Senior researchers, on the other hand, should be involved in forming research groups. Thus although they are expected to produce more publications and receive more citations than research associates, they need not necessarily be the first author on as many publications.

Table 12.4 shows how points are awarded within IMSS for the diffusion of scientific products. This is a good example of biomedical research for international consumption, because Mexican investigators receive almost three times as many points for articles they publish in international as opposed to national journals. Compared to a prior version of this evaluation

Table 12.3 Categories of IMSS Researcher, with Points and Number of Articles Needed to Attain Each Rank

Title	No. of Points	No. of Articles	No. of Citations, last 4 years
Research associate A	12.5	2	0
Research associate B	25.0	3 (1 as 1st author)	0
Research associate C	50.0	5 (2 as 1st)	0
Research associate D	100.0	6 (3 as 1st)	50
Senior researcher A	150.0	7 (1 as 1st)	100
Senior researcher B	250.0	8	150
Senior researcher C	350.0	8	200
Senior researcher D	450.0	9	300

Source: "Instructivo para la Evaluacion Curricular de los Investigadores del Instituto Mexicano del Seguro Social," Mexico City: IMSS, March 1992.

Table 12.4 Points Awarded for Diffusion of Scientific Products, IMSS, Mexico (1992 revised policy)

	Published in English, French, or German (Category I)	Published in Other Languages (Category II)
Articles listed in any of six computerized indices	8 (was 6 until 1992)	3 (was 2)
Book chapter	6	2
Editing book	6	6 (was 2)
Author book	15	7
Citations in Science Citation Index	1	

Source: "Instructivo para la Evaluación Curricular de los Investigadores del Instituto Mexicano del Seguro Social," Mexico City: IMSS, March 1992.

system published in 1987, an article is now given relatively more weight than a book chapter and is worth more than half the points that a book would bring. The system was revised to push researchers to publish articles in non-Spanish journals.

Mexican researchers in the IMSS system are also judged by how often their work is cited in the Science Citation Index (which, as I have noted, includes few journals from Latin America or other developing regions). Receiving three citations from international sources gives one the same number of points as publishing a paper in a Spanish-language journal. The policy has resulted in anecdotal reports of citation trading between colleagues ("I'll cite yours if you'll cite mine") and extensive self-citation. Some analysts have noted that increasing rates of international publication and citation reflect the maturation of Mexico's biomedical research community (Fortes and Lomnitz 1994; Lomnitz et al. 1987).

If the outcome of Indonesia's incentive system is relatively low support for international publication, the outcome of Mexico's incentive system is relatively low support for national dissemination. The IMSS system's reliance on English citation sources to measure the scientific impact of Spanish-language publications has already helped one Mexican journal decide to change its language of publication. The editorial board of the Archivos de Investigación Clínica decided in 1992 that the journal would no longer appear in Spanish, but rather only in English, as the Archives of Medical Research. The editorial board rationalized this as the internationalization of Mexican science (Loria and Lisker 1995; Lozoya et al. 1995), but it also meant the abandonment of a national Spanish-speaking audience (Perez-Padilla 1995). This is a clear example of the conflict between national and international research goals, and of the struggle between local and foreign standards. Mexican researchers who do not speak English can no longer use this journal to learn about the research of their fellow citizens.

The Impact of Policies on Scientific Production: Data from the ADDR Project

We looked at publication policies in the last section to reflect on their intent, and to note differences across sites. To assess whether scientists in different sites ranked publication types differently, a questionnaire was distributed to about three hundred ADDR grantees working on one hundred projects in 1994–1995. Preliminary results received from eighty-nine ADDR grantees revealed many significant differences in rankings across countries, though larger surveys would need to be done to assess how the rankings were influenced by scientific discipline, type of institution, site of investigator training, and the like. These survey results should therefore be taken as tentative and exploratory rather than definitive.

In order to work with larger numbers and to combine institutions with similar policies, I grouped Thailand and Indonesia as Southeast Asian nations, and Mexico, Guatemala, and Peru as Latin American ones (see Table 12.5).

I asked each scientist to rank twelve research outcomes (local, regional, and international articles; citations, reports, books, chapters, policy statements, translations, local and international presentations, and posters) in terms of their importance to career advancement. Significant differences can be seen in the rankings for regional and international journals (more important in Latin America); in reports (more important in Southeast Asia); and in book chapters (more important in Southeast Asia). To control for differences by discipline, I then looked only at clinical scientists in these two regions. When this was done, the same trend was seen, though

Table 12.5 How Southeast Asian (Indonesian and Thai) and Latin American (Mexican, Guatemalan, and Peruvian) ADDR Scientists Ranked the Importance of Various Scientific Products

	Mean rank	
Type	Southeast Asia	Latin America
International journal	5.0	3.2[a]
Regional journal	5.2	3.8[a]
Local journal	5.8	5.2
Books	4.2	5.7[a]
Reports	4.2	7.6[a]
Chapters	5.4	6.0
International talks	5.5	6.2
Local talks	6.3	7.3
Citations	8.4	7.3
Policy summaries	7.9	9.3
Posters	8.9	8.2
Translations	9.0	10.3

Notes: Lower numbers = higher ranks.
a. Statistically significant difference at $p<0.05$.

the smaller numbers in each group meant that "reports" was now the only difference that reached statistical significance, with the Southeast Asian scientists ranking them higher in importance than the Latin American ones did.

These rankings are consistent with the general objectives of the two types of incentive systems described earlier, where the Indonesian type seemed to promote local dissemination, and the Mexican type international dissemination. More problematic for the broader approach to publication outlets espoused in this chapter, production of policy statements was ranked quite low by each group in this survey: second to last among the Southeast Asian respondents, and third to last among the Latin American respondents. This could reflect the absence of incentives to disseminate scientific findings to a broad audience, and the relative unimportance of policy impact as a component of the evaluation process for scientific researchers. It could also reflect cultural differences in the importance science plays in the public arena, or the extent to which publication itself forms an important channel for public discourse. It is unfortunate that we did not inquire about the significance to researchers of other public dissemination efforts such as writing letters to the editor or commentaries for newspapers or magazines, or speaking before organized social gatherings such as religious organizations or neighborhood groups.

The survey also uncovered quite large differences in the amount of time researchers estimated they could spend on teaching and research. Table 12.6 shows that Latin American researchers estimated they spent 17

Table 12.6 Mean Percentage Time Devoted by ADDR Scientists to Institutional Activities in Southeast Asia and Latin America (self-estimated)

Type	Southeast Asia	Latin America
Teaching	32	17[a]
Research	37	63[a]
Service	22	20
Other	10	6

Note: Statistically significant difference at $p<0.05$.

percent of their time teaching, whereas Southast Asian scientists estimated they spent 33 percent of their time on teaching. Moreover, Latin American researchers estimated they spent about 63 percent of their time on research, whereas the Southeast Asian respondents estimated they spent only 37 percent of their time in this way. These proportions remained about the same even when looking only at clinicians in these countries. The differences likely reflect both the incentive systems we have reviewed already, and the types of economic and institutional resources made available to researchers. They may also reflect differences in institutional emphases on creating new knowledge versus transmitting existing knowledge. These, in turn, are products of cultural expectations about the role of researchers and professors in society, and of the relevance of research to politics and policymaking.

I therefore conclude that, at least for the institutions with which ADDR staff were interacting, the types of incentive structures reviewed in the last section of this chapter help to create and manifest real differences in health researchers' perceptions of how they need to disseminate their work. These differences might not be as sharp if one were to include other institutions, other disciplines, or other scientists, but there is some concordance between the institutional incentives and the individual perceptions of researchers working in these and similar institutions.

Different rules about what science is for, and who it is for, help to create different strategies for disseminating research results. These local incentives are missed, or ignored, by health research development programs that assume the pinnacle of success for any researcher is an article published in an international journal. Worse yet, the foundations of this assumption are increasingly tenuous, as papers go uncited, journals unreferenced, and articles unread.

The high cost and slow speed of journal production are two factors driving more research onto the Worldwide Web, but Web access is still quite limited outside the industrialized world. Worse yet, market pressures are reducing the number of full-time academic and research jobs in industrialized countries, increasing the pressure to publish early and often among those seeking to enter or rise in the academic world. This exacerbates the problem of journal pollution in the present, and it is not clear that Web distribution will reduce this problem in the future.

Where Next? Toward Audience, Advocacy, and Application

Recent news from *The Chronicle of Higher Education* in the United States suggests that a few educational institutions are beginning to confront these problems. The glut of articles and expensive journals has caused some U.S. libraries and universities to rethink their incentive structures. An article (Wilson 1998) from the *Chronicle* headlined "Provosts Push a Radical Plan to Change the Way Faculty Research Is Evaluated" describes a proposal to separate peer review from publishing. Panels of certification experts would provide legitimacy and prestige. Publication could be in electronic or paper form, or not happen at all.

Some universities' tenure and promotion policies are also beginning to reflect this reexamination. Medical school faculty at Harvard University saw their tenure and appointment policies change in the late 1980s to combat the growing emphasis on quantity over quality in publications: those up for review in the medical school were asked to include only two principal publications if recommended for assistant professor, five if associate, and ten if full professor, rather than providing a full publication dossier (Harvard Medical School 1989). In 1994 the councils in the United Kingdom that distribute money to universities changed their method of measuring research quality: "They will no longer use total publication counts as a measure of the relative strengths of research departments. Instead, they will take into account only the four best papers individual researchers in each department have published in the previous three years" (O'Brien 1994:1840). These types of measures give some hope that researcher evaluation strategies can be improved in the United States and elsewhere. If evaluation criteria are not changed, we run the risk of producing much information that we cannot read or even find, on topics so trivial that only the author would care.

Being a process of communication as well as a system of production, international health research should not and cannot unfold in similar fashion at all sites. Good communication strategies require that those who seek to disseminate information identify audiences and, subsequently, select appropriate channels to reach those audiences and develop messages for those audiences. Given a single set of applied health results, there is still great cross-cultural variability in the audiences, channels, and messages developed around those results. The following suggestions are offered to expand the list of potential research outcomes beyond articles in English in scientific journals, and to improve researchers' abilities to disseminate their research findings effectively.

Research always has an audience. It is produced for other researchers in one's province, or nation, or profession; for the general public; for policymakers in government or in the private sector; or for some combination of these. Knowledge of audience ideally should facilitate a researcher's choice of dissemination strategy. Therefore, failure to publish locally an important solution to a local problem of applied importance is as lamentable as an attempt to publish that simply local solution at international scale (unless the elegance of that local solution might prompt similar success were it known elsewhere).

Most researchers can learn to think about how their research will be used, and by whom. The notion of stakeholders or interest groups moves one from describing passive consumers of research to active and interested advocacy groups for research. As political concerns about power and resistance become more visible, so also do local forms of dissemination become more appropriate and effective. Researchers advocating the use of needle exchange programs to control HIV in Springfield, Massachusetts, need dissemination strategies quite different from researchers employed in New York City. So also do researchers in Jakarta often need to disseminate their applied findings differently from scientists in Lagos or Caracas.

If the stance of the international donor is that all science should lead to international publication, this can reduce the potential local impact of research even as it can enhance the international reputation of the researcher. It is, therefore, important for donors and researchers to discuss who will use results, how best to reach those who will use results, what might be done to increase the applicability of research results, and how to assess the quality of research. The success of scientific institutions can be measured through numbers of publications or prizes, but it can also be measured through the permanence of institutions through time, their ability to recruit staff and maintain public support, and their ability to "serve local needs or understand local problems" (Stepan 1981:9). This broader list of attributes of research quality was used to describe an important research center in Brazil, the Oswaldo Cruz Foundation, as it functioned half a century ago. But it nonetheless has contemporary relevance, for it suggests ways to assess research quality that go far beyond the publication and citation-based assessment strategies now used by many research institutions. More attention to these other components would, I contend, support more relevant, more effective, and longer-lasting communities of researchers, both in the United States and elsewhere.

The focus to date on quality of the research playing field rather than rules of the research game has a number of important and pernicious implications. First, as long as the "problem" of research quality is defined as solvable through more inputs (whether those inputs are computers, journals, doctorates, or techniques), it is not necessary to ask whether the definition of quality is in any way problematic. Much as the development literature of the 1960s and 1970s cast "underdevelopment" as the issue rather than "overdevelopment," and thereby avoided critiques of Western consumption patterns, so also does the literature on research quality avoid a careful reexamination of the legitimacy and sustainability of the prevailing standards.

Second, the rules that define quality, and the myth that all researchers should and do follow the same rules, systematically exclude some researchers from the field of play. We see this systematic exclusion enacted in the ways that scientific literature is indexed and made available. We also see it in ability of European and American researchers to obtain support allowing them to undertake research in areas that local researchers themselves do not have the resources to enter.

Third, these rules provide barriers to some researchers and some research paradigms (basic versus applied, for example). Those who can follow the publication rules can disseminate their work, not because it is better than work by those who do not disseminate, but because they have the resources to be able to follow the rules, and the rules they follow are usually consistent with outcomes valued by their institutions.

Finally, lack of attention to rules limits the range of creative solutions to the problem of disseminating research. If all researchers seek and measure their success through international publication, we collectively miss opportunities to explore the possible impact of other strategies such as writing policy memos, sending letters to newspaper editors, or hosting television or radio shows. In fact, we discount many actions that could lead to direct policy or public impact, in exchange for actions that may eventually have some impact over the long term (creation of data banks, accumulation of wisdom, contributing to scientific debate). These latter activities are in no sense unimportant, but to the extent that they become actions expected of high-quality science, they potentially reduce the public engagement and applied contribution of scientists.

Conclusion

Although research quality may differ from site to site (and scientist to scientist), it would be wrong to assume that lack of participation in international science can be attributed either to invariant handicaps in projects from developing countries, or their failure to compete successfully in a larger and more open world marketplace of ideas. The third section of this chapter described a set of thick filters limiting scientific journals from developing countries from appearing in so-called "international" indices. The fourth section described institutional incentives for publication that vary across developing countries, pushing some toward international dissemination and others toward national or local dissemination. The fifth section showed that scientists have patterned differences in their rankings of various scientific products, in ways consistent with these incentives. And the sixth section briefly described some alternative dimensions to use in disseminating and evaluating health research, in an attempt to get away from the traditional narrow focus on publication and citation.

Imagine training young researchers to write effective executive summaries of their findings, press releases, letters and commentaries to newspapers, to speak in public, produce plays, or write songs. This might produce more effective communicators than the present emphasis on early publication does. Imagine working with foundations and universities to help them pay more attention to local applicability, appropriate dissemination, and diverse audiences. This might help change the rules of the research game, increasing incentives to communicate results to appropriate audiences. In the meantime, specific cultural rules about evidence and authority should not go unexamined or unchallenged, especially when they systematically exclude specific regions of the globe. Close connections between locally generated data and international policies are possible only when knowledge is broadly disseminated and available to all.

Notes

Portions of this paper were presented at the 1992 Annual Meeting of the American Anthropological Association, the 1993 Research Retreat of the Harvard Institute for International Development (HIID), and at the 1997 Annual Meeting of the American Anthropological Association in a session entitled "The Fallacy of the Level Playing Field: Globalization, Health, and Identity." I am grateful to various staff at HIID for assistance with data collection and processing, especially Heidi Clyne, Charlotte Gnecco, Cynthia Lopez, Bradley Nixon, and Laura Tesler. Andrew Noymer and Camvan Phu provided bibliographic assistance. Richard Cash, Fitzroy Henry, Jonathon Simon, and Johannes Sommerfeld provided collegial support, and Lynn Morgan and the editors gave helpful comments on prior drafts. Funds for the research reported here came to HIID from the United States Agency for International Development, through Cooperative Agreement #DPE-5952–A-00–5073–00. Neither HIID nor USAID has any responsibility for the views expressed here.

1. When citation indices began to be used as a measure of scientific impact, some critics raised questions. One sarcastically gave the following scenario: "Dissemination of weekly changes in citation frequency rates and rankings could provide an extremely sensitive measure of intellectual status. One imagines the eventual establishment of a social science tickler [sic] tape, which would spread citation rates to the offices of deans and department chairmen instantaneously" (Wiener 1974:589).

It is, therefore, particularly interesting to note that the ISI now advertises a part of its Web page devoted to "Hot Data for the Week": "What's really hot in research? Each week, the ISI Research Services Group provides an update based on their Research Performance & Evaluation Tools" (http://www.isinet.com/whatshot/whatshot.html, seen July 2, 1998). Their page also has links to interviews with scientists "conducting the hottest research" as revealed by citation counts. For example, their interview with Walter Willett notes that *"Science Watch's* recent Top Ten lists in medicine have provided ample evidence of the impact of the work by Willett and his colleagues. One example is a hot paper from the Health Professionals Follow-up Study . . . which first appeared last October at #5 on the *Hot Papers* chart in medicine and quickly rose to the #1 spot" (http://www.isinet.com/whatshot/intrvws/willett.html, "Risks and Benefits: Harvard's Walter C. Willett on Epidemiology," reprinted from the ISI newsletter *Science Watch* 6:3–4, June 8, 1995, seen July 2, 1998).

2. I will not discuss how rhetorical expectations limit acceptance rates for nonnative speakers who seek to publish in English-language medical journals—for a discussion of some of these conventions see Segal 1993. Kelly (1993) argues that cultural tradition, not objective standards, is what allows a manuscript's quality to be assessed partly on the size or currency of its literature review.

References

Altbach, P. G. 1987. *The Knowledge Context: Comparative Perspectives on the Distribution of Knowledge.* New York: SUNY Press.

Arends, T. 1975. "Vinculación de Latinoamerica a la literatura científica y tecnológica internacional," *Medicina Buenos Aires* 35: 505–512.

Bottiger, L. E. 1983. "Reference Lists in Medical Journals—Language and Length," *Acta Medic Scandinavica* 214: 73–77.

Campbell, F. M. 1990. "National Bias: A Comparison of Citation Practices by Health Professions," *Bulletin of the Medical Library Association* 78: 376–382.

Clark, D. H., and M. O. Oey-Gardiner. 1991. "How Indonesian Lecturers Have Adjusted to Civil Service Compensation," *Bulletin of Indonesian Economic Studies* 27: 129–141.

Commission on Health Research for Development. 1990. *Health Research: Essential Link to Equity in Development.* New York: Oxford University Press.

Cronin, B. 1984. *The Citation Process: The Role and Significance of Citations in Scientific Communication.* London: Taylor Graham.

Fortes, J., and L. A. Lomnitz. 1994. *Becoming a Scientist in Mexico: The Challenge of Creating a Scientific Community in an Underdeveloped Country.* University Park: Pennsylvania State University Press.

Gaillard, J. 1992. "Use of Publication Lists to Study Scientific Production and Strategies of Scientists in Developing Countries," *Scientometrics* 23: 57–73.

Gibbs, W. W. 1995. "Lost Science in the Third World," *Scientific American* 273: 92–99.

Haiqi, Z., S. Yamazaki, and K. Urate. 1997. "The Tendency Toward English-Language Papers in MEDLINE," *Bulletin of the Medical Library Association* 85: 432–434.

Hamilton, D. P. 1990. "Publishing by—and for?—the Numbers," *Science* 250: 1331–1332.

———. 1991. "Research Papers: Who's Uncited Now?" *Science* 251: 25.
Harvard Medical School. 1989. *Procedures for Making Permanent, Term and Annual Appointments.* Cambridge, MA: Harvard University.
Hull, T. H. 1994. "Institutional Constraints to Building Social Science Capability in Public Health Research: A Case Study from Indonesia," *Acta Tropica* 57: 211–227.
Kaplan, D., and R. A. Manners. 1972. *Culture Theory.* Englewood Cliffs, NJ: Prentice Hall.
Kelly, Martyn. 1993. "Academic Double Standards," *New Scientist* (January 2): 43.
Klein R. 1991. "Risks and Benefits of Comparative Studies: Notes from Another Shore," *Milbank Fund Quarterly* 69: 275–291.
Lezana, M. A., and G. Faba. 1992. *La Producción Científica en Salud en Mexico.* Mexico, DF: Secretaría de Salud.
Lomnitz, L. A., M. W. Rees, and L. Cameo. 1987. "Publication and Referencing Patterns in a Mexican Research Institute," *Social Studies and Science* 17: 115–133.
Loría, A, and R. Lisker. 1995. "Objetivos, Estratégias y Tribulaciones de la RIC," *Revista de Investigación Clínica* 47: 89–93.
Lozoya, X., E. Rivera-Arce, F. Dominguez, et al. 1995. "Archives of Medical Research: An Historical and Subject Coverage Overview," *Archives of Medical Research* 26 (suppl.): S1–S5.
MacLeod, R. 1988. "Introduction." In *Disease, Medicine, and Empire: Perspectives on Western Medicine and the Experience of European Expansion,* R. MacLeod and M. Lewis, eds. London: Routledge.
May, R. M. 1997. "The Scientific Wealth of Nations," *Science* 275: 793–798.
Merton, R. 1988. "The Matthew Effect in Science: II. Cumulative Advantage and the Symbolism of Intellectual Property," *Isis* 79: 606–623.
Nylenna, M., P. Riis, and Y. Karlsson. 1994. "Multiple Blinded Reviews of the Same Two Manuscripts: Effects of Referee Characteristics and Publication Language," *Journal of the American Medical Association* 272: 149–151.
O'Brien, C. 1994. "Quantity No Longer Counts in Britain," *Science* 264: 1840.
Pellegrini, Filho A. 1992. "El Proyecto Regional Sobre la Situación de la Investigación en Salud en América Latina." In *La Producción Científica en Salud en Mexico,* ed. M. A. Lezana and G. Faba, eds. Mexico, DF: Secretaría de Salud.
Perez-Padilla, R. 1995. "El Futuro Incierto de las Revistas Medicas Mexicanas," *Revista de Investigación es Clinicas* 47: 165–167.
Sanberg, P. R., C. V. Borlongan, and H. Nishino. 1996. "Beyond the Language Barrier," *Nature* 384(6610): 608.
Sanz, E., I. Aragón, and A. Mendez. 1995. "The Function of National Journals in Disseminating Applied Science," *Journal of Information Science* 21: 319–323.
Segal, J. Z. 1993. "Strategies of Influence in Medical Authorship," *Social Science and Medicine* 37: 521–530.
Stepan, N. 1981. *Beginnings of Brazilian Science.* New York: Science History Publications.
Susser, M., and A. Yankauer. 1993. "Prior, Duplicate, Repetitive, Fragmented, and Redundant Publication and Editorial Decisions," *American Journal of Public Health* 83: 792–793.
Testa, J. 1997. "The ISI Database: The Journal Selection Process," *Institute for Scientific Information,* online at http://www.isinet.com/whatshot/essays/esay9701.html (viewed November 8, 1997).
Trostle, J., and J. Simon. 1992. "Building Applied Health Research Capacity in Less-Developed Countries: Problems Encountered by the ADDR Project," *Social Science and Medicine* 35: 1379–1388.

Warner, J. H. 1995. "The History of Science and the Sciences of Medicine," *Osiris* 10: 164–193.
Wiener, J. 1974. "Footnote—or Perish," *Dissent* 21: 588–592.
Wilson, R. 1998. "Provosts Push a Radical Plan to Change the Way Faculty Research Is Evaluated," *The Chronicle of Higher Education,* June 22, online at http://www.chronicle.com/colloquy/98/perish/background.shtml.

Selected Bibliography

Aggleton, Peter, ed. *Men Who Sell Sex: International Perspectives on Male Prostitution and AIDS.* London: University College London Press, 1998.

Akin, J. S. *Financing Health Services in Developing Countries: An Agenda for Reform.* Washington, DC: International Bank for Reconstruction and Development, 1987.

Altman, Dennis. *Power and Community: Organizational and Cultural Responses to AIDS.* London: Taylor and Francis, 1994.

Atkinson, M. M., and W. D. Coleman. "Policy Networks, Policy Communities and the Problems of Governance," *Governance: An International Journal of Policy and Administration* 5(2): 154–180.

Baer, Hans A., M. Singer, and I. Susser. "AIDS: A Disease of the Global System." In *Medical Anthropology and the World System.* Westport, CT, and London: Bergin and Garvey, 1997.

Bennett, S., B. McPake, and A. Mills. *Private Health Providers in Developing Countries: Serving the Public Interest?* London: Zed Books, 1997.

Bracken, P. J., and C. Petty, eds. *Rethinking the Trauma of War.* London: Free Association Books, 1998.

Brown, Peter, and Marcia Inhorn, eds. *Anthropology and Infectious Disease.* Newark, NJ: Gordon and Bleach, 1997.

Cardoso, Fernando Henrique, and Enzo Faletto. *Dependency and Development in Latin America.* Berkeley: University of California Press, 1979.

Chetley, A. *A Healthy Business? World Health and the Pharmaceutical Industry.* London: Zed Books, 1990.

Commission on Health Research for Development. *Health Research: Essential Link to Equity in Development.* New York and Oxford: Oxford University Press, 1990.

Coreil, J., and J. D. Mull, eds. *Anthropology and Primary Health Care.* Boulder, CO: Westview Press, 1990.

Cowen, M. P., and R. W. Shenton. *Doctrines of Development.* London and New York: Routledge, 1996.

Davis, P. *Managing Medicines: Public Policy and Therapeutic Drugs.* Buckingham, UK: Open University Press, 1997.

Escobar, A. *Encountering Development: The Making and Unmaking of the Third World.* Princeton, NJ: Princeton University Press, 1995.

———. "Power and Visibility: Development and the Invention and Management of the Third World." *Cultural Anthropology* 3(4): 428–443.

Etkin, N. L., and M. L. Tan, eds. *Medicines: Meanings and Contexts.* Quezon City, Philippines: Health Action International Network, 1994.

Farmer, Paul, Margaret Connors, and Janie Simmons, eds. *Women, Poverty and AIDS: Sex, Drugs and Structural Violence.* Monroe, ME: Common Courage Press, 1996.

Featherstone, M., S. Lash, and R. Roberston. *Global Modernities.* London: Sage, 1995.

Ferrie, J. E., J. Shipley, M. G. Marmot, S. Stansfield, and G. Davey Smith. "The Health Effects of Major Organizational Change and Job Insecurity," *Social Science and Medicine* 46(2): 243–254.

Fisher, J. "Doing Good? The Politics and Antipolitics of NGO Practices," *Annual Reviews in Anthropology* 26: 439–486.

Flemming, Alan, et al., eds. *The Global Impact of AIDS.* New York: Alan R. Liss, 1988.

Giddens, A. *The Consequences of Modernity.* Cambridge: Polity Press, 1990.

———. *Modernity and Self-Identity. Self and Society in the Late Modern Age.* Cambridge: Polity Press, 1991.

Gordenker, Leon, Roger A. Coate, Christer Jönsson, and Peter Sönderholm. *International Cooperation in Response to AIDS.* London and New York: Pinter, 1995.

Gunder Frank, Andre. "The Development of Underdevelopment." In *The Political Economy of Development and Underdevelopment,* C. K. Wibur, ed. New York: Random House, 1988.

Hight-Laukaran, Virginia, et al. "The Use of Breast Milk Substitutes in Developing Countries: The Impact of Women's Employment," *American Journal of Public Health* 86(9): 1235–1240.

Homedes, N., and A. Ugalde. "Patients' Compliance with Medical Treatments in the Third World. What Do We Know?" *Health Policy and Planning* 8(4): 291–314.

Illich, I. *Medical Nemesis: The Expropriation of Health.* London: Calder and Boyars, 1975.

Keane, C. "The Local and the Global: The Anthropology of Globalization and Transnationalism," *Annual Reviews in Anthropology* 12(2): 226–240.

Kearney, Michael. "The Local and the Global: The Anthropology of Globalization and Transnationalism," *Annual Reviews in Anthropology* 24: 547–565.

Kirp, David, and Ronald Bayer, eds. *AIDS in the Industrialized Democracies: Passions, Politics and Policies.* New Brunswick, NJ: Rutgers University Press, 1992.

Kleinman, A., M. Lock, and V. Das, eds. *Social Suffering.* Berkeley: University of California Press, 1997.

Long, N. "Globalization and Localization: New Challenges to Rural Research." In *The Future of Anthropological Knowledge,* H. L. Moore, ed. London: Routledge, 1996.

MacLeod, R. *Disease, Medicine and Empire: Perspectives on Western Medicine and the Experience of European Expansion.* London: Routledge, 1988.

Mann, Jonathan, and Daniel Tarantola, eds. *AIDS in the World II.* Oxford: Oxford University Press, 1996.

Mann, Jonathan, Daniel Tarantola, and Thomas Netter, eds. *AIDS in the World.* Cambridge, MA, and London: Harvard University Press, 1992.

Marsella, Anthony, et al., eds. 1994. "Historical Aspects of Refugee and Immigration Movements." In *Amidst Peril and Pain: The Mental Health and Well-Being of the World's Refugees.* Alan Krant, ed. Washington, DC: American Psychological Association.

McColl, M. A., H. Leui, and H. Skinner. "Structural Relationships Between Social Support and Coping," *Social Science and Medicine* 41(3): 395–407.

Miller, Heather G., Charles F. Turner, and Lincoln E. Moses, eds. *AIDS: The Second Decade.* Washington, DC: National Academy Press, 1990.

Mills, A., and A. B. Zwi. "Health Policy in Less Developed Countries: Past Trends and Future Directions," *Journal of International Development Special Issue: Health Policies in Developing Countries* 7(3): 299–328.

Minear, L., and T. G. Weiss. *Mercy Under Fire: War and the Global Humanitarian Community.* Boulder, CO: Westview Press, 1995.

Minkler, Meredith, ed. *Community Organizing and Community Building for Health.* New Brunswick, NJ, and London: Rutgers University Press, 1997.

Musgrove, P. "The Economic Crisis and Its Impact on Health and Health Care in Latin America and the Caribbean," *International Journal of Health Services* 17: 411–441.

Nichter, M. *Anthropology and International Health: South Asian Case Studies.* Dortrecht: Kluwer, 1989.

Nichter, M., and N. Vuckovic. "Agenda for an Anthropology of Pharmaceutical Practice," *Social Science and Medicine* 39(11): 1509–1525.

Obermeyer, Makhlouf, Carla Castle, and Sandra Castle. "Back to Nature? Historical and Cross-Cultural Perspectives on Barriers to Optimal Breastfeeding," *Medical Anthropology* 17: 39–63.

Pelto, P. J., and G. H. Pelto. "Studying Knowledge, Culture, and Behavior in Applied Medical Anthropology," *Medical Anthropology Quarterly* 11(2): 147–163.

Petchesky, Rosalind P., and Karen Judd, eds. *Negotiating Reproductive Rights: Women's Perspectives Across Countries and Cultures.* London: Zed Books, 1998.

Pigg, S. L. "Acronyms and Effacement: Traditional Medical Practitioners (TMP) in International Health Development." *Social Science and Medicine* 41(1): 47–68.

Rich, Bruce. *Mortgaging the Earth: The World Bank, Environmental Impoverishment, and the Crisis of Development.* Boston: Beacon Press, 1994.

Roth, G., and S. Ekbad. "Migration and Mental Health: Current Research Issues." *Nordic Journal of Psychiatry* 47(3): 185–189.

Sargent, C. F., and T. M. Johnson, eds. *Handbook of Medical Anthropology: Contemporary Theory and Method*, rev. ed. Westport, CT: Greenwood Press, 1996.

Scheper-Hughes, Nancy, and Carolyn Sargent, eds. *Small Wars: Child Survival Revisited.* Berkeley and Los Angeles: University of California Press, 1997.

Sillitoe, P. "What, Know Natives? Local Knowledge in Development," *Social Anthropology* 6(2): 203–220.

Silverman, M., et al. *Bad Medicine: The Prescription Drug Industry and the Third World.* Stanford: Stanford University Press, 1992.

Silverman, M., P. R. Lee, and M. Lydecker. *Prescriptions for Death: The Drugging of the Third World.* Stanford: Stanford University Press, 1982.

Singer, M. "Reinventing Medical Anthropology: Towards a Critical Realignment," *Social Science and Medicine* 30(2): 179–187.

Singer, Merrill, ed. *The Political Economy of AIDS*. Amityville, NY: Baywood, 1997.
Stuart-Macadam, P., and K. A. Dettwyler, eds. *Breastfeeding: Biocultural Perspectives*. New York: Aldine de Gruyter, 1995.
Trostle, J., and J. Simon. "Building Applied Health Research Capacity in Less-Developed Countries: Problems Encountered by the ADDR Project," *Social Science and Medicine* 35: 1379–1388.
Tully, Julia, and Kathryn G. Dewey. "Private Fears, Global Loss: A Cross-Cultural Study of the Insufficient Milk Syndrome." *Medical Anthropology* 9(3): 225–243.
Turshen, M. "The Political Ecology of Disease." *Review of Radical Political Economics* 9: 45–60.
van der Geest, S. "Pharmaceuticals in the Third World: the Local Perspectives," *Social Science and Medicine* 25(3): 273–276.
van der Geest, S., and S. R. Whyte, eds. *The Context of Medicines in Developing Countries: Studies in Pharmaceutical Anthropology*. Dortrecht: Kluwer Academic Publishers, 1988.
van der Geest, S., S. R. Whyte, and A. Hardon. "The Anthropology of Pharmaceuticals: A Biological Approach," *Annual Reviews in Anthropology* 25: 153–178.
Van Esterick, Penny. *Beyond the Breast-Bottle Controversy*. New Brunswick, NJ: Rutgers University Press, 1989.
Waters, M. *Globalization*. London: Routledge, 1995.
Weindling, P., ed. *International Health Organizations and Movements, 1918–1939*. Cambridge, England: Cambridge University Press, 1995.
Whelhan, Patricia, ed. *Women and Health: Cross Cultural Perspectives*. South Hadley, MA: Bergin and Garvey, 1988.
Whiteford, Linda. "Child and Maternal Health and International Economic Policies," *Social Science and Medicine* 37(11): 1391–1400.
WHO (World Health Organization). *Guidelines for Developing National Drug Policies*. Geneva: World Health Organization, 1988.
———. *The World Drug Situation*. Geneva: World Health Organization, 1988.
———. *The World Health Report 1998: Life in the Twenty-first Century: A Vision for All*. Geneva: World Health Organization, 1998.
World Bank. *Investing in Health: World Development Report 1993*. Oxford: Oxford University Press, 1993.
World Health Organization Action Programme on Essential Drugs. *Report of the WHO Expert Committee on National Drug Policies*. Geneva: World Health Organization, 1995.
Young, A. *The Harmony of Illusions: Inventing Post-Traumatic Stress Disorder*. Princeton, NJ: Princeton University Press, 1995.

The Contributors

Harriet Birungi is a senior research fellow at Makerere Institute of Social Research in Uganda. She obtained her degree in anthropology from the University of Copenhagen. She has done extensive research on health care in Uganda, focusing on the use of injections and pharmaceuticals, decentralization, and the changing relation between public and private health care. Her publications include articles on these topics and a technical report on injection use in Uganda for WHO.

Arachu Castro is research associate in the Department of Population and International Health at the Harvard School of Public Health. She is an anthropologist and public health professional, currently working on reproductive health in Latin America, after a few years of research in nutritional anthropology. She is particularly interested in the medicalization of pregnancy and birth, and in the informed consent process for female sterilization and for the recruitment of participants in randomized clinical trials. Castro has developed most of her fieldwork in Latin America and Europe. She has published the book *Saber Bien: Cultura y Practicas Alimentarias en La Rioja* and several articles.

David Craig is a lecturer in social sciences and health in the indigenous health program, Australia Centre for International and Tropical Health and Nutrition, University of Queensland, Brisbane, Australia. His research interests include governance and self-determination in relation to health; local responses to globalization; traveling rationalities, identity, and subjectivity; and partnerships in health and development.

Abdallah Daar is professor of surgery in the College of Medicine at Sultan Qaboos University and Hunterian Professor, Royal College of Surgeons of England. He is a member of the Ethics Committee of the International Transplantation Society, the Asian Society of Transplantation, and the Human Genome Organization. Dr. Daar is the WHO special rapporteur to the working group on genetic manipulations. Recent publications include: "Animal-to-Human Organ Tranpsplants—a Solution or a New Problem?" *Bulletin of the World Helath Forum* 77, no. 1 (1999); "Analysis of Factors for the Prediction of the Response to Xenotransplantation," *Annals of the New York Academy of Science* 862 (1998); with P. Marshall, "Cultural and Psychological Dimensions of Human Organ Transplantation," *Annals of Transplantation* 3, no. 2 (1998); and with I. Kennedy, R. A. Sells, R. D. Guttman, R. Hoffenberg, R. M. Lock, and J. Radcliffe-Richards, "The Case for Presumed Consent in Organ Donation," *Lanet* 351, no. 9116 (1998).

Judith Justice is professor of medical anthropology and health policy, School of Medicine, University of California at San Francisco. Her research interests include international and national health policy, foreign assistance and health development, reproductive and child health, and cultural context of emerging and reemerging infectious disease. Current research includes two multisited comparative studies on child immunization and another on tuberculosis. Publications include *Policies, Plans and People: Foreign Aid and Health Development* (University of California Press). She has worked in South and Southeast Asia, Africa, and the United States conducting research and as a consultant with foundations and international organizations and nongovernmental organizations.

Margaret Kelaher is a Sydney Sax Fellow at the Joseph L. Mailman School of Public Health, Columbia University and the Key Centre for Women's Health in Society, University of Melbourne. She is currently researching the impact of socioeconomic status and transitions in health insurance on health and health care utilization with particular focus on women and minority groups. She completed her Ph.D. on Decisionmaking and HIV Risk Behavior in Gay Men and Injecting Drug Users in 1995 at the National Centre on HIV Social Research and the National Centre for Drug and Alcohol Research, University of New South Wales. From 1995–1998 she was the project director for the indigenous and immigrant cohorts of the Australian Longitudinal Study of Women's Health at the Australian Centre for International and Tropical Health and Nutrition, University of Queensland.

Lenore Manderson is a medical anthropologist and social historian. She has been professor of women's health and director of the Key Centre for

Women's Health in Society, University of Melbourne, since January 1999. Previously, she was professor of tropical health in the Australian Centre for International and Tropical Health and Nutrition, University of Queensland, for 11 years. Her primary research interests and publications relate to infectious disease in poor resource communities, the health of women in immigrant and indigenous communities, and to gender, sexuality, and sexual health. She has worked in Malaysia, Thailand, the Philippines, China, Japan, and Ghana, as well as Australia. Her recent publications include *Sickness and the State: Health and Illness in Colonial Malaya, 1870–1940* (1996), *Maternity and Reproductive Health in Asian Societies*, edited with P. Rice (1996), and *Sites of Desire/Economies of Pleasure,* edited with M. Jolly (1997).

Lauré Marchand-Lucas is a medical and a lactation consultant (IBCLC). She is currently working mostly in France with health care providers as a breastfeeding and community health educator in institutions such as professional schools, hospitals, and well-baby clinics. She particularly focuses on practical aspects of breastfeeding, on relationships between families and providers and between (maternity and infant care) providers in the institutional framework. As a volunteer, she is also a breastfeeding counselor and a resource person for unusual and complicated medical breastfeeding situations coming from mothers accessing La Leche League for help in Africa, Asia, Europe, and Latin America.

Milica Markovic is a research fellow at the Key Centre for Womens Health in Society, University of Melbourne. She has a Ph.D. from the University of Queensland for her thesis entitled Under the Sun of a Foreign Sky: Resettlement of Immigrant Women from the Former Yugoslav Republics. Her research focuses on the sociology of the family, with special interests in womens health and migration.

Patricia A. Marshall is associate director of the Medical Humanities Program and associate professor of medicine at Loyola University, Stritch School of Medicine, Chicago. Her research interests include cultural diversity and bioethics practices, organ transplantation and donation practices in India, informed consent in international health research, and HIV prevention. Recent publications in the area of organ transplantation include: "Organ Transplantation: Defining the Boundaries of Personhood, Equity and Community," *Theoretical Medicine* 17, no. 1 (1996); with D. Thomasma and A. Daar, "Marketing Human Organs: The Autonomy Paradox," *Theoretical Medicine* 17, no, 1 (1996); with A. Daar, "Cultural and Psychological Dimensions of Human Organ Transplantation," *Annals of Transplantation* 3, no. 2 (1998). She is on the executive board of the Society for

Bioethics Consultation and on the advisory board of the Fogarty International Center at the National Institutes of Health. She is a consultant to the President's National Bioethics Advisory Commission on their initiative examining international research ethics.

Richard Parker is a medical anthropologist and a professor in the Department of Health Policies and Institutions of the Institute of Social Medicine at the State University of Rio de Janeiro and the Sociomedical Sciences Division of the Joseph L. Mailman School of Public Health at Columbia University in New York City. He is also director and president of the Brazilian Interdisciplinary AIDS Association (ABIA), a nongovernmental AIDS service and advocacy organization based in Rio de Janeiro. His recent publications include *Beneath the Equator: Cultures of Desire, Male Homosexuality and Emerging Gay Communities in Brazil* (Routledge, 1999) and *Culture, Society and Sexuality: A Reader* (coedited with Peter Aggleton, 1999). He is a founding editor of the new journal *Culture, Health and Sexuality*.

James Trostle worked from 1988 through 1995 as senior social scientist and research associate at the Harvard Institute for International Development, then moved to a position as director of the Five College Program in Culture, Health and Science, and Five College assistant professor of anthropology, based at Mount Holyoke College. Since 1998 he has been an associate professor of anthropology at Trinity College, Hartford, Connecticut. His research has been on the history of collaboration between anthropology and epidemiology, use of health research in policymaking, supporting applied research in developing countries, medication usage, and social aspects of epilepsy in the United States, Ecuador, and Kenya.

Peter van Eeuwijk did postgraduate studies on developing countries at the Swiss Federal Institute of Technology (Switzerland), where he obtained a diploma in development policies. His Ph.D. thesis deals with illness behavior, especially health-seeking behavior, and with cultural dimensions of health and illness. This study is based on four years of fieldwork among the Minahasa (Indonesia). Other regions of interest are East and West Africa and Melanesia. He works as research associate at the Institute of Ethnology.

Linda M. Whiteford is a medical anthropologist, professor, and chair of the Department of Anthropology at the University of South Florida in Tampa, Florida. The focus of her research is infectious disease and international health, and much of her writing has focused on comparative health systems, particularly in the Caribbean and Latin America. Her publications related to comparative health systems are "Children's Health as Accumulated Capital: Structural Adjustment in the Dominican Republic and Cuba," in *Small Wars: The Cultural Politics of Childhood,* and "Sembrando el Futuro: Globalization and the Commodification of Health," in *Crossing Currents: Latin America in Transition;* "Caribbean Colonial History and Its Contemporary Consequences: The Case of the Dominican Republic"; and "International Policies of Child Health." In addition to her work on comparative health systems, Dr. Whiteford has published on infectious and vector-borne diseases such as cholera and dengue fever, and child maternal health.

Susan Reynolds Whyte is a professor at the Institute of Anthropology, University of Copenhagen, with interests in East Africa, health, development, cosmology, and pragmatic anthropology. She is author of a monograph, *Questioning Misfortune*, and coauthor of *Popular Pills: Community Drug Use in Uganda*; and she is coeditor of *Disability and Culture* and *The Context of Medicines in Developing Countries.*

Christina Zarowsky is a physician and anthropologist, lecturer in the Department of Psychiatry, McGill University, and researcher at the Psychosocial Research Division, Douglas Hospital Research Centre, McGill. Her current work focuses on inequality and population health, and critical analyses of trauma and PTSD in war-affected populations.

Suzanne Zhang Gottschang's research interests focus on the intersection of gender, medicine, and health policy in China.

Index

Acute respiratory infection (ARI), 131, 136, 143
Administration for Refugees and Returnee Affairs (Ethiopia), 194
Adome, Richard Odoi, 141
Aedes aegypti, 60, 62, 64, 65; household ecology of, 66. *See also* Dengue fever
Ahmed, Gureh, 180
Aid: bilateral aid, 16, 28; foreign aid policies, 23; humanitarian, 178
Alma-Ata, Declaration of, 80
American Association of Pediatrics, 242
Amharic society, 185
Amin, Idi, 129
Amnesty International, 170
Anthropologists: role of, 134
Appadurai, Arjun, 129
Applied Diarrheal Disease Research Project, 299
Australia: assistance to migrants, 159, 169–170; Commonwealth Employment Service, 159; humanitarian program, 152, 153; from Latin America, 171n7; Migrant Resource Center, 160; migration to, 155–170; Telephone Interpreting and Translating Service, 160; visa categories, 171n6; White Australia Policy, 153, 154; women refugees, 153–154

Badinter, Elisabeth, 247
Bangladesh, 24, 34n1
Batista, Juan, 68
Bellagio, 25, 33, 211, 221
Biomedicine: dissemination of, 291–297; dominance of, 97n9, 128, 236. *See also* Media; Publishing
Biopower, 275
Boltanski, Luc, 178
Bosnia and Herzegovina, 11, 161, 164
Bourdieu, Pierre, 122
Brazil: HIV/AIDS in, 47–48; Ministry of Health, 47; National AIDS Programme, 40, 47
Bread for the World, 29
Breast-feeding: class differences, 248; as health cost, 246; health effects of decline, 233; HIV testing, 244; medicalization, 246, 249–251; representations 270, 271. *See also* Colostrum; Infant feeding; Weaning
Bretton Woods institutions, 16
Broumand, B., 210
Bruenjes, A., 10

Cassanelli, Lee, 197
Castro, Fidel, 61
Catholic Church: support for immunization, 28
Charity, 181–182, 184–185; Christian, 185; under Islam, 184

325

Child survival, 6, 23; in Egypt, 23, 30; in India, 23, 30; in Indonesia, 23, 30–32; in Uganda, 23, 30
Child Survival Revolution, 24–30
Children: international conventions and declarations, 274. *See also* Child survival; Infant feeding; Motherhood; United Nations Children's Fund; World Health Organization
Children's Vaccine Initiative (CVI), 27
China, 2; breast-feeding education, 279–284; Chin dynasty, 61; decline of, 269; economic growth, 268–269; economic reforms, 267; government attitudes toward, 266, 269; hospital practice, 279–282; ideologies of motherhood, 273–276; infant feeding, 14, 265; legislation relating to women and children, 273, 275, 276; marketing of breast-milk substitutes, 277–278; one-child policy, 268, 269, 274–275
The Chronicle of Higher Education, 307
Citations: *Index Medicus,* 294; Science Citation Index, 294; Social Science Citation Index, 298
Colonialism, 12, 68, 97n9; British, 177; introduction of Western medicine, 129; maternal and child health policies under, 13–14; state intervention under, 13
Colostrum, 237–238
Comaroff, John and Jean, 177
Communication, 292; access to, 136; information technology, 1, 3, 83, 88, 95; of research, 307–309
Communications systems, 3, 4, 95
Community-based action, 42, 49, 51, 57, 60, 69, 71; Brazilian Interdisciplinary AIDS Association, 41; and mosquito-borne diseases, 58, 64, 67. *See also* Dengue fever; HIV/AIDS; Malaria
Community participation, 4, 5, 6, 64, 66, 67, 74
Contextual assessment, 5
Cost-effectiveness: of HIV/AIDS prevention and treatment, 45, 46, 47; of immunization, 32

Cuba, 7, 13, 57–64, 67–75; colonial history of, 68; impact of global recession on, 68; infant mortality rates in, 70, 72; primary health care in, 69; Public Health Plan, 69; Soviet Union relations with, 69
Cultural dominance, 3

Danish International Development Agency (DANIDA), 130, 141
De Beauvoir, Simone, 247
Dengue fever, 7, 13, 61–76; distribution of, 61, 62, 63
Dengue hemorrhagic fever, 61, 63, 65
Dengue shock syndrome, 62, 63, 65
Dependency, 44, 197–199; charity and, 190. *See also* Refugees
Disability Adjusted Life Years (DALYs), 16, 45, 52n4
Dominican Republic, 7, 57–62, 65–75; collapse of primary health care in, 69; colonial history of, 68; impact of global recession on, 68; infant mortality rates, 72; infrastructure in, 65–66, 68; population increase in, 65; workforce participation of women in, 68
Drought, 89
Drug resistance, 15, 134. *See also* Medication; Multinational; Pharmaceuticals
Drug sellers: in Nepal, 143; training in Uganda of, 140, 141
Drugs. *See* Medication; Pharmaceuticals
Duffield, Mark, 198

Economic development and health, 15–16
English Poor Laws, 181, 182
Environmental health, 64, 89–90, 97n16; and global warming, 96n3
European Union, 111
Expanded Programme of Immunization. *See* Immunization

Family Welfare Organization (Indonesia), 91
Farmer, Paul, 74
Foege, William, 26

Former Yugoslavia, 4, 11, 96n5; migration from, 155–170. *See also* Bosnia and Herzegovina; Kosovo; Post-traumatic stress disorder
Foucault, Michel, 108, 221, 275
France: breast-feeding in, 14, 233–259; Committee of Public Health, 244; cultural resistance to, 234, 245–246; government attitudes, 243–245, 258; health professionals, 234, 235, 249–251; lobbying by formula manufacturers, 243, 244; National Committee for the Promotion of Breast Feeding, 242; National Committee on Children, 245; rates of breast-feeding in, 234. *See also* Infant feeding; United Nations Children's Fund
Frank, Gunder, 185

Geddes, B., 3, 8, 10
Geertz, Clifford, 79
Gender relations, 41, 171n2. *See also* HIV/AIDS; Inequality; Women
Global Programme on AIDS, 5, 40. *See also* HIV/AIDS; United Nations Joint Programme on AIDS; World Health Organization
Global Network of People Living with HIV, 50
Grant, James, 26, 27
Growth, oral rehydration, breast-feeding, and immunization (GOBI), 25. *See also* United Nations Children's Fund

Haaland, Ane, 144
Harrell-Bond, B. E., 184, 186
Hansen, Art, 186
Harvard Institute for International Development, 299
Hathaway, James C., 197
Health: -seeking behavior, 93; as a supervalue, 80
"Health for All by the Year 2000," 2, 80, 93
Health services: access to 73, 114; privatization, 130; user charges for, 114
Hepatitis B, 27
HIV/AIDS, 2, 5, 39–51; bisexual men and, 41; demographic factors associated with, 5; ethics of, 46; gay men and, 41, 50; and gender relations, 41, 49; and identity politics, 48, 50; and injecting drug use, 41, 49; institutional responses to, 40; international policies, 6; local-level responses to, 48, 50; National AIDS Programmes, 42, 43, 51, 130; risk behavior of, 41; sex workers and, 41; in San Francisco, 49; in Sydney, 49; vulnerability to, 41. *See also* Community-based action; United Nations Joint Programme on AIDS; World Health Organization
Howson, C. P., 15–16
Human rights, 45, 83. *See also* Refugees

Identity: construction of, 60; politics, 48, 50; ethnic, 168–169; local, 59, 67–68, 79; refugee, 190. *See also* HIV/AIDS
Ideology, 81, 82
Idioms: of dependency, 11, 193, 198; of despair, 7, 57–59, 67–72; of empowerment, 12; of globalization, 7, 8; of hope, 7, 57–59, 67–72; of the limits of law, 109; of modernization, 85; of underdevelopment, 84–85
Immunization: Expanded Programme of Immunization, 4, 25, 93; as a technological intervention, 32, 71. *See also* United Nations Children's Fund; World Health Organization
Indonesia, 23, 30–32, 79–96; constitution, 98n20; *era reformasi*, 83; Green Revolution in, 84; in Minahasa, 98n21; New Order, 83, 84, 98n21; Period of National Development, 84; rewards for research and publications, 300–302; state philosophy of *Pancasila*, 81, 97n14; Unity in Diversity, 81. *See also* Child survival; Minahasa
Infant feeding: bottle feeding, 14, 233; insufficient milk syndrome, 239–240; international agreements on, 240–242; lactation consultants, 14, 255; market expansion of formula, 8, 278; policies after

delivery, 258; supplementation, 238–239, 253. *See also* Breast-feeding; China; Colostrum; France; La Leche League; United Nations Children's Fund; Weaning; World Health Organization
Inequality, 40, 41, 50, 51, 52n3; and gender-based persecution, 171n2; migrant women and, 158; power, 225; technological resources, 225. *See also* Gender relations; HIV/AIDS; Women
Injections, 94, 136
Institutional strengthening, 5, 17; and fragility of health systems, 33
International Council of AIDS Service Organizations (ICASO), 50
International Federation of Pharmaceutical Manufacturing Associations (IFPMA), 110
International Labour Organization (ILO), 152
International Monetary Fund, 16, 46, 52n2, 68
International Network for the Rational Use of Drugs (INRUD), 123n3, 144

Jakarta: perceptions of, 85; political influence of, 89
Java: dominance of, 80; mythologies, 98n20
Jordan, Brigitte, 236

Kearney, Michael, 7, 58, 79
Kleinman, Arthur, 259
Kleinman, Joan, 4, 16, 73, 74, 75, 128, 179, 199–200, 266
Knowledge: authoritative, 133, 236, 251–253; dissemination of, 291–297, 306, 307–308; of economics and politics, 2, 12, 17, 128, 136, 141–142; and production, 297–300. *See also* Biomedicine; Communication; Media; Traditional medicine
Kopytoff, Igor, 221
Kosovo, 3, 177

La Leche League, 14, 249, 254–256
the *Lancet,* 15–16
Learned helplessness, 182–183
Lemarchand, René, 184

Leslie, Charles, 135
Levine, N., 272
Lions Clubs, 26
Lock, Margaret, 209
Longitudinal Study of Immigrants to Australia, 156

McNamara, Robert, 26
Mahler, Halfdan, 26
Malaria: control of, 4, 7, 61, 93, 142; effect of, 89, 131; high rates in Uganda of, 136; vector habitat and behavior, 7
Malkki, Lisa H., 186
Mann, Jonathan, 42
Media, 27, 31, 83, 91, 97n19, 112, 122, 309; health education, 64, 67, 269; reports, 192; representations of breast-feeding, 245–246; representations of organ donation, 222. *See also* Communications
Medical pluralism, 81, 94–95, 96, 117
Medical Research Institute (Kenya), 144
Medication: and breast-feeding, 252; compliance with, 109–110; in household practice, 117–118, 122–123, 131, 133, 138; self-, 8, 9, 94, 95, 131; knowledge of, 136–137, 140, 142; legitimation of, 140; use of mnemonics for, 118–119; and polypharmacy, 8, 84, 131, 134, 135; regulation and control of, 121, 128, 130. *See also* Drug sellers; Pharmaceuticals
Megatrends 2000, 81, 82, 91, 97n17
Menjivar, C., 159
Merson, Michael, 42
Merton, Robert, 297–298
Mexico: rewards for research and publications, 302–304
Migrants, 10; friction among, 171nn9–10; from Horn of Africa, 187; identities of, 155, 169; and intermarriage, 169; and mental health, 167; women at risk as, 11, 153–154, 157, 162. *See also* Migration; Refugees
Migration: labor, 71, 152; adjustment following, 154, 163–164; changes in health status from, 166–167;

difficulties in adaptation, 157, 161–167; drought and, 191; economics of, 157; forced, 154; poverty and, 191
Minahasa, 7–8, 79–96; agricultural change in, 86, 87; compliance with *adat,* 87–88; cultural borrowing, 97n18; demographic change in, 90, 98n23; effect of economic crisis in, 86, 98n22; health status in, 89; kinship and power, 87; local co-operatives, 89; logging, 87; mining, 89, 97n16; primary health care, 89; Protestant Minahasa Church, 89; villager perceptions of globalization, 85, 88, 91–93
Mohammed Abdille Hassan, 180, 202n3
Motherhood, 247–249, 268. *See also* Inequality; Infant feeding; Medication; Women
Mothers in New Country (MINC) study, 156
Multiculturalism, 4
Multinationals: and consumer activism, 113; of infant formula, 8; of pharmaceuticals, 8; of tobacco, 7–8
Muturi, John, 144

Nakajima, Hiroshi, 42
Naisbitt, John, 81, 82, 91, 97n17
National Institutes of Health, 44, 299
Nichter, Mark, 135
North Atlantic Treaty Organization (NATO), 3

Organ transplant: American Medical Association and, 208, 209–210; Bellagio Task Force, 211, 221; and brain death, 208–209; cultural and national differences on, 206–211; ethical issues of, 206–225; government committees on, 210; in India, 12, 205–225; Indian Human Organs Transplants Act, 206, 210, 211–214, 222–224; informed consent to, 220; integrity of the human body and, 209; Japanese demand for, 12; kinship and, 224; marketing and sale of, 209, 213; paid donation to, 205–206, 211–217; stigma of, 219; United Network for Organ Sharing, 212
Oral rehydration solution (ORS), 24, 32, 139
Oral rehydration therapy (ORT), 23, 25, 134; in Cuba, 72; in Dominican Republic, 72
Oswaldo Cruz Foundation, 308
Overseas Development Agency (ODA) (United Kingdom), 44

Pan-American Health Organization (PAHO), 60
Patients: treatment of, 137
Pharmaceuticals, 8, 94; deregulation of, 106, 130, 133; quality of, 105, 113; rational use, 120–121, 127; regulation of, 8, 107, 110, 111, 122, 142; sale of, 105–106, 137–138; in Uganda, 127–145; in Vietnam, 105–123. *See also* Drug resistance; Medication; Multinationals
Polio: eradication of, 4
Post-traumatic stress disorder, 161–162, 171n7, 199–200
Poverty: and migration, 191; and organ sales, 213–214, 220–221
Primary health care, 5, 64, 81; compared with immunization, 28; decline of, 59, 69; extension of, 69; selective vs. comprehensive, 27. *See also* Cuba; Dominican Republic; Indonesia
Publishing, 291–310

Radcliffe-Richards, Janet, 220, 221
Rapid assessment. *See* Contextual assessment
Reeler, Anne, 133
Refugees, 10; in Angola, 186; camps, 4, 188, 193–197; dependency, 178–193; Hutu, 186; international governance on, 201n1; mental health of, 199–200; in Somalia, 11, 177–201; in Sudan, 186; women as, 153. *See also* Post-traumatic stress disorder
Research: capacity of, 5, 17, 293–294; consumption of, 300–304; on sustainability of immunization programs, 29–32. *See also* Knowledge

Results (nongovernmental organization), 29
Rockefeller Foundation, 26
Rotary International, 26
Rustow, Walt W., 186

Salk, Jonas, 26
Schensul, Jean, 74
Scheper-Hughes, Nancy, 135
Selassie, Haile, 189
Semantic network, 179–180
Slavery, 221
Smallpox: eradication of, 4, 25
Socialization with neighbors, 163–164
Social networks, 162–165, 168–169
Social suffering, 67, 75, 128, 259
Somalia, 177–201; downfall of, 188; history of war in, 180; Menghistu Haile Mariam of, 187; Siad Barre, 188; and war with Ethiopia, 187, 190
Structural adjustment, 48. *See also* World Bank
Suharto, General, 83, 84, 86, 98n19
Swedish International Development Assistance (SIDA), 112

Tobacco: market expansion of, 8
Traditional healers, 5, 81, 90, 116
Traditional medicine: knowledge of, 80, 119–120; promotion of, 114; in Uganda, 131, 145; in Vietnam, 116–117
Transplantation. *See* Organ transplant
Travel: and increased transmission of disease, 62
Trujillo, Rafael, 68
Technology. *See* Communications; Immunization; Transplants
Tourism, 4

Uganda, 8; Community Drug Use project, 131, 139, 140, 143; depletion of medical workforce, 129–130; Essential Drugs Management Programme, 130–132, 139, 140; expulsion of professionals, 129; health problems in, 130–131; Health Policy Review Commission, 130; introduction of Islamic medicine to, 129; Malaria Control Unit, 142; National Drug Authority, 142; National Drug Policy, 128, 132, 142; National Resistance Movement, 130; Red Cross and Red Crescent in, 139, 140, 141, 183; "time of regimes," 129, 141
Unemployment, 166–167, 171n8
United Nations Children's Fund (UNICEF), 14, 24, 25, 30, 33, 43, 130, 152; Baby Friendly Hospital Initiative, 14, 242, 265, 270–272, 276; in France, 242; immunization, 25; Innocenti Declaration, 241–242; joint World Health Organization/UNICEF statement on breastfeeding, 241
United Nations Development Programme (UNDP), 5, 26, 43, 45, 46
United Nations Economic and Social Council (ECOSOC), 43, 51n2
United Nations Educational, Scientific, and Cultural Organization (UNESCO), 43
United Nations Environment Programme (UNEP), 152
United Nations General Assembly, 42, 43, 52n2
United Nations High Commission for Refugees (UNHCR), 11, 152, 153, 177, 183, 185–186, 189, 194, 196, 201
United Nations Joint Programme on AIDS (UNAIDS), 43, 48, 51
United Nations Population Fund (UNFPA), 43
United Nations Security Council, 152
United States: congress, 28, 29; and demographic indicators, 70; Economic Recovery Act, 68; and HIV/AIDS research, 44; lobbying groups, 29; Uniform Anatomical Gift Act, 207
United States Agency for International Development (USAID): and AIDS Care and Prevention Program, 52n5; and HIV/AIDS, 44, 52n5; and immunization, 24, 30. *See also* United States
United States for Child Survival, 30
Universal Childhood Immunization (UCI), 25, 28; evaluation of, 32. *See*

also Cost-effectiveness; United Nations Children's Fund; World Health Organization
Urbanization, 65

Vector control, 62, 63–64; and environmental surveillance, 64. *See also* Dengue fever; Environmental Health; Malaria
Vertical programs, 5, 112
Vietnam, 7, 105–123; body regulation, 121; consumer complaints, 115; *doi moi* (free market reforms), 106; and Eastern medicine, 116–117; Essential Drugs Policy, 111, 112, 114; jurisdictional boundaries in, 113; Ministry of Health, 113, 114, 123n5; National People's Assembly, 113. *See also* Medication; Pharmaceuticals; Traditional medicine
von Buchwald, Ulrike, 183, 187, 199

Walt, Gill, 16, 17
Weaning, 235–236; and socialization of children, 249, 256–257
Wellcome Trust, 144
Women: and maternity leave in France, 236, 246; prenatal care for, 69; responsibility for family health, 106, 123, 267; workforce participation of, 68, 235–236, 267, 272. *See also* Australia; Gender relations; HIV/AIDS; Refugees
World Bank, 3, 5, 15, 16, 17, 26, 43–48, 52n2, 52n5, 110, 112, 141; *Confronting AIDS,* 43; *Investing in Health,* 15, 52n4, 109. *See also* Disability Adjusted Life Years
World Food Programme, 194
World Health Assembly, 233, 241
World Health Organization (WHO), 4, 5, 9, 16, 25, 26, 43, 48, 51, 60, 80, 110, 111, 151; Action Programme on Essential Drugs, 10, 111, 127, 144; Diarrheal Disease Programme, 42; Expanded Programme of Immunization, 4, 25–26, 130; Global Programme on AIDS, 40, 42, 45; *International Code of Marketing of Breast-Milk Substitutes,* 233, 240–241; Joint World Health Organization/United Nations Children's Fund statement on breast-feeding, 241, 277; *Manual on Mental Health of Refugees,* 199; National Drug Policies, 111; Special Programme on AIDS, 42. *See also* HIV/AIDS; Pharmaceuticals
World Summit for Children, 26, 27
World Trade Organization, 16, 274

Yellow fever, 61, 62

About the Book

International health planners often design programs based on the assumption that recipient nations share the same "level playing field" with regard to conceptions of health, illness, and at-risk populations. This volume challenges that perception, analyzing the outcomes of humanitarian projects that fail to recognize local ethnic and national identities, as well as the tensions between international health agencies' mandates and powerful centralized government agendas. Case studies are drawn from Africa, Asia, and the Caribbean.

Linda M. Whiteford is professor of anthropology at the University of South Florida. She is widely published on social aspects of health and illness. **Lenore Manderson** is professor of women's health at the University of Melbourne. She is author of *Sickness and the State: Health and Illness in Colonial Malaya, 1870–1940* and is coeditor (with Pranee Rice) of *Maternity and Reproductive Health in Asian Societies*.